Nordic Welfare States in the European Context

This important sequel to *Nordic Social Policy* (Routledge 1999) compares welfare state development over the last twenty years in Denmark, Finland, Norway and Sweden with that of Germany, the Netherlands, the United Kingdom and other Western European countries. Topics covered include:

- income distribution, health inequalities and gender equality
- gender policies, health and social care services and policy reaction to family changes
- social security and employment policies
- financing of welfare states

In the context of globalisation, ageing, changing family and employment patterns and rising inequalities, *Nordic Welfare States in the European Context* offers an empirical analysis of welfare state adaptations and a lively discussion of the development of European social policy. It finds a greater ambiguity regarding variation and trends than is commonly suggested. Contrary to expectation, there is little evidence of Europeanisation of the Nordic welfare states, rather the reverse.

The comparable and empirical data used in this study make it a unique contribution to understanding current trends in European social policy.

Mikko Kautto and **Hannu Uusitalo**, National Research and Development Centre for Welfare and Health, Finland. **Johan Fritzell**, Swedish Institute for Social Research, Stockholm University, Sweden. **Bjørn Hvinden**, Norwegian University of Science and Technology, Norway. **Jon Kvist**, The Danish National Institute of Social Research, Denmark.

Nordic Welfare States in the European Context

Edited by Mikko Kautto, Johan Fritzell, Bjørn Hvinden, Jon Kvist and Hannu Uusitalo

London and New York

First published 2001
by Routledge
11 New Fetter Lane, London EC4P 4EE

Simultaneously published in the USA and Canada
by Routledge
29 West 35th Street, New York, NY 10001

Routledge is an imprint of the Taylor & Francis Group

Typeset in Times by BC Typesetting, Bristol
Printed and bound in Great Britain by
TJ International Ltd, Padstow, Cornwall

British Library Cataloguing in Publication Data
A catalogue record for this book is available from the British Library

Library of Congress Cataloging in Publication Data
Nordic welfare states in the European context/edited by Mikko Kautto . . . [et al.].
p. cm.
Includes bibliographical references and index.
1. Social service – Scandinavia. 2. Scandinavia – Social policy. 3. Europe – Social policy. 4. Welfare state. I. Kautto, Mikko, 1965–

HV318.N58 2001   00-062810
361.6′5′0948–dc21

ISBN 0–415–24161–8 (pb)
ISBN 0–415–24160–X (hb)

Contents

Figures

Tables

Contributors

Jochen Clasen is Professor of Comparative Social Research at the University of Stirling, Scotland. His particular research interests are unemployment, employment policies and social security policy in the cross-national European context. His latest publications include *Comparative Social Policy: concepts, theories and methods* (Blackwell 1999), 'Beyond Social Security: the economic value of giving money to unemployed people', *European Journal of Social Security* 1(2), 1999, and 'Motives, means and opportunities – reforming unemployment compensation in the 1990s', *West European Politics* 23(2), 2000.

Johan Fritzell is an Associate Professor of Sociology and a Senior Researcher at the Swedish Institute for Social Research, Stockholm University. His main research interests are social inequality, income distribution research and comparative social policy. He currently directs a research programme on income inequality and health, and is a member of the Swedish Governmental Commission 'A Balance Sheet for Welfare of the 1990s'.

Aksel Hatland is a Senior Research Fellow at Norwegian Social Research (NOVA) in Oslo and a Professor of social policy at Lillehammer College. He is Co-ordinating Research Director for the Research Council of Norway's Welfare Programme. His research interests include social policy, family policy and research ethics.

Matti Heikkilä is a Research Professor at the National Research and Development Centre for Welfare and Health (STAKES) in Helsinki, Finland. His principal research interests are poverty, deprivation and the welfare state. He worked as a Detached National Expert in the European Foundation for the Improvement of Living and Working Conditions, Dublin, Ireland in 1997–8.

Bjørn Hvinden is a Professor of Sociology at the Department of Sociology and Political Science of the Norwegian University of Science and Technology (NTNU), Trondheim. He has carried out comparative research on income maintenance and employment policies, especially for people with disabilities, the administration of social security, and self-organisation among disadvantaged groups. He is currently co-directing a cross-national study of disability policies in a number of European countries. He is co-ordinating a research programme on policies aimed at Travellers in Norway and their counter-strategies.

Ilkka Kankare is a PhD student at the Department of Social Policy of the University of Helsinki. His current research interests are the EU social programmes and their structures of governance.

Mikko Kautto is a Researcher at the National Research and Development Centre for Welfare and Health (STAKES) in Helsinki, Finland and Co-ordinator of the 'Nordic Welfare States in the 1990s' researcher network. His research interest is in comparative welfare state research and welfare state development. He recently authored a comparison of welfare state adaptation in Finland and Sweden during the 1990s. He is one of the editors of *Nordic Social Policy* (Routledge 1999).

Randi Kjeldstad is a Senior Research Fellow and Assistant Director of Research at the Division for Social and Demographic Research, Statistics Norway. Her work includes analyses of employment, income and social policy in a gender and life course perspective. In recent years her main research interest has been single parents.

Jon Kvist is a Senior Researcher at the Danish National Institute of Social Research. His research interests include comparative social policy and welfare state research, methodology, and the social divisions of welfare. He has been a visiting scholar at Bath University and Northwestern University.

Eero Lahelma is Professor of Medical Sociology at the Department of Public Health at the University of Helsinki, Finland. His research includes health inequalities within the Finnish, Nordic and a broader European context, and recently health and well-being in the work setting.

Juhani Lehto is Professor of Social and Health Policy at Tampere University, Finland. He has worked at the National Board of Social Welfare, at the National Research and Development Centre for Health and Social Welfare (STAKES) and at the WHO Regional Office for Europe. He has published research on alcohol and drug treatment systems, alcohol and drug control policies, financing and management of social and health care, reforms in social and health care, and urban social policy.

Olle Lundberg, PhD, is an Associate Professor of Sociology at Stockholm University and an Associate Professor of Medical Sociology, University of Helsinki. He also holds a position as Senior Researcher at the Swedish Institute for Social Research, Stockholm University. His main research interests include health inequalities, general welfare research and gerontology. He is presently a member of the Swedish Governmental Commission 'A Balance Sheet for Welfare of the 1990s'.

Wim van Oorschot is Associate Professor of Sociology at the Department of Sociology and Policy Studies at the Tilburg Institute of Social Security Studies of Tilburg University, The Netherlands. He has published on poverty, welfare state legitimacy, solidarity and equity in social protection, the history of social security, client satisfaction in social security administration, disability benefits and reintegration measures, and on activation of unemployed people. He is currently co-ordinating a study on welfare solidarity patterns among Europeans.

Tine Rostgaard is a PhD student at the Danish National Institute of Social Research. Her research interest is comparative welfare state research, in particular social care systems. She has published on social care systems in Europe, social responsibility of enterprises and the role of the family.

Annemette Sørensen is Director of the Henry A. Murray Research Center at the Radcliffe Institute for Advanced Study, Harvard University. She is a sociologist specialising in the study of gender stratification, the sociology of the family, and the life course of women and men in modern society.

Hannu Uusitalo is Professor and Deputy Director General at the National Research and Development Centre for Welfare and Health (STAKES). His research since the 1970s has focused on level of living studies and income inequality, especially in the

Nordic countries, on Finland in a broader comparative perspective and on causes and outcomes of the welfare state in terms of living conditions. His work in the 1990s has been oriented towards more politically relevant issues in Finland.

Preface

This book is the second product of a Nordic researcher network established in the mid-1990s. The aim of the research project has been to assess changes in the Nordic welfare states from an empirical perspective and employing comparative data. The first goal was to examine developments within the Nordic group of countries and compare their paths in a framework stressing the changing preconditions for the maintenance of the welfare states. The second aim was to examine the recent history of the Nordic welfare states from a broader perspective by including non-Nordic countries in our comparison.

'The Nordic welfare states in the 1990s' this network was created in 1995 when the first ideas for empirical comparative research on changes in Nordic welfare states were presented to a number of Nordic scholars. Idea papers were distributed, and seminars to discuss these and the emerging drafts were arranged. The discussions on research areas, choice of partners and type of co-operation eventually resulted in a research proposal that was granted funding from the Joint Committee of the Nordic Social Science Research Councils (NOS-S) for 1996–97. The research network thus formed set out to be international at the design level, and in the analysis of data and its interpretation.

While the research work on Nordic comparisons was being set in motion, the Nordic Council of Ministers launched a four-year research programme entitled '*Norden och Europa*'. This was motivated by the changing relationship patterns between the Nordic countries and the EU and by the larger political, economic and cultural upheavals happening in the integrating Europe and after the collapse of the Soviet bloc. The programme invited research on areas identified to be under pressure for change. One of the four themes was the future of the 'Nordic welfare state'. Not surprisingly, the idea soon emerged for a second phase of research to build on the work in the pipeline. A larger European comparison in terms of number of countries was envisaged, but with a closer targeted research focus. The Nordic Council of Ministers and NORFA, the Nordic Academy for Advanced Study secured funding for this endeavour.

The project was divided into two phases. The first phase results were published by Routledge in 1999 under the title *Nordic Social Policy*, and the second appear in this follow-up volume *Nordic Welfare States in the European Context*. Twenty-one scholars contributed to the first book, and sixteen to the present publication, which marks the completion of this five-year-long process. We express warm gratitude to our Nordic financers and to all those who have participated in the work of the network in one way or another, be it for a shorter or longer term. We also want to thank the language editor Richard Burton for his professional skills. We hope this project and its results will prove useful for students of social policy, welfare studies and sociology as well as for academics, policy makers and analysts of social policy.

The editors

1 Introduction: How distinct are the Nordic welfare states?

Mikko Kautto, Johan Fritzell, Bjørn Hvinden, Jon Kvist and Hannu Uusitalo

The aim of the book

This volume explores the issue of whether the Nordic welfare states have become more like other Western European welfare states in the past twenty years. Are there still notable and systematic differences, or has the distinctiveness of the Nordic welfare states evaporated over time? We address changes in social policies and living conditions from an empirical perspective using comparable data.

In our earlier volume, *Nordic Social Policy* (Kautto *et al.* 1999), we examined the so-called 'Nordic model of welfare states' by looking at variations across the Nordic countries of Denmark, Finland, Norway and Sweden. We demonstrated how close scrutiny sometimes reveals substantial variation and even divergent trends between countries, but also how the latter may nevertheless result in less variation within a group of countries. We adopted a framework that encompassed the major upheavals in the economic and employment situation in these four Nordic nations during the early 1990s. Against expectations, the empirical analysis of welfare state adaptation to changing circumstances showed more stability than change, both in terms of social policy measures and living conditions. A central conclusion of the book was thus that even in differing economic situations the Nordic welfare states seemed to have developed in a relatively similar manner; if there was Nordic unity in the early 1980s, it seemed to have persisted into the mid-1990s.

This follow-up title continues from where *Nordic Social Policy* ended by shifting from an intra-Nordic focus to a larger Western European comparison. A broader perspective and the opportunity to update some of the data allow us to ask two important questions. First, how different are the Nordic welfare states as a group when contrasted with certain other Western European welfare states? Second, are such differences narrowing or widening over time? In other words, when we examine differences between the Nordic welfare states in a Western European comparison, taking account of recent policy developments and signs of growing inequalities in the Nordic countries, is talk of a distinct Nordic variety of welfare states still justified?

Most of the existing research indicates that it does make sense to talk about a Nordic model of social policy, or, models aside, it at least suggests that Nordic countries often group together when compared with other countries. With its roots in the mid-1970s and gaining renewed momentum in the 1990s, this strand of thinking has spawned such concepts as typologies, welfare state models or welfare regimes, welfare clusters and families of nations. Despite the variety of terms and criteria a common denominator in formulating typologies is the recognition that countries have qualitatively different types of social policies that to a large extent result from diverse social structures, and historical and political processes. Furthermore, the characteristics of welfare regimes are believed to explain much of the variation in outcomes for the population. Another suggestion is that countries associated with a particular welfare regime tend to follow similar development paths.

This position of regime–specific development is challenged by ideas in which convergence is expected to occur, either explicitly or implicitly. Such beliefs offer another interpretation for the development of social policy by questioning the permanence of contrasts between countries. While a common denominator here is the notion of narrowing disparities, the different views do not gather comfortably beneath a common label because of their varied assumptions about the mechanisms behind these convergent trends. One prevalent assumption is that convergence is stimulated by similar challenges, be they internal and/or external. For instance, external challenges are said to subordinate social policies to economic policies, and to confine autonomous national decision-making. Also, political actors with growing numbers of international contacts are believed to seek broadly similar types of solutions to similar pressures and problems. As a result, institutional arrangements and provisions are expected to become more uniform. Another view is that some countries pioneer policies that are later adopted by others; in this sense countries are reckoned to learn from each other's policy innovations and good experiences. Previously, ideas about policy learning were often underpinned by notions of a more or less uniform evolution from simpler to more advanced policy arrangements, but such views are rarely articulated any longer. Today, regardless of what the underlying mechanisms are believed to be, convergence implies that the welfare arrangements of different countries will gradually become more similar.

In our attempts to judge whether the distinctiveness of Nordic social policy is lasting or dissolving we are here dealing with both of the above lines of thinking. Accordingly, the first general aim of the comparative studies that follow is to address *variation,* and especially to consider distinctive characteristics of the Nordic welfare states. What features of social policy distinguish the Nordic welfare states from others? To what extent does the level and distribution of welfare[1] as measured by outcomes separate the Nordic countries from others? The second general aim is to address the issue of *convergence* and *divergence* by scrutinising European trends within certain important policy areas and in the light of established indicators on living conditions. Are policy solutions becoming more similar? How are the level and distribution of welfare developing?

In thinking about the distinctiveness of the Nordic welfare states it is necessary to consider *both* the similarities *and* the differences. To be distinct the Nordic welfare states should have features in common, but they should also be different enough as a group to stand a certain distance from other countries. Obviously the reference group and time period adopted are crucial for such judgements. The overall set of countries compared in this volume is formed of the Nordic countries and the other member states of the European Union. There are thus fifteen EU countries and Norway, or to put it in another way, four Nordic countries and twelve non-Nordic EU countries. As in the earlier volume Denmark, Finland, Norway and Sweden feature in all our analyses. In addition, we decided to incorporate three non-Nordic countries in the study analyses of all chapters. Germany,[2] the Netherlands and the United Kingdom were chosen because welfare state arrangements and their consequences in these three non-Nordic countries are generally believed to be very different from each other and the reason these countries are often associated with distinct welfare state models.[3] Other countries have been included in the analyses and discussions when the study design has allowed this. As in the previous volume we start from the 1980s but place most emphasis on changes during the 1990s. In all chapters we have stretched our analyses to include the most recent data, but there are inevitably differences in the choices of reference year depending on the research questions or dictated by data limitations.

Having now specified the focus of the book, the countries to be compared and the time period for our studies, we next discuss issues that are crucial to all the chapters, namely the controversial ideas on differing

European welfare models and pressures for convergence in European social policy. Finally, we present the common approach behind the comparative studies that form this volume and the research questions pursued in individual chapters.

The Nordic welfare model

While the notion of a 'Nordic' or 'Scandinavian model' has existed for some time, it was only in the 1990s that the research community entered into deeper discussions on the pros and cons of thinking in terms of 'types', 'models' or 'regimes' of welfare. Much of this discussion has centred around – for and against – the approach adopted by Esping-Andersen (1990, 1999), who suggested that the typically different relations existing between welfare states, labour markets and families can be characterised as three 'welfare regimes'. These Liberal, Social Democratic and Conservative welfare regimes result from different historical forces, are organised according to their own logic, produce different outcomes, and follow qualitatively different development trajectories (Esping-Andersen 1990: 3, 1996 and 1999; for earlier writing see e.g. Titmuss 1958, 1974; Wilensky and Lebeaux 1958; Mishra 1977; Korpi 1983; for overviews see Kvist and Torfing 1996; Abrahamson 1999).

Some scholars have criticised typology thinking in the first place (Baldwin 1990; Ringen 1991), while others engaged in discussion with Esping-Andersen have sought to identify the most crucial criteria for the establishment of welfare regimes (e.g. Lewis 1993; Orloff 1993; Sainsbury 1994; Anttonen and Sipilä 1996). Others have presented views on the appropriate number of welfare regimes (e.g. Castles and Mitchell 1990; Leibfried 1992; Ferrera 1993). Some have compared the extent to which measures of outcomes between different countries vary systematically with the regime type (e.g. Fritzell 1991; Bianchi *et al.* 1996). Ultimately, many of these studies have aimed to empirically test the validity of the theoretical framework pertaining to welfare regimes.

Among the potential problems in using typologies is that they easily lead one to think in deterministic terms and to homogenise cases across areas and time. For instance, it may be tempting to argue that determinants of all welfare policies are the same within countries having more or less the same regime, or that countries believed to be close to a given regime are close in all respects. Yet within a country policies may have different determinants. The determinants of policies and policy outcomes may also differ between countries, and factors influencing policy may vary over time as has recently been shown by Francis Castles (1998). Moreover, similar aims or outcomes may sometimes be achieved through different policies (cf. 'functional equivalents' in Merton 1968). Evidently, then, if there is a 'Nordic model' there also seems to exist a varying number of other models, depending on the focus of studies. For instance, it has been argued that we can distinguish between five models of social insurance (Korpi and Palme 1998), five social care models (Anttonen and Sipilä 1996), four family policy models (Millar and Warman 1996), four gender policy approaches (Chamberlayne 1993) and three unemployment insurance regimes (Gallie and Paugam 2000), while there may exist only two health care models in Europe (Saltman *et al.* 1998).

One paradox when using welfare regime theory is that while social policy schemes are in a state of constant flux, the regimes themselves are mostly thought of as being stable. Yet it has been shown that countries' associations with regimes are not carved in stone, because their welfare systems do develop over time, and countries may move from one regime to another (Kangas 1993). Sometimes development paths may be similar but with a different timing (Kangas 1994). It is thus not surprising that instead of a single Nordic model some prefer to talk about several Nordic models. For example, a number of authors have noted intra-Nordic disparities in the balance between economic and social goals (Mjøset *et al.* 1986; Kosonen 1998), in social policy schemes (e.g. Alban and Christiansen 1995; Ploug and Kvist 1996; Korpi and Palme 1998), in the balance between cash transfers and services, between private and public solutions, as well as institutional (e.g. Baldersheim and Ståhlberg 1999) and political variations (Marklund and Nordlund 1999). It is easy to expose differences between the Nordic countries, but harder to place them in perspective.

In other words, numerous objections against typologies have been raised from various viewpoints, and currently there is certainly no watertight typology covering the various dimensions of the welfare state that everybody agrees upon. Nevertheless, it is still plausible to think that differences in policy choices lead to differences in outcomes and that countries, as the important policy-making units, cluster around varieties of policy options and policy outcomes. This situation is not necessarily an impasse as it is possible to distinguish between empirically created models and theoretical ideal-types. In addition, and in contrast to empirical clustering of countries, the 'Nordic model' may be understood as an ideal-type in the Weberian sense, meaning that no country will embody all the characteristics of this model. An ideal-type model represents a standard against which empirical cases can be compared. It can be a helpful tool for empirical comparisons, as it allows researchers to study the degree of proximity or conformity of countries to the model (Weber 1949: 90).

In our previous book, the list of Nordic welfare state characteristics included elements that characterised both policies and their outcomes (see Kautto *et al.* 1999). Accordingly, a Nordic welfare model is associated with a broad scope of public social policy and political commitment to full employment, accompanied by active labour market measures. Universal flat-rate basic security and an earnings-related component for those with a work history are the elements of a fairly generous income security system. Another feature is local and publicly funded service provision to cater for all needs and the whole population (see also Erikson *et al.* 1987; Kolberg 1991; Hansen *et al.* 1993; Sipilä 1997; Kvist 1999). These characteristics mean that the 'Nordic model' has a greater share of public expenditure and a higher share of social expenditure of the GDP than other models, accompanied by higher taxation. With regard to outcomes, the ideal–typical Nordic model should achieve low income inequality, low poverty rates and small differences in levels of living and gender equality. What is more, these various aspects are thought to interact and reinforce each other: only together do they constitute the whole that we may describe as the 'Nordic model' (Esping-Andersen and Korpi 1987).

The above characteristics do not represent an exhaustive listing, but do help us to understand the crucial elements in an ideal–typical Nordic model, and these we aimed to include in our empirical comparisons. It is clear that in reality, and as mentioned above, no one country will display all, if any, of these characteristics perfectly. And to be sure, countries are more or less close to or distant from a standard. A common starting point is that countries are the key unit of comparison and it is up to the individual chapter studies to show whether and how clustering of countries occurs in certain key dimensions. The authors also examine whether the Nordic characteristics located in different dimensions in previous research have persisted.

Is there convergence between the Nordic and other Western European welfare states?

Whereas welfare models are often portrayed as institutionally resilient to change, and even as 'immovable objects' (Pierson 1998), another strand of current comparative welfare state research focuses on pressures for change. This literature is of particular interest for the purposes of this book as it argues that welfare states are prone to change in response to pressures, and furthermore in a way that will ultimately lead to convergence of different types of welfare models. Again this is a controversial argument and we need to clarify our standpoint here.

Despite the recent growth of interest in convergence, the hypothesis itself is not new. In the context of societal development in general, early sociologists like Herbert Spencer and Auguste Comte advocated the idea that societies develop and modernise along a similar path in response to common causal factors and that this adjustment may ultimately lead to narrowing differences between nations. In the context of welfare state development the idea of convergence was formulated most explicitly in the 1960s and 1970s. This so-called first generation of comparative welfare state studies typically saw welfare state development as a response to changing societal processes, although there were different variants to this general functionalist hypothesis. The most influential school of thought is often labelled the logic of industrialism (e.g. Kerr *et al.* 1960; but see also Wilensky and Lebeaux 1958; Wilensky 1975). The basic underlying mechanism here is that technological and economic rationality engenders convergence in all advanced industrialised societies regardless of historical and political tradition, not only in terms of the institutions of the welfare state but more generally. According to this functional logic, all societies and their institutions were expected to evolve towards 'pluralistic industrialism'. Within welfare state research this basic idea is sometimes embedded within modernisation theory (Flora and Alber 1981). As pointed out by Palme (1990), among others, the functionalist orientation was also prevalent in more Marxist-oriented writings, in which the development of the welfare state was largely seen as a necessary feature of modern capitalism (see e.g. O'Connor 1973).

In several branches of research these ideas were subjected to severe criticism, and for a decade or two the convergence hypothesis was abandoned (see e.g. the volume edited by Goldthorpe 1984). Few would then have foreseen that the notion of convergence would receive renewed attention in the 1990s. When the convergence hypothesis is spelled out today, it is usually accompanied by arguments stressing factors such as internationalisation, geopolitical transformations, technological revolution, liberalisation of money and capital markets and globalised culture. What is common to past and present convergence thinking is the tendency to portray the pressure factors as irresistible forces that will lead to increased similarity of welfare states. Another common element is the limited attention given to partisan politics. Despite many similarities one profound difference between the 'old and new hypotheses of convergence' (Montanari 2000) should be stressed: the former theories were mainly occupied with historically understanding how and why the growth of welfare states occurred in the twentieth century, whereas the latter are basically dealing with the necessity of welfare state restructuring.

Much of the current discussion on convergence in the context of social policy and welfare revolves around the twin themes of the effects of globalisation and European integration. In the literature the concepts 'globalisation' and 'integration' are often intertwined and their interrelationships are rarely specified precisely and explicitly. While analytically globalisation can be divided into different dimensions, *economic* globalisation, which is seen to result chiefly from unconstrained capital flows and operations of multinational enterprises, is clearly the dimension attracting most interest (e.g. Hirst and Thompson 1996). Those focusing on European integration, on the other hand, have directed attention to the *political* constraints created by the European Union and deepening European integration (Streeck 1995, 1996; Scharpf 1999), although the birth of EMU has added an economic flavour to the existing literature (see e.g. Pochet and Vanhercke 1998). To some extent these two aspects have been bound together in discussions of the role of international or supranational agencies as precursors for the development of 'epistemic communities' that share perceptions of current challenges and how they should be met (Deacon, B. 1998, 1999).

Globalisation is regarded as including processes that by-pass or at least affect autonomous decision-making, and some actually fear that nation–states have lost their ability to remain sovereign. One measure of sovereignty is the possibility of implementing fiscal policies and it is here that much of the discussion of welfare states is located. A key argument in the globalisation literature is that in a globalised world production forces have become so mobile that firms wanting to avoid high taxation, and especially labour costs, can shift their operations from one country or part of the world to another. Exposure to this threat forces nation–states to tax competition, or at least to modify their tax systems to prevent substantial emigration of firms and jobs. The fact that 'tax evasion' has become easier than before threatens tax bases, and thereby also the prospects of the welfare states to implement their present redistribution policies (Mishra 1999; Perraton 2000; Swank 2000). Because of its impacts on financing, globalisation is perceived as a threat to welfare states, particularly so in countries with high taxation, the Nordic countries being the prime example. (e.g. Kosonen 1994; Strange 1996; Scholte 1997; Gough 1999; Tanzi 1999.)

However, alternative views have also been presented. Attention has been drawn to the fact that many of the countries that have long been highly exposed to international trade competition, such as the small and open Nordic economies, also tend to have 'larger' welfare states. One could even argue that the Nordic welfare states historically developed as responses to outside pressures, rather than being threatened by international economic liberalisation (e.g. Katzenstein 1985; Mjøset *et al.* 1986). Furthermore, as small and 'enabling' nation–states they may be faster and more fit to adjust to global competition and other challenges than countries elsewhere in Europe (Garrett 1998; Stephens *et al.* 1999). Several scholars express scepticism about the impact of globalisation on the abilities of national governments to pursue their own social and welfare policies and argue that the welfare states of Western Europe are likely to survive globalisation (Hirst and Thompson 2000; Kuhnle 2000).

A more tangible issue is the effect of European integration, or more specifically of the EU, on the policies of member states. While globalisation is supposed to impact on welfare states mainly through unintended consequences, here it is more a question of intentional efforts at a supranational level to achieve 'harmonisation' and 'co-ordination' between the member states. There is a growing and heterogeneous body of literature devoted to the impact of the EU on the freedom of member states to implement their policies. Most agree that in the social dimension nation–states remain sovereign actors, but views are at variance regarding the spillover effects from economic integration. Some authors believe that fiercer competition indirectly exerts pressure towards greater similarities in institutional arrangements and levels of provision in the EU member states (Streeck 1995, 1996; Hagen 1999; Scharpf 1999; Leibfried and Pierson 2000). Unless the governments of the member states manage to agree on some joint objectives and standards in this area, this pressure may make it difficult for the countries with the most generous provisions to sustain them.

Convergence may simply be defined here as a process where dispersion among countries decreases. Sometimes this is interpreted to mean a move towards a European average, or even towards a European minimum. If this were the correct interpretation, convergence from a Nordic perspective would mean a 'Europeanisation' of the Nordic welfare states. However, convergence may occur in more than one way and the fate of the Nordic countries is not a foregone conclusion. As already suggested, it may also be that other Western European countries start to adopt policies and arrangements already institutionalised in the Nordic countries, e.g. in the areas of gender equality and active employment policies. 'Catch-up convergence', long discussed in economics (see e.g. Dowrick and Ngyuyen 1989; Alber and Standing 2000), is a term used to depict the situation where countries at the low end of any given scale move closer to the others without a corresponding fall in standards in countries at the top end of the scale. For instance, the fact that Southern European countries have developed their social protection schemes rapidly has led to such catch-up convergence (Greve 1996). In fact, in contrast to non-empirical writings, empirical research into the fate of the Nordic welfare states has not produced gloomy verdicts. Empirically, there remain few clear signs that welfare state development in the Nordic countries has been 'Europeanised' (Hagen 1999). Our earlier study confirmed that, despite economic and other pressures, actual changes in the welfare state machinery – its outputs and people's living conditions – appear limited in the Nordic countries (Kautto *et al.* 1999). More generally, social and political institutions still explain much of the difference among national welfare states (Bonoli *et al.* 2000).

In sum, whether convergence is taking place (or merely parallel trends, stability or even divergence), and if so, what kind of convergence and why, are all open questions. Moreover, as convergence is not an encompassing process we may find it in some areas but fail to recognise it in some other dimensions; for instance, convergence could occur in certain outcomes despite continuing differences in policies. In this book all chapters analyse trends, and they also provide more specific material to assess the direction of trends and various manifestations of convergence or divergence in European social policy.

Framework of the book and research themes

The focus and unit of analysis in comparative research differ. Some researchers examine welfare *regimes* and intend to include all major institutions in their holistic analysis, while others compare welfare *states*, i.e. the state-component of regimes, and still others limit themselves to examining particular *social policies* of the welfare states. And while it could be argued that analysis of various *outcomes* is embedded in regime thinking, the institutional focus may still vary. In this book the changing nature of welfare states is the ultimate concern, but the framework for the chapters is based on the belief that to understand current changes in welfare states we need to recognise the constant interplay between the different institutions in society, and that social policies reflect changes in the interplay between the state, the market and the family. Welfare states react and adapt to changing circumstances, but they also aim to exert a proactive impact on the development of other institutions. Thus while changing labour markets and family structures put pressure on welfare state adaptation, welfare state programmes may actively influence the working of labour markets and choices within families. Instability in one institution may spill over into another, and there may be problems of integration between various institutions. The studies in this book investigate these relationships between institutions from a welfare state perspective, concentrating on certain aspects or programmes of the welfare state.

In addition to relationships between institutions, this book examines changes in people's living conditions. While institutions may be specified and defined analytically, in market economies their interplay is inherently complex and their combined effects may prove inseparable in practice. The literature on welfare production terms the effects of the welfare state as 'outcomes', but scholars struggle to explain how much of such outcomes should be attributed to the functioning of the welfare state and/or to other factors. Production and consumption in the market, participation and rewards from the labour market, care and support from the family and welfare state programmes all have implications for individual welfare. Separately and in combination they influence resources at the individual's disposal, their available options and behaviour. And conversely, the situation and behaviour of individuals may contribute to changing institutions.

Hence crucial policy challenges can be interpreted as concerning changes in the institutions and in the interplay between markets, families and the welfare state. They also concern the welfare state's ability to respond to people's changing needs. The numerous common policy challenges identified include globalisation, mobility of capital and production, competitiveness, changes in the nature of work and employment patterns, unemployment and social exclusion, gender equality, provision of care, changing family and household patterns, ageing, ethnicity and balancing of budgets. There is no doubt that all European countries seek ways to better address these challenges. But it is equally true that due to the variation in their institutional set-ups their starting points differ, and that the pressures for change are not equally severe for all countries. Moreover, the extent to which policy makers actually perceive and prioritise the challenges, and the way they address them, may vary considerably. Welfare states may also differ in their desire to affect other institutions. Despite the widespread rhetoric stressing common challenges and common responses, empirical scrutiny exposes significant differences in the degree and form of adaptation and policy responses (see, for example, Ferrera *et al.* 2000).

Therefore, rather than addressing and analysing policy challenges *per se*, we decided to concentrate on the interrelationships between the welfare state and other institutions. Thus the chapters address the interplay between the welfare state and one or other institution with reference to one or more important policy challenges in a certain dimension of the welfare state. The remainder of the book deals with a number of themes that are generally seen as acute policy challenges particularly relevant for all Western European countries. These topical themes concern the level and distribution of some essential aspects of living conditions and the impact of the welfare state on them (Chapters 2, 3, 4 and 5), the interplay between the family and the welfare state (Chapters 6 and 7), the relationship between the labour market and the welfare state (Chapters 8 and 9), and pressures on financing of welfare states arising from the relationship between the market and the welfare state (Chapter 10).

In the Scandinavian research tradition welfare tends to be analysed as the various resources that enable the individual to determine his or her own life (Johansson 1970; Erikson and Uusitalo 1987). Although welfare is generally accepted to be composed of different elements, there is no commonly accepted way of weighing the relative importance of these and, here too, the method is to study welfare in different dimensions separately. Also, as it is easier to reach a common understanding of what constitutes 'bad circumstances' than of 'welfare' (Allardt 1999), in practice, research on welfare has studied lack of resources and concentrated on themes such as the extent of poverty, inequality and ill-health, and their distribution across social categories.

Ultimately, welfare states should be judged on their ability to contribute to the overall welfare of their citizens, and in particular to prevent inferior conditions. Over recent years there has been growing criticism that welfare states fail to achieve this goal. For example, increased levels of inequality in most countries is taken to imply that welfare states have failed to serve their original and prime objectives, or that they do so inefficiently. This theme is an acute one in all European countries, but for the Nordic countries, where the goal of equality has long been high on the political agenda, such a development would certainly raise serious problems of legitimacy for the Nordic model. We know from previous research that the Nordic countries have been among those with the most equal income distribution (Atkinson *et al.* 1995); but we also know that income inequality has been on the increase lately, with the possible exception of Denmark (see SOU 2000 for Sweden; Ministry of Health and Social Affairs 1999 for Norway; Uusitalo 1999 for Finland; Hansen 1995 for Denmark). In Chapter 2, *Johan Fritzell* clarifies the issue of whether increases in income inequality have led to a blurring of differences between the countries. Can we still identify a Nordic pattern of low inequality in disposable incomes? Fritzell studies cross-national differences in income inequality and examines whether we can discern any tendency towards convergence over time. He also questions the extent to which cross-national variation in income inequality is a result of the functioning of the welfare state. Finally, he compares the situation of specific social groups, i.e. the young, the old, and single parents, in order to elucidate whether specific vulnerable groups still fare better in the Nordic countries than elsewhere.

While income is a widely used indicator of welfare, health – or more precisely lack of good health – is another and in many senses a more fundamental indicator. To be able to perform daily routines and pursue one's ambitions and goals is a fundamental resource for a good life. In welfare state research, however, health aspects have often been sidelined as not part of the 'social' sphere. Although there are many studies that show the existence of health and mortality differences in the Nordic countries, and also some comparative analyses, this field of research is largely unknown outside medical sociology and social epidemiology. It is also the case that very little is known about the role of the welfare state and welfare state regimes for variations in public health and health inequalities. Do the Nordic countries have a better level of health? Is health distributed more equally than elsewhere? In their chapter, *Olle Lundberg* and *Eero Lahelma* focus on inequalities in health from a comparative perspective. They estimate the level and distribution of ill-health and mortality and show cross-national differences in how socio-economic positions are linked to health risks. With the help of a recent European comparative study, in which the authors participated, they also address the difference between absolute and relative differences and discuss the policy implications of their findings.

Obviously gender equality is another aspect of equality generally thought of as very pronounced in the Nordic countries. Gender equality is often a stated objective in national and supranational policy documents designed to modernise social protection (see e.g. COM (1999) 347 final). The Nordic countries are implicitly exemplified in such documents, and this is one more reason for taking a closer look at processes leading to increased gender equality and its implied consequences for social life.

In her chapter *Randi Kjeldstad* first emphasises the development of gender policies and the process towards gender equality. She investigates the differences between European countries in these respects with the help of a typology of gender equality. Kjeldstad examines the historical process and the current predominant gender approach in the countries compared and then considers to what extent these may be connected to various levels of documented gender inequality.

Annemette Sørensen pursues the topic of gender equality further by analysing earnings differentials between women and men. She asks whether more balanced participation in the labour market has resulted in more even earnings equality in the Nordic countries. First, she examines cross-national variation in gender differences in earnings at an aggregate level, both absolutely and relatively. Second, she addresses women's economic dependence on the men they live with, before moving on to consider the consequences of a more pronounced earnings equality pattern for partnerships, i.e. the interdependence of spouses and the inequalities related to sharing economic risks in the event of losing one income. In her intriguing analysis Sørensen, contrary to conventional wisdom, makes a case that economic independence for women may in fact lead to greater economic interdependence between spouses.

The relationship between the family and the welfare state is two-way in the sense that changes in family patterns create new demands for the welfare state while social policy arrangements may lead to changes in people's behaviour, both intentionally and unintentionally. In Chapter 6 *Aksel Hatland* concentrates on this relationship by first outlining how conceptions of family status differ between national social security programmes. Whether one is married or not has formed an important dividing line for policies as needs are believed to differ largely according to family status. New family forms and the spread of cohabitation present a serious challenge to the traditional policy goal of redistribution between families. Hatland examines differences and similarities in the spread of cohabitation in the European countries and in national policy responses.

Another perspective on the relation between the welfare state and families is given by *Tine Rostgaard* and *Juhani Lehto,* who address social and health care services in Chapter 7. Care services as an alternative to family-based care have often been identified as a factor contributing to the realisation of gender equality (e.g. Hernes 1987a). Arranging care is also topical in view of the ageing of European societies and because the availability of child care services has been seen as crucial to the potential for combining work and family life (OECD 1999c: 88–90). Some view the absence of sufficient and affordable care services in certain countries as one of the factors underlying declining fertility rates (Esping-Andersen 1999). Welfare states may choose to respond to these needs by arranging care differently or even providing alternative forms of support to parents. Traditionally, the Nordic countries are portrayed as 'service heavy', implying that they have an abundance of care services compared to the 'cash heavy' income transfer countries in continental Europe (Kohl 1981; Sipilä 1997). Rostgaard and Lehto examine different national mixes of care from the perspective of 'functional alternatives' (Merton 1968), which leads them to consider the situation and development in health and education sectors in addition to the social care sector.

The next two chapters examine the interplay between the welfare state and the labour market. The contribution by *Bjørn Hvinden, Matti Heikkilä* and *Ilkka Kankare* concentrates on differences in policy emphasis in activation, while that by *Jochen Clasen, Jon Kvist* and *Wim van Oorschot* discusses prevailing differences in the role of work in unemployment insurance. Both chapters address the link between welfare and work; they discuss whether we are witnessing a change in welfare state policies targeted to ensure a flow 'from welfare to work', and to what extent this may lead to convergence or divergence in this area of the welfare state.

Employment and employability are probably the central political theme in current European social policy reform debates. Hvinden, Heikkilä and Kankare first consider the views of supranational bodies like the OECD and the EU, which stress that social policy measures should more deliberately direct non-employed people to employment and address employability issues. They then investigate the empirical support for such a shift in policy emphasis and question how far activation has become a practical reality in Western European countries. They present an analysis of measures and provisions targeted at people out of work and examine the possibility of identifying some distinct profiles of activation policies rather than just a general move in one direction or another.

In Chapter 9 Clasen, Kvist and van Oorschot investigate how work plays a different role in unemployment insurance across countries with regard to access to benefits, their level and duration, and the requirements expected of benefit recipients. Besides comparing countries across these various dimensions of work-conditionality they also consider the interplay of the various dimensions. For example, some countries may have easy access to benefits, but which are small and only paid for short periods, whereas others may have easy access to generous benefits, but coupled with strict conditions on accepting available work and participating in activation programmes. Such configurations of work-conditionality, the authors argue, constitute distinct policy responses towards the unemployed and represent regime–specific welfare states. The authors also examine how work-related conditionality has changed over the past fifteen years.

The interplay between the market and the welfare state is the fourth and final relationship addressed in this book. Globalisation is often used as a catch word to capture processes linked to increased mobility of capital, investments, goods, services and labour. Along with political integration and economic deregulation in Europe, the internationalisation of market forces is seen as a key factor forcing governments to reconsider their financing structures to ensure competitiveness in the global market. In Chapter 10, *Mikko Kautto* addresses this pressure on welfare states. Since levels and ways of financing are linked to the redistribution strategies adopted, limits to financing have potentially far-reaching consequences for welfare state measures, and thence for the targets of redistribution. Kautto starts by summarising the literature on the supposed potential of external forces such as globalisation, European integration and the EU to affect financing of welfare states. The Nordic countries, characterised as they are by higher costs for social protection and high shares of tax financing, should be especially vulnerable to such pressures. Kautto continues by investigating responses in the light of empirical data on financing social protection. The results are used to discuss whether we may detect convergence in financing patterns and if clustering of countries according to specific financing arrangements is apparent.

Each chapter stands alone as a contribution to a specific field of welfare state research. The Conclusion gathers the main strands of all the chapters to discuss the distinctiveness of the Nordic countries and the variety of options different welfare states have been pursuing. We also assess whether there are common or group-specific tendencies, and if policy adaptation has resulted in converging or diverging trends in the various sub-areas of welfare state development in Europe.

Notes

1 We are aware that the notion 'welfare' has negative connotations in some countries. However, from a research perspective there are good reasons to use welfare rather than 'well-being', as the former notion refers more

to objective indicators, whereas the latter also embraces subjective elements that are not analysed in this book.

2 In Chapter 4 Germany is not included in the comparison.

3 In addition to standard distinctions, these three countries are among the closest to the Nordic countries from both historical and geographical perspectives. They are also the countries that have been the main sources of experience when inspiration for reforms has been sought. Other practical and important reasons for the choice were the availability of comparable data and contacts.

2 Still different? Income distribution in the Nordic countries in a European comparison

Johan Fritzell

Introduction[1]

Underlying the interest in welfare state programmes and cross-national variations in the pattern, size and structure of various social policies, is that we regard the welfare state as an institution exerting great influence on our lives and well-being. A further assumption is that this impact differs between individuals and social categories, and accordingly that the degree of inequality in the distribution of societal goods and resources has scope to be affected. Hence, in so far as there is cross-national variation in these programmes, 'outcome' inequality may systematically vary between nations.

One characteristic of the Nordic welfare states is said to be that they pursue a different conception of equality from others, with a particularly strong focus on equality of result (or outcome), as opposed to equality of opportunity or different equity conceptions (for a discussion see e.g. Esping-Andersen 1996). This chapter sets out to examine a central outcome in this respect, namely economic resources or to be more precise the distribution of annual income. Without embarking on a thorough review it seems safe to say that earlier research on income distribution and poverty has by and large confirmed the view that the Nordic countries have a low degree of income inequality and also very low poverty rates (see e.g. Atkinson *et al.* 1995; Rainwater and Smeeding 1995; Gottschalk and Smeeding 1997 and 2000; Korpi and Palme 1998; OECD 1998a; Jäntti and Danziger 2000). In fact, in the late 1980s, Finland, Sweden and Norway (mostly in that order) emerged with the lowest inequality levels among the OECD countries according to most of the inequality estimates presented by Atkinson *et al.* (1995) in their thorough study for the OECD.

The overarching question raised in this chapter concerns whether or not we still find proof of a specific Nordic model when looking at the distribution of income from a variety of perspectives and comparing the outcomes with those in three other European countries. Do we find evidence of convergence, divergence or similar trends? Within this general issue four questions are raised and analyses of each of them conducted. The first question concerns the level of inequality. Were the Nordic countries in the mid-1990s really so different from other European countries in terms of overall income inequality? Second, to what extent do we find commonality and variation with regard to recent changes in inequality? Is there any evidence for convergence with respect to the degree of inequality? Third, what is the role of cash benefits of welfare states in the income distribution process? This will be studied by comparing the size and distributional profile of income transfers and the extent of inequality before and after cash benefits are taken into account. Fourth, to what extent do we find cross-national similarity and variation with regard to the relative income position and poverty risks for more specific social categories when comparing their situation in the mid-1990s with that prevailing about a decade earlier? Is it still the case that specific vulnerable groups fare relatively better in the Nordic countries, as indicated by earlier research?

The data will be based exclusively on the Luxembourg Income Study (LIS), which has been the source of most of the ample evidence on comparative income poverty and inequality estimates among the world's richer nations during recent decades. The next section discusses some earlier and recent argumentation concerning why and how we should expect convergence to take place. The empirical section following thereafter consists of three parts. The first presents an overview of levels and trends in inequality among the countries included in the study. The middle section explores the role of welfare state redistribution – cash benefits – in producing the outcomes presented in the first section. The third delves into more detail on the relative positions of some social categories, with regard to changes in both average incomes and relative poverty rates. All analyses are based on comparisons between the four Nordic countries, Denmark, Finland, Norway and Sweden, and on data from Germany, the Netherlands and the United Kingdom. The data cover the period from around the mid-1980s to the mid-1990s. The chapter ends with a summary and a concluding discussion of whether or not the presented results are supportive of Nordic uniqueness in this respect.[2]

Convergence, similarity or cross-national variation?

The idea that a convergence of various social phenomena would take place across nation–states was a basic feature of most post-World War II theories of societal change. It is perhaps most commonly referred to in relation to what is often phrased the 'logic of industrialism', a theoretical perspective of pluralistic modern societies evolving according to the law of the system (see, e.g. Kerr *et al.* 1960). This school of thought, with a clear functionalistic approach, emphasises cross-national similarity rather than variation, and the path supposedly followed by industrial societies gives rise to a convergence (of attitudes, power structures, levels of inequality, etc.). The assumed underlying mechanism is that technological and economic rationality engender convergence among all industrial societies, despite differences in historical and political context. It is important to note that proponents of this school did not necessarily claim that welfare state redistribution as such was unimportant, but rather: 'taxes and benefits taken together have a highly egalitarian effect on income distribution' (Wilensky 1975: 94). What was claimed was more that welfare state development followed in the general pathway of industrialism and could be explained in terms of this logic. Accordingly, any cross-national variation could largely be explained by cross-national variations in economic and industrial development.

Going back even further, and focusing more specifically on the distribution of income, it is notable that the idea of income distribution as a 'natural law' has a much longer history. The first theories on the degree of inequality and the shape of an income distribution were solely based on mathematics and statistics. To give but one example Pareto, about 100 years ago, thought he had found a law (a coefficient) that could summarise the shape of the distribution of income, and several other scholars elaborated on his work with more sophisticated models, but solely based on stochastic processes and probability theory (for a review see e.g. Pen 1971).

From a social science perspective the extremely influential work of Kuznets (1955, 1963) is more interesting. Once again the outcome, the degree of inequality, would obey a more or less universal law (the inverted-U curve) according to Kuznets' hypothesis. As societies move from agrarian to industrial production, income inequality first increases, then stabilises on a fairly low economic level, and from then on decreases. Although based on both historical data and economics, Kuznets's hypothesis once again stresses cross-national similarity and convergence, in which the level of economic development is the basic factor for understanding both long-term trends and differences between nations in the size distribution of income. As long as economic growth continues, this hypothesis basically suggests that the long-term trend should be towards a more compressed income distribution. It should be stressed that Kuznets was primarily investigating the societal change leading *towards* industrialism, not the societal changes we are witnessing today across the affluent world. Moreover, Kuznets himself was not so deterministic in his writings, in which he discusses several counterbalancing forces. It is rather the many followers of Kuznets who have tended to regard the inverted-U curve as a law.

Ideas about similarities and convergence have more recently been reshaped, and this, of course, forms one of the basic points of departure for this whole volume. However, it is now the widening of income differentials that is postulated to be inescapable. The main empirical evidence for such an opinion is the experience of the UK and the US, which led Atkinson to so eloquently label the hypothesis 'the Transatlantic Consensus' (Atkinson 2000). It is important to note that several of the suggested contenders for why income inequality has increased so dramatically in the United States, for example the technological change explanation and the deindustrialisation thesis, are to a large extent global theories and tend to imply a more or less inevitable type of change that nation–states cannot escape.[3] In the new global economy multinational firms can more easily move labour-intensive production to countries with lower wage costs levels, which thereby, together with technological changes, creates a shift in the relative demands for high skilled vs. low skilled workers. This in turn will lead to higher wage inequality and/or increasing unemployment. Further, it is a commonly held view that the higher degree of internationalisation of our economies means that the scope of action for national welfare states has diminished. The growing importance of multinational organisations such as the EU is also believed to foster convergence. And indeed, these ideas have some face validity in the light of research on trends of rising income inequality. There is no doubt that income inequality increased dramatically in the UK and US after around 1980. Moreover, few, if any, countries have experienced a substantial decline in inequality since then.

What, then, has empirical research more generally unearthed about similarities and convergence? It seems safe to say that these theories and hypotheses of convergence have so far been strongly refuted by comparative income distribution research. The findings can rather be seen as quite supportive of the fact that income inequality as such differs substantially among the richer nations. Moreover, the provisions of the welfare state and its influence on the distribution of income and relative poverty rates show a high degree of cross-national variation. In other words, instead of support for any notions of convergence, profound cross-national variation has been noted both with regard to level of inequality and changes in it. Consequently, on the most general level it is, at least indirectly, the idea that 'politics and institutions matter' which has gained support.[4] However, it should also be mentioned that Gottschalk and Smeeding (forthcoming) claim that in a longer time perspective we tend to find a U-shaped pattern of inequality in many countries; in other words they make a case for 'similar trends', at least with regard to the longer term.

It is of course beyond the scope of the present chapter to mount a full challenge to any of the major hypotheses discussed above. What can be scrutinised is to what extent the results of the empirical analyses are congruent with explicit or implicit suggestions in different theoretical discussions. Is it still the case that we can distinguish a specific Nordic model when looking at a central outcome such as the distribution of income, or have the Nordic countries finally converged into a more European-type level and structure of inequality?

Data and methods

The analyses in the empirical sections are solely based on the comparative database of the Luxembourg Income Study (LIS). This database consists of harmonised cross-national microdata on income for about twenty-five countries (with three to four waves for most of them), thereby providing the best comparative source for analysing levels and trends of income distribution, income poverty, etc. (for a presentation of the data and the national data sources used see e.g. Atkinson *et al.* 1995, or the homepage at *http://www.lis.ceps.lu*).

In this study data for seven countries are analysed, ideally from the mid-1980s to the mid-1990s. However, since LIS-data do not cover annual observations there is a slight cross-national variation in years between observations. The four Nordic countries (Denmark (1987/1992), Finland (1987/1995), Norway (1986/1995), and Sweden (1987/1995) are contrasted against three non-Nordic countries: Germany (1984/1994), the Netherlands (1987/1994) and the United Kingdom (1986/1995).[5] The first empirical section, depending on availability of data, also includes inequality estimates from survey years in the middle of these observation periods. The choice of countries is partly practical, but also consistent with most of the other chapters in this volume, which include countries usually characterised as belonging to different welfare state regimes. If we were to find no substantial cross-national differences, we would surely have a rather good case for the convergence thesis. It should be noted that we only have two or three observation points at our disposal in the empirical investigation. Ideally we should have *comparable* yearly data to more carefully examine trends. We therefore cannot fully rule out the possibility that changes depending on, for example, the business cycle could have had some impact on the results presented.

Income and equivalence scale

Most of the analyses are based on the disposable, i.e. post-tax and transfer, income of the income unit, which in this case is the household (though slight variation exists in defining households). However, when studying the role of cash benefits the comparison is instead between market (i.e. pre-tax and transfers) income and gross income (i.e. pre-tax and post-transfers). In order to be able to compare income between households of differing size and structure all incomes are adjusted with an equivalence scale. However, since there is no objective superior way of constructing an equivalence scale, a simple one-parametric scale that has quite recently become common in cross-national research is used. If y denotes disposable income and n the number of persons in the household, the equivalent disposable income (EDI) is:

$$\text{EDI} = y/n^{e}$$

It has been shown that most equivalence scales in use with reasonably high accuracy can be estimated by the factor *e* (Buhmann *et al.* 1988). The lower one sets *e,* the higher economies of scale assumed. If *e* is set to zero, one basically assumes that it is irrelevant how many persons are living in the household. If, on the other hand, *e* is set to 1, no economies of scale are assumed and thus all incomes are calculated per capita. If *e* is set to 0.5, which it is here, it means that the equivalence scale is the square root of the number of persons in the household. Thus, a four-person household in this case must have twice the disposable income of a single-person household in order to have the same equivalent income. Although the household is the income unit, the unit of analysis is the individual living in each household; in other words we count persons rather than households (for a discussion on the theoretical backgrounds, see e.g. Cowell 1984).

It should also be mentioned that the Swedish household definition means that individuals are regarded as separate households from the age of 18, regardless of whether or not they are living with their parents. This obviously presents a comparability problem since their income will be grossly underestimated (and somewhat overestimated for the parents). In order to avoid most of this problem, all results will, for all countries, refer to persons living in households headed by someone aged 20 or above, except for the general overview in the first section.[6]

Empirical results

Levels and changes of income inequality

Unlike the situation prevailing some twenty years ago we now have substantial evidence that rather profound cross-national differences exist in the degree of inequality in income distributions among the rich (post-)industrialised nations (see e.g. Fritzell 1993; Atkinson *et al.* 1995; Gottschalk and Smeeding 1997 and 2000). Do the LIS data then support the uniqueness of the Nordic countries so often assumed in the welfare state literature? A first glance at this issue is presented in Figure 2.1, which shows how the overall level of inequality in the distribution of equivalent disposable income in our seven-country sample according to LIS data changed from the mid-1980s onwards. For all countries except Denmark and Germany we have three observation points, the middle one referring to the years around 1990.[7]

The upper part of the figure gives the level of inequality according to the perhaps most widely used measure, the Gini coefficient, whereas the lower part presents the so-called 90/10–percentile ratio. The latter measure shows the relative distance in terms of the ratio between the upper and lower end of the distribution of equivalent disposable income. For example, if this ratio equals three it means that someone located at the 90th percentile of the distribution lives in a household in which the equivalent income is three times higher than for someone located at the 10th percentile.

A first glance at Figure 2.1 reveals that the Nordic countries indeed had a comparatively low degree of inequality, regardless of on which time period or which of the two inequality measures we are focusing. Further, the relatively low degree of income inequality occurred in all four countries and at least a simple visual inspection of the estimates and changes appears quite supportive of the view of Nordic distinctiveness in terms of overall inequality in the distribution of income. As regards changes of inequality in these seven countries, from the

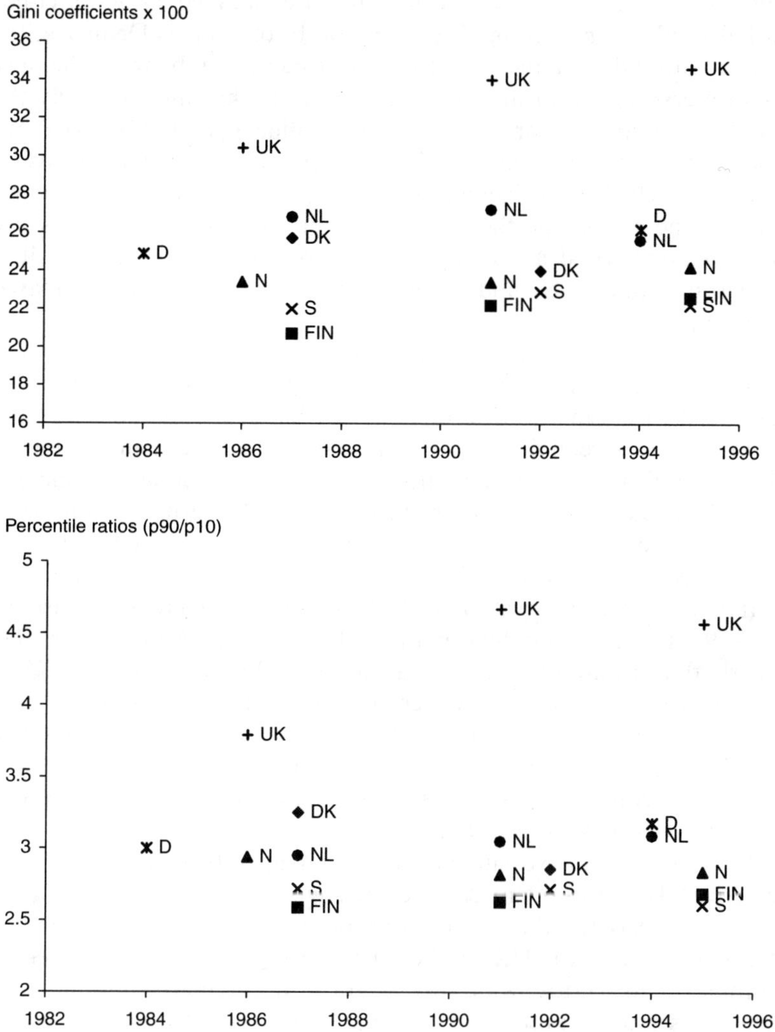

Source: Luxembourg Income Study.
Notes: Income refers to equivalent disposable income. Equivalence scale: square root of household size. Person weights adopted.

Figure 2.1 Income inequality in seven countries from 1984 to 1995

mid-1980s to the mid-1990s the data indicate that inequality was either rather stable or increasing. The exception to this rule is Denmark, for which both indices indicate a decrease of inequality between the only two observations that are available (but note that unfortunately the latest observation year we have for Denmark is 1992).[8] Without going into details it seems as if the data are supportive of a conclusion already reached when inequality trends during the 1980s were compared. The degree of the increase differs and some countries are better characterised as having roughly constant inequality, but it is rather uncommon to find countries in which inequality decreased substantially.[9]

From the viewpoint of single countries it is notable that the increase was remarkably high in the United Kingdom, but inequality also increased in Germany. One obvious candidate for this development in Germany is reunification, but at least a superficial inspection of the data fails to support this since the increase of inequality remained roughly at the same level when the citizens of Eastern Germany were excluded from the analysis. An increase in the United Kingdom would perhaps be expected, but its size is still surprising. Few countries within the OECD experienced such a dramatic increase up to the mid-1980s, notwithstanding that the LIS inequality estimates for 1986 clearly did not imply that the peak of inequality in the United Kingdom had been reached. However, after the early 1990s it seems as if inequality became fairly stable in the UK too, as indicated by the fact that both inequality indices in Figure 2.1 are fairly similar in 1991 and 1995 (this conclusion is also supported by national series, see e.g. Jenkins 1999, Atkinson 2000).

How, then, can we summarise the changes from a Nordic perspective? To what extent can we see signs of similarity, in terms of inequality, between the Nordic countries on one hand and Germany, Netherlands, and the UK on the other? In Figure 2.2 this is presented graphically in the following way: if, for both the mid-1980s and mid-1990s observation points, we treat the Nordic countries as one group and calculate the unweighted average Gini coefficient and percentile ratio and then compare these with each of the three non-Nordic countries in terms of relative distance, we obtain a rough indication of convergence or divergence.[10] As seen in Figure 2.2 the outcome of such an exercise is, for example, that the Gini coefficient in the UK, compared to the Nordic average, was 32.4 per cent higher in the mid-1980s, whereas it was 48.8 per cent higher in 1995. Even though we clearly see that our inequality measures behave somewhat differently, it is evident that the distances between the Nordic countries on one

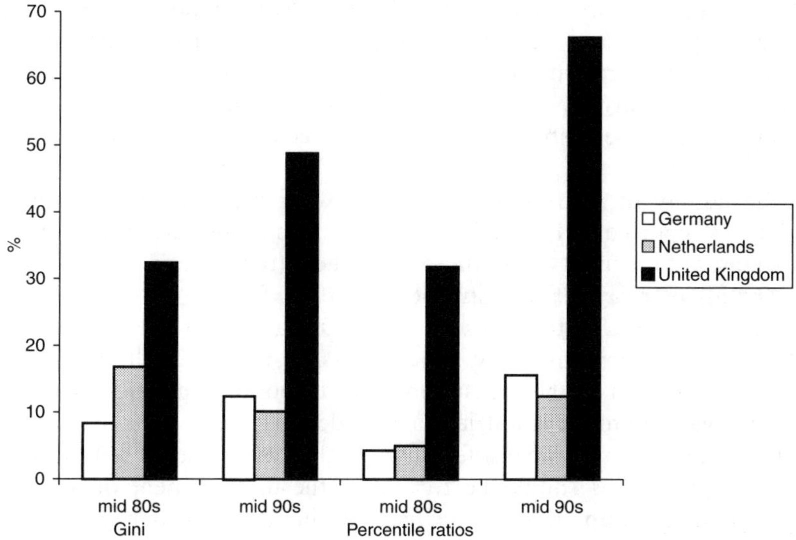

Source: Luxembourg Income Study.
Notes: Equivalence scale: square root of household size. Person weights adopted.

Figure 2.2 The relative difference in inequality between the Nordic countries and Germany, the Netherlands and the United Kingdom around mid-late 1980s and mid-1990s

hand and Germany and the UK on the other increased between the mid-1980s and mid-1990s. The outcome in the Netherlands comparison is less clear, reflecting the fact that our inequality indices report a slightly different direction of change in the Netherlands. Still, according to both indices the Nordic countries in the mid-1990s all had a lower degree of inequality, even compared to the Netherlands.

In sum, we find no evidence that the Nordic countries in terms of levels of inequality became more, so to speak, European. Given the macroeconomic background these results are quite startling. Between our measurement years unemployment skyrocketed in Finland, increased to unprecedented rates in Sweden, and also rose substantially in Denmark and Norway. Despite this there are no signs whatsoever of any convergence between the groups of countries studied here with regard to income inequality. Finally, one should of course be aware here of the small-n problem. The choice of comparison countries might certainly be of utmost importance for the impression given. Still, the total lack of support for the general idea of convergence is overwhelming, whereas the Nordic countries, if anything, seem to have become more alike. The lack of a clear relationship between unemployment and income inequality in the Nordic countries is confirmed in a recent study by Aaberge *et al.* (2000), in which they thoroughly analysed the impact of the marked increase in unemployment on income distribution during the economic recession of the early 1990s.

Scandinavian readers might be somewhat confused by the small changes reported in Figure 2.1. National studies tend to report larger increases of inequality than those found here (for Finland see Uusitalo 1999; for Norway see Ministry of Health and Social Affairs 1999; for Sweden see SOU 2000). One of the main reasons for this is that the LIS data for comparability reasons do not include realised capital gains (or losses) in the measurement of disposable income. Realised capital gains in many countries have tended to become a more important component over the last few decades. It is by no means self-evident how capital gains should be treated in the measurement of income distributions. Capital gains realised during a particular year may refer to an accumulation over several years. Recent comments on this issue, basically following the Haig-Simons definition of income, seem to suggest that ideally both realised and unrealised capital gains should be included, but only the part referring to the particular period for which the analysis is done (see Everaers *et al.* 2000). In any case, most national reports in the Scandinavian countries do include realised capital gains, which then increase the level of income inequality but more importantly also tend to lead to widening income differentials over time. A second issue is that the end year of the data presented in Figure 2.1 is 1995. In at least Finland and Sweden the above-mentioned sources indicate that income inequality increased in the second half of the 1990s. In other words, no or only a minor change of inequality is reported during the worst recession years, whereas it seems to be the case that during the subsequent up-swing of the economy inequality has been increasing. In both countries capital income (including realised gains) has been a major driving force in explaining this recent increase in national trend data.

Welfare state redistribution: the influence of cash benefits

It is, of course, of great interest to focus specifically on the role of the welfare state in producing the cross-national variation reported above. For that purpose the extent to which welfare state benefits influence cross-national variation of inequality needs to be studied. The analysis is conducted by comparing inequality in equivalent market income with equivalent gross income, that is the change as we move from the pre-transfer to post-transfer income distribution.[11] It should be stressed that the analysis has a static character, which does not detect any feedback effects of redistributive programmes. It is solely what has been called the first-order effects of the welfare state that are under scrutiny (Dodge 1975; Uusitalo 1989). Further, it should be noted that some of the transfers are taxed and ideally one would only take the net benefits into account.

The analysis has a two-fold focus. First, do the cash benefits of the Nordic countries have a more distinct redistributive pattern that distinguishes them from the other European countries? The changes of inequality as we move from market income to gross income (i.e. including cash benefits) are basically dependent on two factors: the redistributive size of transfers and the degree to which transfers are directed towards those with low income, often referred to as targeting. Second, what are the changes in the role of cash benefits when comparing the situation in the mid-1990s with that prevailing in the mid-1980s? The second question is of course related to the overall issue of whether or not we still find proof of a distinct and unique Nordic model. What is to be expected as regards the changes in the 1990s in the Nordic countries? There are arguments both for and against an outcome of 'less distinctiveness'. On one hand, the reduction of inequality could decrease because the economic recession led to various cuts in benefit schemes; on the other hand, the fact that more people in the 1990s could no longer rely solely on the market to maintain their living standard will presumably lead to a stronger impact of welfare state redistribution in the income distribution process. How much these forces will counterbalance each other is also dependent upon changes in the 'redistributive profiles' of various cash benefits, i.e. to what extent cash benefits are focused on those with low market income.

This analysis is performed only for those between 20 and 64 years of age,[12] because otherwise the results would be strongly dependent on the relative number of pensioners, who almost inevitably have very low market income. However, it should be remembered that one major cash benefit is thereby excluded from the analysis. Otherwise households are included in the analysis irrespective of whether or not they have any market income.

The measure of dispersion is the percentile ratio, but this time focusing on the 80th/20th percentile ratios.[13] Figure 2.3 gives the percentile ratios for both the pre- and post-transfer income distributions, and thereby indirectly the reduction of this ratio before and after taking cash benefits into account. If we start with the Nordic countries we

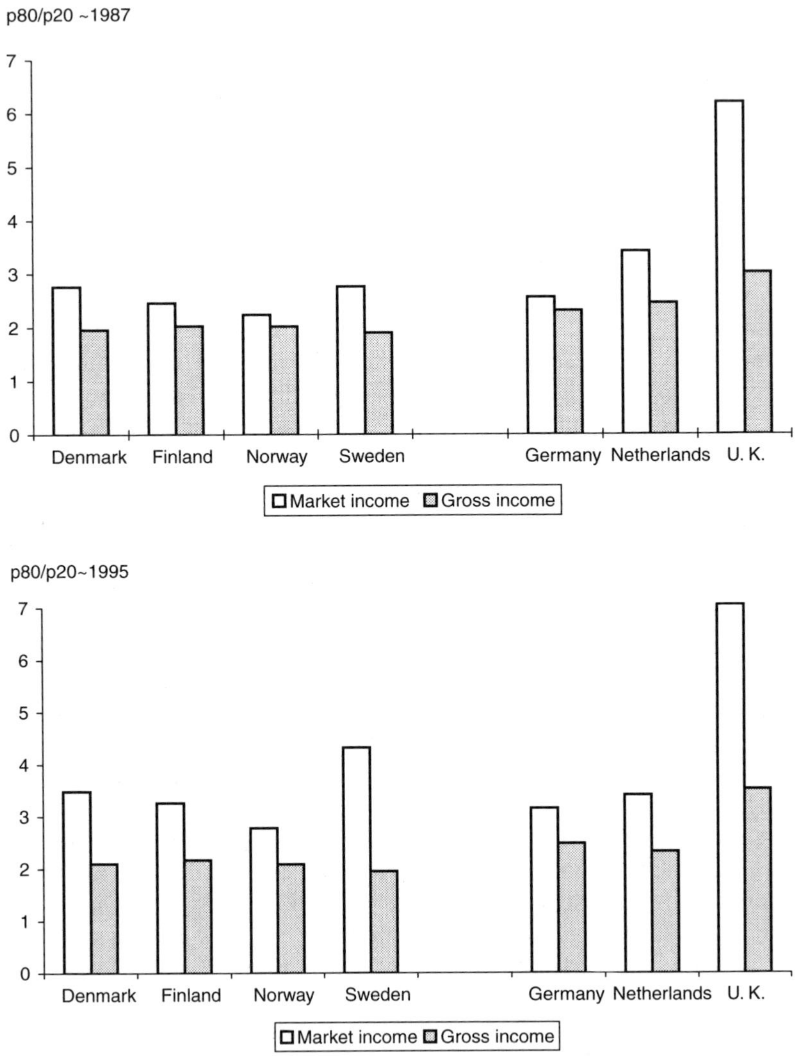

Source: Luxembourg Income Study.
Notes: Equivalence scale: square root of household size. Person weights adopted. The percentile ratio for market income in the U.K. in 1995 is in reality 12.2.

Figure 2.3 Income inequality in equivalent market and gross income in mid-late 1980s and in mid-1990s

note several interesting changes over time. First, the recession in the early 1990s obviously led to a quite substantial increase of market income inequality, no doubt largely caused by increased unemployment and an even larger decline in labour force participation. Second, the reduction of inequality when cash benefits are included strengthened quite dramatically in all four countries. This in turn means that the importance of cash benefits increased and this impact was obviously much more marked than any cuts in benefit levels, etc. Third, this led to an outcome of only minor increase in the percentile ratios of gross income, so in this respect it can be claimed that the Nordic welfare states acted according to intentions. There is remarkable congruence in this general picture among the four countries, notwithstanding minor variations.

As for the three non-Nordic countries, it is notable that the inclusion of cash benefits again led to a clear reduction of inequality in all cases. This is indeed a general finding in all income distribution research (but note the feedback effect argument above). In fact, nowhere was the reduction of inequality so large (according to this measure) as in the United Kingdom. However, it should be said that this primarily reflects the huge percentile ratio of market income (note that the bar in Figure 2.3 for the UK should actually be much taller).

In sum, one could say that what is evident from this analysis is a similar trend, although from different starting points. In all countries market income inequality increased between the mid-late 1980s and the mid-1990s. The welfare state modification of this increase varied strongly, however, and produced an overall picture with a clear Nordic cluster. The general impression of very small changes of inequality in the Nordic countries basically resembles the results presented earlier, even though the focus this time was solely on the potential working population and only on the role of cash benefits.

We now turn to the issue of how these changes in inequality when including cash benefits came about. This was examined by studying both the size of cash benefits and how they were distributed over the income distribution, but this time restricting the analysis to the latest available year of observation for each country. Table 2.1 reports how total transfer income, for the same age group as earlier, was distributed over income groups divided by quintiles. That is, we divided the distribution into five equal groups sorted by equivalent gross income. We then calculated how the large fraction of total transfer was located within each income group. As is seen for all the countries, a larger sum of cash benefits was distributed to those at the lower end of the distribution, but some cross-national variation is evident. In general,

Table 2.1 Distribution of transfers by income quintiles and average transfer income as a fraction of median equivalent gross income, households aged 20–64, percentages

Country and year	*Lowest*	*2*	*3*	*4*	*Highest*	*Total*	*Average transfer income*
Denmark, 1992	30.1	26.7	16.9	14.7	11.7	100	16.7
Finland, 1995	29.8	24.3	19.9	15.2	10.7	100	18.3
Norway, 1995	35.0	23.6	16.5	13.5	11.3	100	12.9
Sweden, 1995	27.2	27.5	19.0	15.4	11.0	100	24.0
Germany, 1994	38.9	23.4	15.9	13.1	8.7	100	9.7
Netherlands, 1994	29.1	22.6	16.4	14.3	17.6	100	15.2
United Kingdom, 1995	37.0	29.5	14.5	10.6	8.4	100	13.9

Source: Luxembourg Income Study.
Notes: Equivalence scale: square root of household size. Person weights adopted. Classification of income quintiles from equivalent gross income. The proportion of transfers refers as well to equivalent transfer income.

the picture to emerge is that transfer in the Nordic countries was to a *lesser* extent concentrated towards the lower income groups. However, it seems as if the Netherlands had a distributional profile fairly similar to Denmark, Finland and Sweden, whereas the distribution of cash benefits in Norway was not that different from Germany. So the country grouping is less clear in this analysis.

The reason why Finland and Sweden in particular still show such a strong reduction as we move from market to gross income is apparent in the last column of Table 2.1, where the average transfer income is reported in relation to gross income. Once again Norway deviates from the other Nordic countries. Thus the average transfer income was higher in both the Netherlands and the United Kingdom compared to Norway. Similar analyses have been presented by Atkinson *et al.* (1995) and by Korpi and Palme (1998), among others. In both cases, however, they also included old-age pensioners. A comparison with their results shows that the profiles generally tend to be less targeted towards the bottom of the income distribution when the elderly and their income are included. However, as far as cross-national variations in profiles are concerned, most results here are similar to ones presented by the above-mentioned sources.

In summary, then, we could say that the relative size of cash benefits is one important factor explaining why gross income inequality has been relatively low in Denmark, Finland and Sweden. The low inequality in Norway seems neither dependent on extremely high targeting of transfers, nor on the size factor. Instead, as already seen in Figure 2.3, the distribution of market income was much more compressed in Norway than anywhere else. It should be said that this probably does not merely reflect low earnings inequality among the working population, but also the high employment rate. A totally different picture emerged for the UK, where the reported redistributive budget size was not particularly low and the extent of targeting seemed to be highest of all the countries studied. The outcome in the UK therefore seems rather to be the reverse of the case in Norway. The high degree of inequality in the UK was mainly caused by the unequal distribution of market income, which is by far the most severe among these seven countries. In other words, this fairly crude analysis has highlighted that in order to understand the relatively high degree of income inequality in the UK we need to consider why market income inequality is so high, and particularly why market income is so poor at the bottom end of the distribution. This conclusion is consistent with a recent analysis by Bradbury and Jäntti (1999) of why the poverty rates of children in the UK and some other English-speaking countries are so high. Their findings show that a major difference between the UK and the Nordic countries is not the amount of social transfers to low-income families with children but rather the much lower market income in the UK families.

Similarly, Kangas and Ritakallio (1999) in a comparison between France and the Nordic countries report that differences in what they label 'social structure' strongly affect poverty rates and poverty alleviation. Labour force participation rates within the household were the dominant part of that structure distinguishing France from the Nordic countries. In other words, their study, too, indirectly singles out differences in market income as a major factor. The above-mentioned results should not, however, be taken as proof that welfare state actions are unimportant. In fact, several of the plausible mechanisms for such findings have to do with how welfare state programmes influence the possibility for people to support themselves via the labour market, such as the provision of child care programmes.

Income changes and relative poverty rates among vulnerable groups

Although the Nordic countries have traditionally ranked low in overall inequality, the most marked disparities in earlier comparative income and poverty research have been for specific social categories often regarded as particularly vulnerable. For example, it was found that Sweden differed more in terms of relative poverty rates among the elderly and single mothers than was the case in overall poverty rates (Fritzell 1992).[14] Cash benefits were seen as a major explanatory factor for this finding among both of these groups (Smeeding 1992; see also Sørensen 1994). However, it is no longer clear that these differences are as profound as they were in the 1980s. It is to this issue we now turn. Old age, at least since the days of Rowntree's classical study, has been associated with a higher risk of poverty (Rowntree 1901). Nowadays, however, with more generous pension levels and maturity of various pension plans, this association is less obvious. A 'new' vulnerable group often highlighted in policy documents on poverty is single parents.

Besides the elderly and single parents, the income situation of a third category is examined here, namely the position of the relatively young adults in each country and how their income levels and relative poverty rates have changed over recent times. Many studies have found that the young rather than the old have a high risk of relative poverty in modern societies, suggesting that Rowntree's life cycle of poverty curve should be redrawn quite drastically to adjust to today's situation (cf. Kangas and Palme forthcoming). The focus on the young is also motivated by earlier findings within this project (Fritzell 1999). The most striking change in relative income when comparing average incomes in the mid-1980s to the mid-1990s by different social categories (age, class and gender) referred to the relative deterioration of the younger segments of the populations in all three countries for which data were available (Finland, Norway and Sweden).[15] A recent OECD report also highlighted the younger segments of the population as a new prime vulnerable group in the OECD countries (OECD 1998a).

So to what extent is this a general feature of the countries included in this study? Table 2.2 reports relative poverty rates for those aged 20–29, those between 60 and 74, and those aged 75 years and above (age of head of household), as well as the relative poverty rates for single parents. The adopted poverty line, i.e. 50 per cent of the median equivalent disposable income, is a common one in comparative research. This threshold is arbitrary, as is basically any income poverty line, and there is of course no real qualitative difference between someone just below the threshold and someone just above. When contemplating these numbers one should bear in mind that the exact location of the poverty threshold can be very important for distinguishing how large a fraction falls into relative poverty. This is perhaps especially true among the elderly and single parents, the latter also being a relatively small population group which makes the estimate less precise. Still, the percentages give us a hint about cross-national differences on the size and composition of the bottom end of the income distribution.

As for the Nordic countries, the overall picture given by Table 2.2 is obviously that the risk of relative poverty over time changed in favour of the elderly at the expense of the young, in line with the maturity of pension plans and cohort replacement. In these countries we find a substantial decline in relative poverty rates among both of the elderly age categories distinguished. In fact, for both these age groups it was more than halved in all countries but Norway, where the decline was by roughly a third. Conversely, we find that relative poverty rates among the younger segments of the populations increased in all seven countries, although the relative deterioration compared to the elderly is less obvious in the non-Nordic countries since poverty rates in some cases actually increased among the elderly, too.

The relative poverty rates for the age group 60–74 represent perhaps the best example of the fact that old age nowadays has less association with poverty. Indeed, in the mid-1990s this age group in all seven countries studied here had a lower prevalence of relative poverty than in the population at large (not seen in Table 2.2). One could argue that cohort

Table 2.2 Relative poverty rates for those aged 20–29, 60–74, 75+ years of age and for single parents, percentages

Country and year	*Aged 20–29*	*Aged 60–74*	*Aged 75+*	*Single parents*
Denmark, 1987	12.0	16.8	41.5	6.6
Denmark, 1992	16.5	5.6	16.3	11.6
Finland, 1987	10.1	7.8	18.1	4.9
Finland, 1995	14.0	3.6	7.6	6.6
Norway, 1986	14.1	8.7	33.5	12.6
Norway, 1995	18.1	5.2	21.9	11.9
Sweden, 1987	12.1	4.8	12.4	5.8
Sweden, 1995	15.7	2.3	3.9	6.8
Germany, 1984	17.2	5.4	15.4	2.9
Germany, 1994	20.6	6.1	8.7	41.7
Netherlands, 1987	12.7	3.4	–	8.4
Netherlands, 1994	15.3	6.5	5.9	24.4
United Kingdom, 1986	16.3	6.4	8.0	18.6
United Kingdom, 1995	22.8	8.1	18.7	39.1

Source: Luxembourg Income Study.
Notes: Poverty threshold 50 per cent of median equivalent disposable income. All households with household head aged at least twenty. Equivalence scale: square root of household size. Person weights adopted. Age categories refer to age of household head.

replacement in the future will make this also true for the oldest elderly in many countries. In the mid-1990s only the Swedish rate among those aged 75 and above was lower than the overall average within each country. However, this hypothesis is not so self-evident as, due to gender differentials in mortality, the vast majority of the oldest elderly tend to be single women who often have low pensions.

The last column in Table 2.2 reports the fraction of single parents with equivalent income below the poverty threshold. Here we find startling differences between the Nordic countries and the other three European nations. In the UK close to four out of ten had incomes below 50 per cent of the median, and the percentage was even slightly higher in Germany. In contrast it remained relatively low in the Nordic countries.

The relative poverty estimates reported above obviously do not tell us how the average income situation evolved for these categories. We therefore turn to this issue next. Figure 2.4 shows how the equivalent income for those aged 20–29, 60–74 and those above 74 *changed*

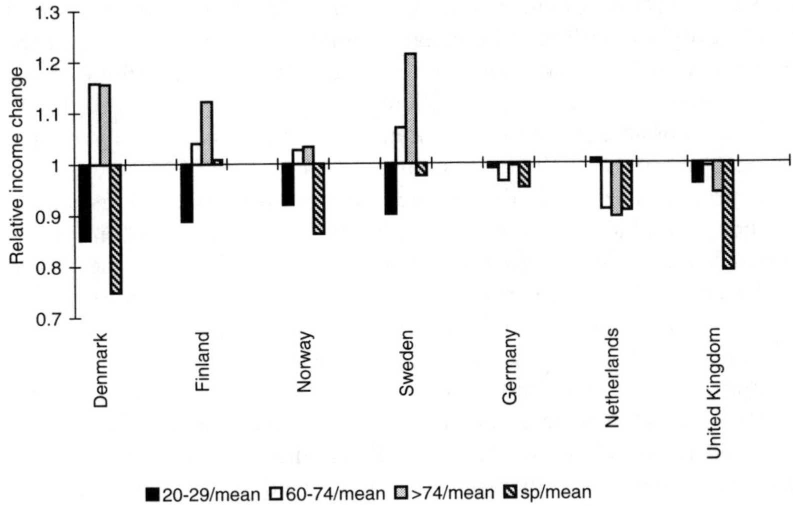

Source: Luxembourg Income Study.
Notes: Age refers to age of household head. Average change is set to 1.0. Equivalence scale: square root of household size. Person weights adopted.

Figure 2.4 Relative income change between the mid-late 1980s and the mid-1990s for three age groups and for single parents

between our observation points in relation to the change of the overall mean (set to 1) within each country. Hence, a number below 1 implies that the group lost ground, relatively speaking, and a number above 1 the opposite. Note that only relative changes appear in Figure 2.4; nothing can be concluded about cross national differences in levels, nor whether or not the young or the old had the lowest level within each country. The focus on change is motivated by the fact that it is less influenced by the particular choice of equivalence scale.

A very distinct pattern emerges for the Nordic countries in this figure. In all four the young lost ground and the elderly gained, thereby confirming the picture given by Fritzell (1999). However, this pattern is not evident in any of the other three European countries. In fact, and somewhat surprisingly, we can detect a slight decrease in relative income for the elderly groups in Germany, the Netherlands and the United Kingdom. However, this observation confirms the changes in relative poverty rates presented above.

Accordingly, once again we find a distinct Nordic pattern. But how is the economic deterioration of young adults in the Nordic countries to be explained? One obvious candidate is the educational expansion that has taken place, although in an earlier analysis focused on three of the Nordic countries it was shown that the relative income loss of the young persisted even when students were excluded (Fritzell 1999). Another possible mechanism behind this finding is certainly related to a characteristic of the Nordic model. One feature of Nordic welfare state programmes is that they are generous, with many earnings-related systems available to those within the labour market. Many of the young found it increasingly difficult to become 'insiders' during the period under study, due to generally poorer employment opportunities. This in turn was related to labour market regulations which basically favour elderly versus younger workers. One hypothesis would therefore be that there is a so-called 'floor-problem' in the social insurance systems of the Nordic countries that we perhaps do not find to the same degree in other welfare states. It remains to be seen whether the growing economic vulnerability of young adults is a mere period effect or a more permanent feature of modern societies; also, what impact this will have both for the well-being of individuals and on a societal level. In both respects this is an issue with long-term consequences. In other words, it will no doubt depend upon whether a substantial fraction of the younger generations will also have more long-term difficulties in becoming insiders as they grow older.

The last bar for each country in Figure 2.4 shows how relative incomes changed for single parents in the same manner as for the age groups. The most negative change is reported for single parents in Denmark, UK, Norway and the Netherlands. The only country in which the relative income for single parents did not decline from the mid-1980s to the mid-1990s is Finland. Despite the fact that the precarious economic position of single parents has for some time now been high on the socio-political agenda (see e.g. discussion in Lewis 1997), we find no evidence that these European countries have been able to substantially improve their economic conditions.

Since the focus of attention in this analysis has been solely on change rather than level, it should finally be mentioned that the relative income level for single parents in all four Nordic countries was markedly higher than in the three non-Nordic countries, which confirms the picture on relative poverty rates presented earlier. Above all, in the United Kingdom there was a huge difference between the relative income level of single parents and the overall average. In 1995 single parents' equivalent income was only slightly above half of the national mean when using this equivalence scale.[16]

Concluding discussion

This chapter has examined the distribution of income in the Nordic countries in comparison with three other European countries, namely Germany, the Netherlands and the United Kingdom. The time period covered was roughly from the mid-1980s to the mid-1990s. The main question raised concerned whether or not we find support for the existence of a Nordic model at the end of the twentieth century. Within this framework some more specific questions were initially asked. First, is a low degree of overall income inequality still a feature of the Nordic countries? Second, do we find any evidence that the Nordic countries are becoming more like the other European countries when comparing recent changes of inequality? Third, what is the role of the cash programmes of the welfare state in producing the cross-national variation in inequality? Fourth, when looking at specific vulnerable groups, like the young, the old, and single parents, do we find a specific Nordic pattern?

The empirical evidence presented in this chapter makes it fairly easy to answer the first two questions. *Yes*, the Nordic countries do still have a low degree of inequality in the distribution of income and *No*, we find no support for a convergence. However, one should qualify these conclusions somewhat. First, national studies in three of the Nordic countries – Finland, Norway, and Sweden – have concluded that income dispersion widened in the latter years of the 1990s. It should also be pointed out that capital income, including realised gains, has been an important factor in this increase, and this source of economic well-being is not fully captured by the LIS data. Still, it seems highly unlikely that including a few more years and a more inclusive measure of capital income would produce a radically different conclusion. More plausible is the argument that over a much longer period we could see widening income differential, i.e. a continuation of the trend most countries are presently witnessing.

Cash benefits, here analysed only for those potentially working, seem indeed to be important. But we find a more complicated pattern when looking cross-nationally. Sweden, Finland, Denmark, and also the Netherlands, are roughly characterised by having large cash benefits which are less concentrated on low income groups and reduce inequality mostly due to their large size. On the other hand, Norway, Germany and the United Kingdom have a different distributional profile of cash benefits, which are more targeted towards those with low income. It is also noteworthy that the size of the redistributive pie in the mid-1990s was in fact higher in the UK than in Norway. The reason that these countries appear so different in terms of inequality is dependent on the distribution of market income, which was by far the most unequal in the UK in the mid-1990s, and the most equal in Norway.

The fourth question concerned the income position of specific socio-demographic groups. The results for single parents do indeed support the Nordic case. Both with regard to risks of poverty and changes therein, we found a marked difference between the Nordic countries and the three others. For young adults, too, we discovered that the Nordic countries stand out, but less in the manner expected from the usual welfare state debate. Accordingly, it was found that in all four Nordic countries the relative income position of young adults deteriorated quite dramatically between the 1980s and the 1990s. This outcome was seen with regard to the risks of relative poverty, but even more visibly when looking at the changes in average incomes for those below thirty years of age.

It was initially argued in this chapter that the Nordic welfare states have tended to be strongly focused on equality of outcome and that such a perspective is no longer sustainable in a global economy. However, as has hopefully been shown in this chapter, it is also evident that at the end of the twentieth century the Nordic countries were characterised as having low income inequality, in accordance with their type of equality focus.

Notes

1 The author wishes to thank Anders Björklund and Hannu Uusitalo for valuable comments on earlier drafts of this chapter.

2 The issue of gender equality seen from an income distribution perspective is thoroughly analysed in Chapter 5 of this volume and therefore not discussed in this chapter.

3 These explanations, however, have been forcefully critiqued, see e.g. the discussions and reviews in Levy and Murnane (1992), Gottschalk and Smeeding (1997).

4 Atkinson (2000) has recently put forward the concept of social norms as an important explanatory factor behind changes of income differentials. Since what are regarded as acceptable pay norms may vary both over time and between countries, and also be influenced by politics, this could still be seen as a hypothesis in line with the 'politics matter' tradition.

5 The years within parentheses refer to the two data points that are mostly under study. The starting year thereby coincides with the ending year in most of the analyses presented in the OECD study by Atkinson *et al.* (1995), which is the most thorough descriptive study of recent data on cross-national variation in the degree and trends of income inequality.

6 In a recent report from a Swedish government commission we have been able to show that the inequality trends, which are the focus in this first section, remain fairly unchanged when using a household definition more in line with that prevailing in other countries, even though the level of inequality becomes somewhat lower (SOU 2000: 3).

7 The numbers reported in Figure 2.1 are basically the 'semi-official' estimates reported on the homepage of LIS. However, the data of some countries, in particular Germany, have recently undergone some revisions. The estimates presented here are based on the corrected data. In the Dutch case I also follow the 'LIS recommendation' of only including households for which full income information is available.

8 Although somewhat surprising, this result was also presented by Aaberge *et al.* (1999). However, as also pointed out by Gustafsson *et al.* (1999) different national series give contradictory indications with regard to inequality trends in Denmark from the mid-1980s.

9 In their review of national studies on income distribution trends, Atkinson *et al.* (1995, Ch. 5) only found two out of sixteen countries in which there was a fall in inequality in the 1980s, namely Italy and Portugal.

10 On several occasions I refer to the two observation points as being in the mid-1980s and the mid-1990s. One should remember that some cases deviate strongly from that. In particular, Denmark, for which the measurement years are 1987 and 1992.

11 The difference between these two income concepts is accordingly that the latter includes various social insurance transfers and also universal and income- and means-tested cash benefits and assistance.

12 From hereon all analyses are conducted with households in which the head is aged at least 20, in order to minimise the definition problem of Swedish households.

13 The rationale for using this ratio is that a fraction in each country has zero market income and in fact this fraction is above 10 per cent in the UK, which makes all ratios meaningless.

14 However, it should be noted that other countries also seem to provide a reasonably good economic situation for single mothers, despite the fact that they are usually categorised into other welfare state models, as a recent comparison between Belgium and Sweden shows (Morissens 1999).

15 The data used in that analysis were the so-called Scandinavian level of living surveys.

16 Household heads below 20 years of age are also excluded in this analysis. Since teenage motherhood is extremely unusual in all these countries except for the United Kingdom (see e.g. Wertheimer and McRae 1999), it seems likely that the relatively worst off situation for single parents in the UK is, if anything, underestimated in this analysis.

3 Nordic health inequalities in the European context

Olle Lundberg and Eero Lahelma

Introduction[1]

The general goal of the welfare state is to improve its citizens' possibilities of leading a good life, which is often understood as being able to avoid bad conditions. To be able to perform one's daily activities, i.e. to enjoy reasonably good health, is certainly a fundamental prerequisite for leading a good life (Allardt 1975; Johansson 1979; Erikson 1992). It may therefore be argued that levels and trends in morbidity and mortality provide essential evidence for evaluating the performance of welfare states. This is also reflected in the frequent use of infant mortality rates and life expectancies in broad international comparisons of welfare. The fact that people's social positions are linked to their morbidity and mortality risk in a systematic way means that it is not sufficient to study overall levels of ill health only. There must be additional focus on health inequalities as revealed by the distribution of ill health between population groups.

Health inequalities, as indicated by morbidity and mortality differences between social classes, educational groups or income strata, can be viewed as a very extreme form of inequality. Not only are people's positions in the social structure important for their daily living conditions, but they also systematically affect their morbidity and mortality risks, resulting in disproportionate levels of illness and death before old age among the least well off. In this way the social structure of society affects people's life chances quite literally.

Since health inequalities are defined as systematic differences in morbidity and mortality between groups of people who occupy different positions in the social structure, the focus in many empirical studies of health inequalities has been on occupational social class differences. In addition, educational, income, regional or ethnic groups, as well as gender differences, have been examined to capture health disparities between socioeconomic positions. The essential finding is that the social positioning of people and their life chances and living conditions emerging from this positioning are linked to their morbidity and mortality risks. This is the main reason why levels of health and health inequalities are not primarily determined by the provision of health services and medical treatment, but rather depend on people's broader social structural and psychosocial environments.

It is important to note that the levels of morbidity and mortality, as well as the size and pattern of health inequalities, are linked to a range of factors contributing to the life potentials of people, and not only to the health care sector (see McKeown 1976). In fact, the health care sector may be much less involved in the production of health inequalities than most other sectors of society, such as the labour market or the family. This is not to say that the organisation of health care or sickness benefit schemes is unimportant. On the contrary, these welfare state arrangements may well diminish or enhance existing health differentials between population groups (see e.g. Keskimäki 1997). The origins of health and ill health are rather to be found in people's environments, living conditions and available resources in general. The challenge for policy, then, is how to manage these broad social and political fields in order to give all citizens the possibility to be as healthy as those at the higher socioeconomic levels.

Compared to other European nations the Nordic countries are often regarded as more equal in terms of the level and distribution of various dimensions of life potentials, such as those related to gender, education, social class and income. One example of this is income inequalities, which in the Nordic nations are smaller than in other European countries (e.g. Atkinson *et al.* 1995; see also Chapter 2). However, it is less well known to what extent the advantageous position of the Nordic countries in certain dimensions of welfare is reflected as individual and group outcomes within some other dimensions, for example, as morbidity and mortality and their distribution across the social structure. One might expect that such major welfare outcomes as health and death would not only show better levels in the Nordic countries, but also be more equally distributed than elsewhere. Whether this is so is the focus of this chapter, where we examine systematic differences in morbidity and mortality, i.e. health inequalities, between different social classes, educational groups and income strata in the Nordic countries compared to a number of other Western European countries. The main aim is to assess the absolute and relative size of health inequalities in these countries in general, and to contribute to the understanding of the positioning of the Nordic countries in particular.

Due to lack of comparable data it was not possible to analyse trends in health inequalities cross-nationally.

The focus on health inequalities

The examination of health as it affects people's life chances has a very long tradition, particularly in Britain, ranging from Petty and Gaunt through Chadwick and Rowntree to Beveridge and Titmuss (see e.g. Webster 1992; Greenberg 1997; Dickerson 1998; Ashton 1999). In addition to the overall levels of morbidity and mortality, emphasis in this tradition has been placed on the health of the worst off as well as on the distribution of health between social classes and other socioeconomic groups. A more recent impetus to health inequalities research was given by the Black Report on Health Inequalities (Townsend and Davidson 1982), which 're-found' socioeconomic differences in morbidity and mortality in the affluent countries. As the latest documentation shows, much research on health inequalities has been carried out since the Black Report, but explanatory and comparative research remains sparse (Davey Smith *et al.* 1990; Macintyre 1997).[2]

The high priority of (poor) health among the various sub-areas of welfare has also been recognised by the United Nations, as well as by leading scholars in the field of welfare research (Allardt 1975; Johansson 1979). Health in these approaches is understood both as a resource and as an intrinsic good. The high priority of health arises from the fact that in order to take part in and enjoy most areas of life one has to be in reasonably good health, in other words, free from disabling illnesses and diseases. Accordingly, health, illness and death need to be included as central outcome indicators in the analysis of the consequences of welfare state arrangements to the individual, population groups and society at large.

We therefore present and discuss data from recent comparative studies on the size and pattern of health inequalities in the Nordic nations compared to other European countries. We also raise some issues concerning the interpretation of such data in terms of policy implications. In order to do this, however, we will start by discussing contemporary analyses of inequalities in morbidity and mortality, as well as some of the key issues relating to whether such studies are likely to be of importance to policy evaluation.

Our analysis of comparative European data on health inequalities sets out to illuminate several issues. In order to assess the effect of welfare state policies on public health two types of health outcomes are important: 1) The overall level of ill health within a country, and

2) the distribution of ill health between population groups. The level of a nation's health may be indicated, for example, by the infant mortality rate, life expectancy (at birth or at a later stage), or by prevalence percentages of various dimensions of illness and disease. The distribution of the burden of ill health can be measured as the pattern and the size of morbidity and mortality inequalities across the social structure. For both the overall level and the distribution of morbidity and mortality the position of one country can be compared with other countries at one time. However, comparative analyses of trends in inequalities are not possible at the moment due to lack of comparable data, although trends in the size and pattern of inequalities can be followed for particular countries.

Thus four aspects of the state of public health in a population can be distinguished: 1) The overall level of morbidity and mortality at one point in time; 2) trends in overall morbidity and mortality; 3) the size of inequalities in morbidity and mortality; and 4) trends in inequalities in morbidity and mortality. However, the production of ill health and of health inequalities is a complex process, and health inequalities and welfare state activities within other areas are not necessarily directly related to each other, as will be discussed below. Throughout the analysis we devote attention to absolute as well as relative health differences between countries and socioeconomic groups, as these have an important bearing not only on people's life chances and their social positioning, but also on policies aimed at improving their health.

Methodology

Health, illness and mortality

In health research, as in Scandinavian welfare research in general, the main emphasis tends to be on bad conditions, that is ill health. At least three dimensions of ill health may be distinguished, namely 1) disease of the organism; 2) illness as perceived by a person; and 3) sickness disabling a person's functioning in the social environment (Blaxter 1989). As a rule, to be healthy equals being free of any form of ill health. Having a disease, an illness or a sickness signifies the negative concept of health.

In addition to the negative concept of health, a positive one can be distinguished. The most famous positive characterisation of health is that presented in the Constitution of the World Health Organisation (WHO) in 1946: 'Health is a state of complete physical, mental and social well-being and not merely the absence of disease and infirmity.'

This extremely broad concept of health does not easily allow such measurement as is needed in an empirical examination, and the concept of positive health rather expresses ideals for life and health policies to be used in individual and community goal-setting (Karisto 1984: 57; von Wright 1972: 87). The negative concept of health, in contrast, involving health problems, allows us to better identify such states as diseases, illnesses and sicknesses of an individual. These negative states can be defined and measured in empirical research, and are also more easily treated theoretically. This is even more true when causes of diseases, illnesses and sicknesses are searched for. Positive health, which is difficult to identify as a state, may not be caused in the same way as negative states of health, i.e. diseases, illnesses and sicknesses (von Wright 1972: 56; Karisto 1984: 59; Allardt 1999).

How, then, should health problems be measured in populations? First of all, it is important to note some fundamental differences between measurement of ill health in populations and medical examinations of individuals. In the latter case, a medical doctor carries out a medical examination in order to make a diagnosis of a disease using symptoms (as told by the patient) and signs (e.g. as measured by clinical or laboratory tests) (Twaddle 1974; Jensen 1985). However, the main purpose of the whole process is for the diagnosis to guide the treatment of the health problem of the patient. Thus it is important to note that treatment of disease is the objective of medical practice, not the study of health and well-being at the population level. This is also a major difference between health measurement in medical practice and that in public health research. Although the latter has to be relevant to the former, individual treatment is not in focus when the health of a population is being measured. The purpose of health measurement within the population is to capture the total burden of disease, illness and sickness, and to examine the whole panorama of illness rather than to identify particular bodily diseases and be able to establish distinct medical diagnoses.

Data describing people's health usually derive from broad population surveys. Sydenstricker and colleagues initiated systematic health surveys in the USA back in the 1920s (see Jaco 1958), since when surveys have been abundantly utilised to accumulate scientific understanding of health and illness, and to monitor the population's health for the purposes of health and welfare policies. Standard measures to examine health in the survey setting have been developed, including simple generic indicators as well as complex summary inventories (see e.g. Blaxter 1989; Bowling 1991, 1995).

Commonly used generic indicators include (limiting) long-standing illness and (self-)perceived health, which the World Health Organisation has also suggested for comparative use (de Bruin *et al.* 1996). These simple health indicators have turned out to be reliable and valid measures of people's general health in research on living conditions. The picture of a population's overall health obtained on the basis of the long-standing illness question comes close to that obtained using medical examinations (Heliövaara *et al.* 1993). The perceived health measure is a broad indicator of health which reflects primarily the negative side of health, but captures the positive sides as well (Manderbacka *et al.* 1998). This measure has been found to be a reliable health indicator in the test–retest setting (Lundberg and Manderbacka 1996; Martikainen *et al.* 1999). Perceived health is also a good predictor of mortality according to a number studies (e.g. Idler and Benyamini 1997).

Although death does not qualify as an indicator of health among people currently alive, mortality calculations do give important information at the population level. Therefore, mortality is a major indicator of ill health used in all societies. Mortality data do have particular advantages from the point of view of inequality studies. For example, class differences in mortality cannot be explained in terms of differential reporting, which is an inherent issue in studies using data on ill health. Mortality, and especially premature mortality at the group level, is the most extreme form of disadvantage. Mortality data from death records are reliable and valid with regard to the 'true' mortality in most countries, particularly so in advanced welfare states. The main drawback with mortality data is that they do not adequately reflect the disease burden among the living population (Macintyre 1986). In other words, there are health problems that cause a lot of pain and suffering among individuals as well as great costs in terms of sick leave, medication, medical treatment and care, but that are not fatal. Major examples include musculo-skeletal diseases and most forms of reduced mental well-being. Therefore, from a welfare perspective we cannot rely entirely on mortality data despite their importance, but need manifold data sources that also include various aspects of health and illness.

Mortality studies use data from death records, which provide information on total mortality as well as cause of death. In the Nordic countries universal personal identification codes have provided a unique opportunity to link death records to census data as well as to data from other public registers. This procedure has allowed socio-economic mortality differences to be studied and followed up more reliably and comprehensively than anywhere else (see Valkonen and Martelin 1999).

European data sources: comparability potentials

A recent broad European study assessed the patterning and size of health inequalities in several Western European countries. This study was made by the EU Working Group on Socio-economic Inequalities in Health directed by Johan Mackenbach, and the group included the present authors (Kunst *et al.* 1996; Mackenbach *et al.* 1997; Cavelaars 1998; Cavelaars *et al.* 1998a, 1998b). The study was more comprehensive than any previous comparison on health inequalities. Since it was based on the utilisation of existing data sources, serious efforts were made to improve the comparability of the national datasets in terms of social class coding, educational coding, harmonising health outcomes as well as measurement of health inequalities (Kunst *et al.* 1996). The results of the study have provided an incentive for further debate and analysis of health inequalities (Vågerö and Erikson 1997). Next, we draw upon analyses made using data as they are found in the main reports (Kunst *et al.* 1996) as well as in other major reports from this comparative study (e.g. Kunst 1997; Mackenbach *et al.* 1997; Cavelaars 1998).

The EU comparative study in fact used a large variety of data sources, including surveys and mortality datasets as comparable as possible from a number of countries. Mortality data based on register linkage could only be obtained from the Nordic countries. In general, the surveys used as data sources for ill health contain more problems than the mortality data. The included surveys were based on interviews as well as mailed questionnaires. Of necessity, there were disparities in both the health and socioeconomic indicators. The sampling frames and response rates also varied from one study to another.

Comparing different countries is always challenging and our examination includes data from a broad set of Western European countries, although the main emphasis is on the more similar northern countries. For example, social and educational structures as well as income distributions vary a lot between European countries, but less so within the Nordic region (Kautto *et al.* 1999). The disease panorama, as for example expressed in the distribution of deaths from different causes, varies across the European countries. The emphasis on the Northern European countries limits the potential variation but helps systematic comparisons and interpretations of the results. Thus, these comparisons are rather closer to maximal similarity than to maximal dissimilarity between countries (Allardt 1975).

The results of the EU comparative study compare health differences between population groups for 25–69-year-old men and women. This age band is a broad one. As ill health and mortality are very much age-related, the analysis must take account of this. Therefore, differences in the age structure of the compared population groups have been eliminated by calculating age adjusted figures for ill heath as well as mortality in Tables 3.1–3.4.

Measurement of health inequalities

Health inequalities can be measured in a number of ways, and this is likely to have a bearing on the picture to emerge. First, patterns of inequalities can be looked at, i.e. can differences in health between population groups be found, and if so, what is the ranking of the groups? Can hierarchies be detected and, if present, how consistent are they? What are the worst off and best off groups in terms of ill health and mortality?

Second, the size of health inequalities can be scrutinised. How large are differences between socioeconomic groups, particularly the extreme ones? Can a gradient be found and, if so, how steep is it? From a public health policy perspective, the total burden of disease imposed by health inequalities is a major concern. From this point of view the size of the groups and not only their distance from each other should also be included in the measurement.

The indices to be used in the measurement of health inequalities include rate ratios, odds ratios, and diverse inequality indices such as the index of dissimilarity, the concentration index and the relative index of inequality (RII) (see Wagstaff *et al.* 1991; Kunst and Mackenbach 1994; Kunst *et al.* 1996). The relative index of inequality is a regression-based measure requiring ordinal level measurement. It takes into account whether high morbidity or mortality is found in the lower, intermediate or higher socioeconomic groups. Thus, this index embodies both population size and the relative socioeconomic position of groups. It does so by regressing the morbidity or mortality rate of socioeconomic groups on a specific measure of their relative position, namely the proportion of the population at a higher position in the socioeconomic hierarchy. The resulting figure can be interpreted as the ratio of the morbidity or mortality rates of those at the bottom of the socioeconomic hierarchy to those at the top, based on the systematic association between morbidity or mortality and socioeconomic status for all groups. A high RII score indicates large health inequalities between high and low positions in the socioeconomic hierarchy. A high score can be attributed either to a large effect of socioeconomic hierarchy on morbidity or mortality, or to large differences between high and low positions across the socioeconomic classification in itself (Kunst and Mackenbach 1994). In the present assessment of the relative health inequalities by socioeconomic groups between countries the RII scores are used.

The absolute and relative differences between populations and socioeconomic groups constitute a fundamental methodological question in all examinations of inequalities, including health inequalities: when measuring the size of health inequalities across socioeconomic groups and making comparisons between countries, should one focus on relative or absolute differences in morbidity and mortality? We present both types of measure, since we believe that one should always be aware of the distinction between absolute and relative measures and their use in different contexts. Thus, absolute measures have a special bearing on health policies, whereas relative measures are particularly useful when examining the aetiology of ill health, i.e. causal research of health and health inequalities (Lahelma *et al.* 1994). However, in contrast to absolute levels of mortality, absolute levels of ill health are more difficult to interpret in international comparisons. Absolute levels of ill health vary by country due to 'true' differences in ill health, in the propensity to report ill health, between national survey methodologies, and in the quality of data used. Such limitations in the use of data on ill health make comparisons of absolute levels of ill health a particularly complicated task and encourage the use of relative approaches in international comparisons of health inequalities. The significance of absolute and relative health inequalities will be raised further in the discussion of the European picture.

Analysis

Previous research and comparisons of health inequalities

Health inequalities as measured by diverse socioeconomic indicators have been found for a number of dimensions of ill health throughout the developed countries, including the Nordic nations (see Fox 1989; Illsley and Svensson 1990; Vågerö and Illsley 1992; Lahelma and Rahkonen 1997). Although equalisation has sometimes been predicted (Kadushin 1966), there is no single country where health inequalities have not been found when studied. Thus health inequalities are universal, and concern not only the worst off groups but rather extend along the whole social ladder: the truism 'the higher the social position, the better the health' applies in a very consistent way in different countries and for numerous health as well as socioeconomic indicators. Moreover, the available evidence rather suggests widening than narrowing inequalities in relative terms, particularly for mortality (Marmot and Dowall 1986; Valkonen *et al.* 1993; Martikainen and Valkonen 1995; Borgan 1996; Vågerö and Gullberg 1996).

In the influential British Black Report (Townsend and Davidson 1982) based on data from the 1970s, Norway and Sweden were singled out as countries with significantly smaller mortality inequalities than others. Although the empirical underpinning of this statement was not entirely convincing, later attempts to make direct comparisons between Sweden and Great Britain led to a similar conclusion (Lundberg 1986; Vågerö and Lundberg 1989). More precisely, these studies showed that the size of inequalities, particularly for mortality, was larger in Britain than in Sweden, despite the hierarchical socioeconomic pattern being fairly similar.

Another study (Lahelma and Arber 1994) addressing inequalities in ill health found that relative differences in limiting long-standing illness by occupational class were larger in Finland, Norway and Sweden than in Britain in the mid-1980s. Furthermore, measuring the size of relative educational differentials in limiting long-standing illness between the three Nordic countries showed that among men the differences in the size of health inequalities between the countries were negligible (Lahelma *et al.* 1994). For women the inequalities were smaller in all three countries, with Swedish women having the largest relative differentials. The order of countries was similar using rate ratios and concentration indices.

A comparative study assessed mortality differentials by education in six European countries in the 1970s (Valkonen 1989). Inequalities in mortality were assessed by a regression-based measure. The largest relative mortality differences by educational groups were found for France, and the smallest for Denmark, Sweden and Norway. Finland occupied an intermediate position, together with Britain.

EU comparative study on health inequalities

The EU comparative study was set up because the evidence from previous comparisons of health inequalities in different countries was only patchy, and covered only a limited set of countries as well as varying time periods. To facilitate systematic comparisons the EU study was designed to cover as many European countries as possible. The morbidity analyses used existing national survey data from 1985–93 for 25–69-year-old subjects. The mortality data ranged from 1975 to 1990 (Kunst *et al.* 1996).

The main aim was to obtain a comprehensive overview of health variations between Western European countries with respect to the size of socioeconomic differences in morbidity and mortality; in other words, to find out whether relative inequalities in morbidity and mortality were smaller in some countries than others. The second aim was to examine potential determinants of the socioeconomic health inequalities (see Cavelaars 1998). Due to limitations in the available data only a few potential determinants could be included, and even these were not available for all countries. We therefore focused mainly on the first aim of the study.

Comparable data on ill health could be found for eleven countries in the European study (Kunst *et al.* 1996; Mackenbach *et al.* 1997; Cavelaars 1998). Although the European study intended to look particularly at relative differences in ill health between socioeconomic groups, it was informative to start with absolute overall prevalence rates among men and women, and between countries. Table 3.1 gives a summary of the level of ill health for perceived health and long-standing illness in ten Western European countries.

Data on perceived health as less than good (or equivalent) are presented for ten countries. For both men and women the highest prevalence of all was found for West Germany (54/56 per cent) and the next highest for Finland (41/42 per cent). Sweden, Norway and Denmark had fairly low prevalences (20–23 per cent). Gender differences in the levels of perceived health were very small in the northern European countries. Data on long-standing illness were available for four countries only. For men and women the highest prevalence was for Finland (42/43 per cent). The rates for the other countries were lower and varied from 30/31 per cent for the Netherlands to 34 per cent for Britain.

The prevalence range between countries was particularly wide for perceived health. For men the highest prevalence of all was 4.1 times greater than the lowest one, and for women 3.6 times greater. The reasons for such large variations are not obvious. Even between the Nordic countries we find substantial prevalence differentials due to a very high prevalence of poor health among Finnish men and women. Nevertheless, the Nordic variation is less than that between the extreme European countries.

Table 3.1 Prevalence rates of less than good perceived health and long-standing illness in ten European countries, men and women aged 25–69

	Perceived health		*Long-standing illness*	
Country	*Men*	*Women*	*Men*	*Women*
Denmark	19.8	22.8	31.2	32.6
Finland	40.9	41.5	42.1	42.9
	(7.4)	(6.5)		
Norway	21.2	23.3	–	–
Sweden	22.0	23.3	–	–
France	22.1	30.0	–	–
Great Britain	31.6	37.7	34.0	33.7
	(10.1)	(11.6)		
Italy	20.0	25.6	–	–
Netherlands	20.8	22.0	30.8	22.9
Spain	28.8	38.7	–	–
	(7.2)	(9.6)		
West Germany	54.1	55.7	–	–
	(13.7)	(15.0)		

Source: Cavelaars *et al.* 1998a.
Note: Cut-off points other than 'less than good' perceived health in parentheses.

Perceived health as rated by the respondents themselves is a valid and reliable health indicator, which would seem to mean that the public health significance of perceived health may be fairly similar across countries, despite variations in the level of ill health captured by that indicator. However, the question may be raised as to whether the considerable variation in ill health between countries affects the absolute as well as relative socioeconomic health differentials. This is discussed below.

Education and morbidity

Turning to the comparison of socioeconomic differences in ill health, we start with differentials by educational level. Educational differences in less than good perceived health could be covered for eleven countries (Mackenbach *et al.* 1997; Cavelaars *et al.* 1998a). Completed education was classified into three levels using standard ISCED categories: 1) secondary education or less; 2) intermediate level of education; and 3) university level or other higher education (Kunst *et al.* 1996).

The main results of the comparison are presented as relative differences between educational and other socioeconomic groups using the

Table 3.2 Relative educational differences in perceived health (Relative Index of Inequality, RII) with 95% confidence intervals (95% CI), men and women aged 25–69

	Men		*Women*	
Country	*RII*	*95% CI*	*RII*	*95% CI*
Denmark	4.60	2.76–7.66	6.80	3.95–11.7
Finland	4.45	3.37–5.88	3.86	2.93–5.09
	(4.70)	(2.67–8.29)	(3.08)	(1.72–5.53)
Norway	6.98	4.55–10.7	4.76	2.92–7.73
Sweden	4.84	3.09–7.57	7.27	4.55–11.6
France	4.23	2.55–7.03	4.18	2.82–6.21
Great Britain	4.06	3.24–5.10	4.02	3.24–4.98
	(4.36)	(3.01–6.32)	(3.92)	(2.76–5.56)
Italy	4.36	3.79–5.01	3.14	2.75–3.59
Netherlands	5.42	4.03–7.29	3.51	2.59–4.75
Spain	2.74	2.11–3.55	3.32	2.47–4.46
	(3.33)	(1.99–5.59)	(4.90)	(2.58–9.33)
West Germany	2.25	1.81–2.79	2.51	1.99–3.17
	(2.86)	(2.08–3.93)	(2.14)	(1.56–2.94)

Source: Cavelaars *et al.* 1998a.
Note: Cut-off points other than 'less than good' perceived health in parentheses.

regression-based relative index of inequality (RII). The picture emerging from Table 3.2 shows that there is a clear tendency for the Nordic countries to have larger relative inequalities in perceived health by education than other European countries: for men, Norway had the largest of all inequalities (RII 6.98) while Sweden had the third largest (RII 4.84). Denmark and Finland had slightly smaller but still fairly large inequalities within the Western European context. The smallest inequalities among men were found for Germany (RII 2.25) and Spain (RII 2.74).

Among women, Sweden had the largest inequalities (RII 7.27) and Denmark the next largest (RII 6.80). Norway (RII 4.76) had smaller and Finland (RII 3.86) even smaller inequalities. The smallest inequalities among women were again found for Germany (RII 2.52), with Italy close behind (RII 3.14).

The results of this comparison exemplify one of the major unexpected findings of this European study, i.e. that the Nordic countries, particularly Norway, Sweden and Denmark, do not have smaller relative inequalities in perceived health by education than other European countries. In fact, the pattern suggested by the results is rather the opposite, i.e. that health inequalities measured in this way may be larger in the Nordic countries than in the other Western European countries studied. However, confidence intervals are large and tend to overlap between countries, so while cross-national differences may seem great, few of them reach statistical significance. Evidence from health indicators other than perceived health was much more limited, but gave some – albeit fairly inconsistent – support to the order of countries.

Income and morbidity

Income differences in perceived health could be covered for six countries, including Sweden and Finland (Cavelaars *et al.* 1998b). Net household income was adjusted for the size of the household by dividing the total household income by household size$^{0.36}$. Respondents in the national studies were grouped into decile groups according to their net household equivalent income.

Relative differences in perceived health by income as measured by the RII (Table 3.3) were again smallest for German men and women (RII 2.84/2.92). However, the most striking result of these income analyses compared to those by education was that health inequalities for Swedish men were the second smallest (RII 3.21), and for Finnish men the third smallest (RII 3.74). The largest inequalities among men

Table 3.3 Relative income differences in perceived health (Relative Index of Inequality, RII) with 95% confidence intervals (95% CI), men and women aged 25–69

	Men		*Women*	
Country	*RII*	*95% CI*	*RII*	*95% CI*
Finland	3.74	2.90–4.81	3.11	2.43–4.00
	(4.45)	(2.86–6.92)	(2.28)	(1.44–3.59)
Sweden	3.21	2.16–4.68	3.82	2.57–5.66
France	3.92	2.70–5.68	3.66	2.70–4.95
Great Britain	4.62	3.65–5.84	4.39	3.53–5.44
	(7.19)	(4.96–10.4)	(6.45)	(4.63–9.00)
Netherlands	5.42	4.00–7.35	3.07	2.32–4.07
West Germany	2.72	2.21–3.34	2.92	2.36–3.61
	(4.02)	(2.98–5.44)	(2.70)	(2.02–3.58)

Source: Cavelaars *et al.* 1998b.
Note: Cut-off points other than 'less than good' perceived health in parentheses.

were found for the Netherlands (RII 5.42) and among women for Great Britain (RII 4.39). These results are also largely in accordance with another broad international comparison of health differentials by income (van Doorslaer *et al.* 1997).

Although the analyses of health inequalities by household income leave out many central and south European countries, it is obvious that these results partly contrast with those obtained from the analyses using education as the socioeconomic indicator. Here, the position of the Nordic countries, notably Sweden, differs from the education finding, i.e. income inequalities in ill health were not larger in Sweden or Finland than in the other countries studied. It is known that these two countries have had particularly small income inequalities compared to other European countries, notably Britain (Atkinson *et al.* 1995, see Chapter 2).

Evidence from health indicators other than perceived health was very patchy in the analyses of health inequalities by income, and cannot be taken as supporting or invalidating the results from perceived health. Taken together, the inequalities in ill health by education and household income show that adding socioeconomic indicators as well as health indicators to the analysis further contributed to the heterogeneity of the results of this European comparison.

Social class and mortality

Next, we point to some interesting evidence on mortality. These analyses present the risk of dying between the 45th and 65th birthday for men in eleven European countries for two broad social classes, namely the working (manual) class vs. other (non-manual) social classes (see Kunst 1997). Table 3.4 presents the mortality risks in these two broad classes as well as the relative mortality risk and risk difference.

The risk of dying during mid-life varies quite dramatically between different countries in both of the two broad social classes. A working-class Irish man runs a risk of dying ten percentage units higher than that of his counterpart in Sweden (29.1 per cent vs. 19.7 per cent). An Irish man from the non-manual social classes has a seven percentage units larger mortality risk compared to a corresponding man in Sweden (21 per cent vs. 14.1 per cent). Apparently, Ireland is a country with relatively poor life expectancy for middle-aged men.

However, when looking at the relative risk of workers vs. other classes Ireland does not stand out in a similar way. On the contrary, Ireland belongs to the majority of countries where the excess mortality risk among male workers relative to other classes falls to just below 40 per cent. France, with a high mortality risk among workers and an average mortality risk in the non-manual social classes, has the highest relative mortality risk of all (1.70). Comparing Denmark and Norway it becomes evident that the public health situation underlying the relative risk of 1.33 can differ dramatically; although these two Nordic countries share first place in the relative equality league (together with Italy), absolute mortality levels in Denmark are more than 20 per cent higher.

The Swedish case is also worth closer examination. Although mortality levels are very low in both broad classes, the relative mortality risk for working-class men is as high or higher than in most other countries. The reason for this anomaly is to be found in the extremely low mortality risk among Swedish non-manual men. Although Swedish working-class men have the lowest mortality risk among the countries compared, the relative risk is boosted by the small death rate among middle-aged Swedish non-manual men.

Some countries also show a fairly consistent picture across the four measures of mortality inequalities presented in Table 3.4. Finland, for example, shows a high mortality risk for both broad social classes, and a large excess mortality risk for workers in both relative as well as absolute terms. Despite this, the methodological conclusion from the mortality analyses by social class presented in Table 3.4 is that

Table 3.4 Risk of dying between 45th and 65th birthday, relative mortality risks (RR) of working classes compared to other classes, and absolute differences between working classes and other classes among men in ten European countries (national rankings according to each indicator in parentheses)

Country	*Working class*	*Other classes*	*RR*	*Difference*
Denmark	25.4 (7)	19.1 (9)	1.33 (1)	6.3 (6)
Finland	28.8 (9)	18.9 (8)	1.52 (9)	9.9 (9)
Norway	20.9 (2)	15.7 (3)	1.33 (1)	5.2 (1)
Sweden	19.7 (1)	14.1 (1)	1.40 (7)	5.6 (2)
England & Wales	24.0 (5)	16.5 (6)	1.45 (8)	7.5 (7)
France	27.6 (8)	16.2 (4)	1.70 (10)	11.4 (10)
Ireland	29.1 (10)	21.0 (10)	1.39 (5)	8.1 (8)
Italy	24.6 (6)	18.5 (7)	1.33 (1)	6.1 (4)
Portugal	22.5 (4)	16.4 (5)	1.37 (4)	6.1 (4)
Spain	21.1 (3)	15.2 (2)	1.39 (5)	5.9 (3)

Source: Kunst 1997.

inequalities as measured exclusively by relative differences are probably a dubious indicator in a comprehensive examination of health inequalities. Particular problems arise when using relative differences only to discuss different policy options to reduce health inequalities.

Discussion

This chapter has given an overview of inequalities in morbidity and mortality in the Nordic countries compared to a broader European context. For this purpose we reviewed and re-analysed results from the first large-scale European comparative study on health inequalities (Kunst *et al.* 1996; Mackenbach *et al.* 1997).

On the basis of our examination three main conclusions may be drawn. First, the size and pattern of health inequalities in the Nordic countries are very similar to those found in most Western European countries when health inequalities are studied as differences in health between social classes and educational groups. Earlier findings of narrower differences between social classes and educational groups in the Nordic countries than in other European nations could not be confirmed. Second, when analysing health inequalities by household income, there actually seems to be a difference between Sweden and Finland on one hand and Great Britain and the Netherlands on the other. In other words, the hypothesis of smaller health differentials in the Nordic countries than elsewhere in Western Europe receives some support when people's economic situation is used as a basis for the analysis, whereas it is not supported when class or education is used for stratification. Third, the choice of the inequality measure – i.e. whether relative or absolute differences across the social structure, or absolute level among the least well off only, are examined – is likely to be crucial both for the evaluation of the size and trends in health inequalities and for policy evaluations.

The last point is actually the one we would like to discuss in more detail below. In addition, we think it is necessary to further clarify the problems of comparative research that may have had a bearing on the findings concerning health inequalities in the European countries. Finally, we would offer some potential explanations for the observed health inequalities and their variation across the countries.

Methodological issues in comparative research

The European comparative study on health inequalities utilised in our analyses was based on available mortality data and surveys conducted in each participating country. It must be stressed that huge efforts were made to cope with the large volumes of data and the comparability problems that arose from this (see Kunst *et al.* 1996). The latter included corrections for differences in non-response rates as well as for the lack of socioeconomic data on non-employed people for some countries. Sensitivity analyses were made to assess the size of the potential bias, as well as parallel analyses using various health and socioeconomic indicators to cross-validate the findings. However, a number of methodological problems which are likely to affect the results and their comparability may have remained. It is likely that morbidity data are more subject to such problems than mortality data.

Morbidity data were derived from a variety of national surveys on health and living conditions (Cavelaars 1998). The coverage of these surveys varied in terms of time periods, age limits and sampling frames. Non-response varied in the studies from 10 to 43 per cent (*ibid.*). Non-response consists of full refusals as well as partial non-response to particular questions. The former affects the overall quality of the survey, while the latter biases delicate questions such as income. To the extent that the non-response is systematic by socioeconomic indicators, this may also bias the results on health inequalities. Information on income in the Finnish and Swedish surveys was derived from tax register linkages with negligible missing data, whereas in other countries income data were based on responses to survey questions.

The wording of the questions measuring health outcomes also varied between the national surveys, which may affect the levels of ill health captured. As the levels of ill health, particularly of perceived health, show considerable variation between countries, the question is, how does this affect the absolute and relative socioeconomic differences? For perceived health, the commonest available health indicator, the wording of the question as well as the response alternatives varied (Kunst *et al.* 1996). However, the measure of perceived health has turned out to show good reliability (Lundberg and Manderbacka 1996; Martikainen *et al.* 1999). It also predicts mortality in all countries where studies have been made (see Idler and Benyamini 1997). This can be taken to indicate that the public health relevance of perceived health is fairly similar across countries despite variations in the question wording and the levels of ill health captured by that indicator.

Mortality data avoid some of the difficulties faced with the morbidity data. However, the mortality data also varied in the European comparative study (Kunst *et al.* 1996). Time periods for each country were not identical, regional coverage varied, and in some countries only data on limited cross-sectional samples were available compared to other cases with longitudinal data only. Socioeconomic indicators were linked at the individual level in the Nordic countries, but were unlinked in most others. In general, the Nordic mortality data sources are of high quality and contain fewer sources of potential bias than in other European countries.

Finally, variations in cultural and structural factors should be considered. For data on ill health we usually have no yardstick to indicate the 'true' morbidity. In any case, 'health cultures' affecting the disposition to experience and report health problems may vary between countries. To be able to better deal with these issues complementary in-depth data on the context in each country would help in the interpretation of the findings. In addition to variations in the overall levels of morbidity and mortality, there are differences in social structures, such as labour markets, allocation to classes and educational systems, which are seen in distributions of the population across the structural variables. This may further affect comparability as the social structures between countries may differ considerably. One example is labour market participation, which varies greatly between men and women, and complicates the examination of occupational class inequalities, particularly among women. However, measures of the extent of inequalities, such as the relative index of inequality, were used to control for the sizes of the socioeconomic groups in order to better compare the relative health inequalities across countries.

In summary, then, the European comparative study has provided important new evidence on health inequalities in Europe. The fact that Nordic survey data may carry more precise information on, for example, income due to the potentials of record linkages represents a remaining comparability problem, especially since higher precision in measurement generally leads to larger inequality estimates. Although these first broad comparisons need follow-up work to clarify and corroborate or falsify the findings presented here, the data represent the most comprehensive effort so far in terms of compiling comparable data on socioeconomic health inequalities across European countries.

Explanations for health inequalities

Several distinct processes may underlie the observed health inequalities, which contribute to the size of absolute and relative differences in morbidity and mortality within and between countries. Such explanatory processes are operative at the individual as well as at the welfare state regime level, and their origins may be in the recent as well as more remote past. Individual level factors contributing to the international patterning of health inequalities include material and non-material living conditions, such as childhood living conditions (Lundberg 1991a, 1993; Rahkonen *et al.* 1997b), current working conditions (Lundberg 1991b), and health behaviours such as smoking (Lynch *et al.* 1997; Cavelaars *et al.* 2000). Also, the European countries operate different welfare state regimes, which implies contrasting structural arrangements – for example in the labour market – as well as different health and welfare policy orientations. A related issue is that European countries, even the Nordic nations, share dissimilar historical backgrounds in terms of their welfare state development, for example, the timing and forms of social structural and demographic transformations (Alestalo and Flora 1994).

The main aim of the European comparative study was to examine the pattern and size of health inequalities in different countries. Explanations for the differences were only a secondary aim and the data did not permit broad explanatory frameworks to be tested.

However, efforts were made to examine health behaviours as determinants of health inequalities. The examination of the impact of smoking offers an example of explanatory analysis that may help understand the production of health inequalities in different European countries and the observed differences between them. The socio-economic distribution of smoking in the Nordic countries is much more unequal than in Southern Europe. Within the European study it was suggested that the southern countries are still at an earlier phase of the 'smoking epidemic', implying negligible or reverse socio-economic differences in smoking (Cavelaars *et al.* 2000). In contrast, the negative atmosphere towards smoking in the Northern European countries, particularly in the higher socioeconomic positions, may imply that people in these positions are less likely to start smoking and more likely to quit than those in lower positions. Whether this kind of unequal distribution of health risks can be found for other forms of health behaviour remains largely unresolved (see Lundberg 1991b; Lynch *et al.* 1997).

In addition to health behaviours, unequal distributions of material living conditions and resources have been regarded as the most important, if not the sole, reason for health inequalities by some scholars (Davey Smith *et al.* 1994; Kuh *et al.* 1997). Strong emphasis has also been placed on the significance of relative income inequalities and their psychosocial impacts (Wilkinson 1996). However, structural causation such as the association between income and health is not likely to be straightforward (see Lundberg and Fritzell 1994). As already noted above, despite small income inequalities in Finland

(Atkinson *et al.* 1995) the inequalities in mortality are very large (Valkonen *et al.* 1993).

Social causation of health, and of health inequalities, is sometimes emphasised as a one-directional process in which unequal material conditions produce health inequalities (see Davey Smith *et al.* 1994; Kuh *et al.* 1997). However, reverse causation must also be taken into account. Selective recruitment to social positions resulting from social mobility between and within generations may contribute to health inequalities (Lundberg 1991a; Rahkonen *et al.* 1997a). It is even possible that in the Nordic countries social mobility plays a particularly important role since they may be more open and meritocratic compared to Central and Southern European countries. Therefore, past living conditions and social mobility are a potential explanation for part of the international patterning of health inequalities.

Partly related to social mobility one should take account of the historical background as well. Industrialisation, urbanisation and related processes of modernisation in terms of economic, occupational and demographic transformation took place in the Nordic countries, particularly Finland, much later than in other Western European countries (Alestalo and Flora 1994; Alestalo and Uusitalo 1986). Accordingly, people in the older birth cohorts may still carry with them the burdens of rural poverty and physically strenuous working and living conditions. On one hand, the effects of this background can be seen among current older cohorts. On the other hand, due to the late modernisation regional and social mobility have probably shaped the social structures of the Nordic countries more than in other Western European countries, which may also have contributed to the production of health inequalities.

Finally, recent evidence from Norway suggests potential new selective processes were effective in the mid-1990s (Dahl and Birkelund 1999). This study found an absence of health inequalities among the economically active Norwegian adult population. However, health among the non-employed differed from the employed more than before. The authors interpret this as indicating increasingly strict selection in the Norwegian labour market: only the fit are allowed to survive within the competitive labour market. Whether similar processes emerge in other countries remains to be seen in subsequent studies. Preliminary observations from Finland (Manderbacka *et al.* 2001) and Sweden (Lundberg *et al.* 2001) would suggest rather dissimilar changes, i.e. stable or even slightly declining health inequalities among both the employed and non-employed.

Policy implications

In order to be of interest for public policy, as well as for any attempt to evaluate such policies, health inequalities have to be of a certain magnitude. There are two reasons for this. First, large health differences between population groups are usually seen as relatively more important than small ones, even if both are equally unjust in principle. Second, large differences in health between population groups represent a larger potential for general improvements in public health.

The magnitude of health inequalities is even large enough to be important from a public health point of view in the Nordic countries. Two examples may illustrate our point. In Finland, the difference in life expectancy at 35 years between the higher educated and the basically educated group is 5.7 years for men and 3.3 years for women (Martikainen and Valkonen 1995), while in Sweden the mortality among those with basic education would decrease by more than 40 per cent if reduced to the level of those with a university degree (Lundberg 1998). Obviously, these figures show that the health differentials found between broad segments of the population in Finland and Sweden are large in an absolute as well as relative sense. It is also clear that such large differentials represent a substantial potential for improving public health in both countries.

Thus differentials in morbidity and mortality between socioeconomic groups are large for both sexes, particularly men. Bringing the morbidity and mortality of the worst off groups closer to the best off groups would result in considerable public health benefits. The fact that the size of health inequalities varies between countries and over time suggests that the potential exists to reduce differences in mortality and morbidity between socioeconomic groups, particularly in the countries where the greatest disparities are found.

The socioeconomic differences in morbidity and mortality found in the European context are very consistent and, although varying in size, are substantial in each country studied. In fact, health inequalities are so large that it may be hard to find any other options with the potential to bring about equally great public health benefits.

Cross-national comparisons of health inequalities such as those referred to above may lend themselves to evaluations of policies already implemented, as well as to discussions on future policies targeted at reducing inequalities. For both these purposes it is extremely important to choose proper measures of inequality and trends in inequalities. Otherwise, we would argue, it is easy to jump to problematic conclusions.

Take the case of Sweden in Table 3.4 (see p. 57). On the basis of relative risks it would be possible to draw the conclusion that more than half a century of egalitarian policies have failed, since inequalities in mortality among middle-aged men are as large in Sweden as elsewhere in Europe. This sort of simplistic conclusion would ignore the fact that Swedish working-class men have extremely good survival rates compared to similar men in other European countries, which in turn may very well result from the wide range of welfare state policies implemented since the 1930s. Therefore, a proper discussion on policy implications must be informed of both the differences between population groups and the absolute levels of health and mortality in these groups.

Summary and concluding remarks

The comparative research on health inequalities in Western Europe reviewed in this chapter reveals that in the 1980s the picture was a varied one. The size of inequalities in mortality and morbidity shows substantial disparities between the studied countries. The ranking of the countries does not accord with expectations that health inequalities would be smaller within the Nordic welfare regime than in those prevailing in the Central and Southern European countries. In fact, some of the evidence suggests that health inequalities in the Nordic countries may be larger than elsewhere, whereas other evidence suggests that the Nordic countries have smaller than average health inequalities.

Our analysis in this chapter also shows that comparing health inequalities across several countries is a very complex task. In future examinations we need to be more specific than has been possible so far in terms of the multiple dimensions of socioeconomic as well as health status, since these are likely to affect the size of health inequalities. In addition, the issue of absolute and relative health differences between socioeconomic population groups has to be taken very seriously.

The data used in the European comparison examined above derive mostly from the 1980s. Later comparative data on the European level is needed *per se*, but also for analyses of trends, since current research does not contain information on the changes over time of health inequalities in a broader European perspective, i.e. whether inequalities are widening or narrowing. However, further work is being done in the Nordic countries. This is particularly important, as the deep economic recession of the early 1990s, which affected Finland

and Sweden most severely, posed a huge challenge to the traditional Nordic welfare state regime and forced changes in its functioning (Kautto *et al.* 1999). During periods of social and economic crisis it is of particular interest to monitor the development of public health and its distribution with regard to the role of the welfare state.

Notes

1 The authors would like to thank the participants of the 'EU Working Group on Socioeconomic Inequalities in Health', particularly the director of the group professor J.P. Mackenbach, as well as doctors Anton Kunst and Adriënne Cavelaars of the Department of Public Health, Erasmus University, Rotterdam. Although this chapter examines some of the main results of that project, the selection of results and the opinions expressed reflect the views of the authors only.

2 Inspired by the Nordic approach to welfare research (Erikson and Uusitalo 1987), a number of cross-national comparisons on health inequalities have been made since the 1970s. Such comparisons have focused on Nordic countries alone (Allardt 1975; Karisto *et al.* 1978; Karisto 1984; Valkonen 1989; Lahelma *et al.* 1993) or included other countries, too (Lundberg, 1986; Vågerö and Lundberg 1989; Lahelma and Arber 1994; Rahkonen *et al.* 1998; Lahelma *et al.* 2000).

4 Gender policies and gender equality

Randi Kjeldstad

Introduction[1]

The Nordic countries are often looked upon as pioneers in the promotion of equal opportunities for women and men. Among the 163 countries included in the gender-related development indexes of the UN Human Development Report, all the Nordic countries range at the very top.[2] This leading position in gender equality is partly related to the strong representation of women among the political elites, as Sweden, Norway, Finland and Denmark are actually the first four countries in the world in terms of the proportion of female national parliamentarians, and among the top six for the percentage of women government ministers. Moreover, Nordic women have a higher participation in education and the labour market than women of most other countries. As a consequence, Nordic women have gained an increasingly independent position in society and the economy over recent decades. The gender-sensitive public policies of the region are generally given the credit for women's relatively independent economic position. These policies include the provision of social services relieving women of some of their care responsibilities, and the integration of women and mothers into the labour market and political system.

This chapter discusses the relationship between gender equality and political priorities. The main questions raised are, on one side, whether inter-country differences in gender equality and the status of women may largely be traced back to national policies and political priorities and, on the other side, whether the success of various policy approaches differs across society. The questions are discussed by comparing and contrasting gender equality policies and the level of attained gender equality in the Nordic countries with two other European countries, the Netherlands and the United Kingdom. As a framework for the analysis the chapter uses a typology of policy approaches to gender equality developed by Prue Chamberlayne. The discussion is illustrated and supplemented by descriptive statistics on women's and men's position in significant social arenas during the last two to three decades although the main emphasis is on the 1990s.

The institutionalisation of gender policies: state versus grass roots engagement

The policy areas closely related to the status of women and gender equality in Western welfare states are not only policies explicitly labelled as gender equality policies. Those labelled as labour market policies, family policies and welfare policies tend to have, for example, a significant influence on the development of women's position as compared to men's in society. Today it is not possible in the Nordic or most Western European countries to clearly distinguish between gender equality policies and other policies aimed at family or individual redistribution. However, countries do differ in the extent to which gender equality has been a significant issue in the process of adopting and implementing policies at state level. As will be shown later in this chapter, there is a tendency for countries with a strong central engagement in gender equality to develop policy approaches which comprise institutional arrangements and regulations.

The concept 'state feminism' is often used to characterise the wide range of gender equality policies, which include state institutions set up specifically with the goals of furthering women's interests and improving their position in the public sphere. Most Western European countries manifest some features of state feminism today, although those most commonly associated with this concept are the Nordic countries (Howell 1998). In comparison to the latter, the Netherlands and the United Kingdom are characterised by weak or scattered elements of state feminism. A common feature of the current institutionalised gender equality policies of the Nordic countries is that they all developed through an interplay of commitment from both the 'top' and the 'bottom', i.e. an interaction between political elites and grass-roots mobilisation (Bergqvist *et al.* 1999). Despite the significant similarities of the political process across the Nordic countries, however, this interplay has taken different forms. While Danish feministic mobilisation has been mainly 'movement oriented', feminists in the other Nordic countries have to a much larger degree been mobilised through the political parties. Finland represents the most developed 'party oriented' model (*ibid.*). In Finland, the women's movement and other social movements have played only moderate roles in the gender equality process. The same is true for other organisations, for example, the labour market organisations. In Sweden and Norway these organisations are central bodies in the bargaining over gender equality issues in both labour market and welfare policies. In Sweden, like Norway, gender equality and woman's issues throughout recent decades have become gradually institutionalised and affirmed as political goals by successive governments. To be sure, prolonged periods of social democratic rule in both Sweden and Norway have meant great support for gender equality. But centre and conservative governments have also included gender equality in their programmes. Of the Nordic countries, Sweden has the longest and strongest tradition of institutionalised gender equality policies.

These days, however, gender equality is a core element of the political and cultural ideals of social equality in all the Nordic countries. However, the broad spectrum of historical conditions has led to a variety of political and institutional frameworks for gender equality among the Nordic countries. These conditions are partly economic, geographic and demographic, and partly cultural (Skrede 1986). Bergqvist *et al.* (1999) highlight religion, maintaining that this has probably had a stronger influence in Norwegian politics than elsewhere in the Nordic region. There is reason to assume a certain coherence between fairly strong Protestant family ideals and a relatively persistent housewife tradition in Norway. In contrast, the fact that Denmark and Sweden are among the more secular countries of the Western world may explain the earlier expansion of public child care and female employment in these countries (as discussed later in this chapter, see also Chapter 7). Denmark stands out from the other Nordic countries in having a somewhat more liberal social and political culture (*ibid.*). Danes are traditionally more sceptical of political authorities organising and controlling their lives than Swedes, Finns and Norwegians. Thus the Danish development towards gender equality is more a result of grass-roots pressure and changing individual perspectives than political enforcement and sanctions. The anti-authoritarian ideal seems to have a strong position in the Dutch discourse, too. These are important cultural characteristics that over the years have brought about considerable inter-country variations in policies. There are reasons for believing, for example, that relatively liberal attitudes towards the sex industry and prostitution in both Denmark and the Netherlands are related to the strong elements of liberal political traditions in the two countries. This – in the Dutch case – in spite of long traditions of religious influence, too. As Joyce Outshoorn puts it: 'While social democratic Sweden optimistically believes that all bad and suppressive behaviour can be abolished by law, Dutch Calvinism believes that human evil cannot be abolished. The best one can do is to regulate it.'[3] Accordingly, Sweden forbade prostitution by law in 1999, while the Netherlands and Denmark aim at regulating the business.

While *gender equality* has been a widely used (and misused) concept within the Nordic political discourse, the core concept of Dutch gender policies has been *emancipation*. The political goals of Dutch emancipation policies include not merely a gender perspective, but aim rather at a multiform society in which everyone, regardless of sex, marital status, ethnicity, sexual orientation, age, religion, etc., has the opportunity to create for him or herself an independent life (SZW undated). During the 1990s, however, gender issues came more and more to the fore in Dutch policies, and state functions and obligations were increasingly formalised. Nevertheless, alliances between non-governmental organisations and the political elites have traditionally been weaker on gender issues in the Netherlands than in the Nordic countries. This is even more true in the case of the United Kingdom, where attempts by grass-roots organisations and individual lobbyists to place the public position of women on the agenda have often been thwarted by the political institutions. Because the British women's movement has been characterised by local and limited objectives and has never managed to combine its grass-roots nature with close co-operation with 'friendly' political forces, it has been vulnerable to counteraction (Chamberlayne 1993). Since the installation of a Labour government in 1997, however, certain attitudinal changes have emerged, and the new government policies are tending to involve initiatives to communicate and co-operate with non-governmental organisations.

Summing up so far, the Nordic countries have had a longer tradition of broad political engagement with the issue of gender equality than the Netherlands and United Kingdom, and a more persistent commitment to pursue this goal at all political levels. This is one important reason why the Nordic countries have commonly been viewed as prototypes of 'woman-friendly states'. 'Woman-friendliness' is generally related to a social and political process that helps free women from economic dependence on their husbands and towards self-support through paid work or public support through economic and welfare transfers. However, Bussemaker and van Kersbergen (1994) criticise the tendency to see the Nordic countries as some kind of *norm* for comparative research on gender and welfare. They maintain that the very idea of 'woman-friendliness' in the Nordic countries is based on somewhat restricted values, and that gender equality should not refer only to economic stratification and economic independence through employment and public child care. Independence should also be understood as the possibility to make choices and to develop insulation from emotional or psychological dependence. Although the Nordic discourse has also included critical and pessimistic views, most Nordic feminists tend to be optimistic (see e.g. Bergqvist *et al.* 1999), claiming that state feminism has improved women's general position and given them new resources for mobilisation, protest and political influence (Dahlerup 1987; Hernes 1987a,b).

A typology of gender equality approaches

The definitions of basic concepts underlying gender equality policies, such as *gender equality, equal status, equal opportunities, women's emancipation* and *feminism,* vary across social groups and time, and the changing perception of gender roles in society has brought about significant policy shifts during recent decades. To clarify the content of some of these concepts in relation to national policy differences, I shall use a typology of gender policy approaches developed by Prue Chamberlayne (1993). In Chamberlayne's analysis, gender policies in France, West Germany, Italy and Britain are compared during the 1970s and 1980s. This chapter argues that Chamberlayne's typology is also a useful frame in relation to the group of countries compared here. Moreover, the typology can contribute to understanding changing gender roles and policies across a longer time-span than suggested by Chamberlayne. The policies of the 1990s can just as well be analysed from the same perspective, and new countries included.

The first of Chamberlayne's four gender equality approaches, *the gender neutral approach*, is characterised by no account being taken of the specificity of women's position, and such policies may be identified as liberal reformist 'equal rights' gender equality policies. Gender policies of equal rights seek the rights of women to operate as free individuals on equal terms with men. Important policy areas are the right to be elected to influential positions, and the right to paid work and equal pay. The main aim of equal rights policies in this area is to attain equal *opportunities* for all citizens – women and men – to participate in society and to determine their own livelihood and future. Whether the *outcome* is equal for women and men is more or less irrelevant to this approach. However, because women and men facing the same opportunities often occupy different social positions and belong to different social contexts, women may experience citizens' rights differently. Consequently, the assumption of gender neutrality of citizenship has been highly disputed in recent years, with many feminist writers advocating that citizenship is and always has been gendered (see e.g. Waylen 1998 and Randall 1998). As Orloff (1993) states, the ideal–typical citizen in classical liberal democratic theory and in the literature on social rights is the independent male householder or the male worker. She argues for a 'gendering' of the concepts of 'citizen' and 'social rights'. Lister (1995) maintains that the identification of women mainly with the private sphere has weakened their position as citizens, and that accordingly the process to attain full citizenship for women must begin with a re-articulation of the public/private divide. This is no 'easy match', however, as the division between public and private is one of the cornerstones of liberal democratic policies.

The second gender equality approach of Chamberlayne's typology is the social feminist *gender recognition* approach, focusing on the particular obstacles women meet in the gender equality process. Recognising the underachievement of the gender neutral approach, the aim is gender equality of *outcome* more than equal opportunities. Policies adapted to this approach often make use of positive discrimination measures, including quota systems, gender equality training programmes and public child and elderly care to ease women's burden in the household.

The third approach, the *gender reconstruction* approach, emphasises the reciprocity in women's and men's roles in society. Policies aiming to change the male role, especially the father role within the family, are viewed as a precondition for real equality between women's and men's status in all spheres of society. The gender recognition and the gender reconstruction approaches are closely related. Actually, as Chamberlayne maintains, the latter presupposes (rather than is replaced by) the former. However: 'Whereas the gender recognition approach assumed spontaneous changes at the interpersonal level, gender reconstruction considered modifications at the structural level a precondition to change at the personal level' (Chamberlayne 1993: 173). In contrast to the gender neutrality approach, the gender recognition and gender reconstruction approaches aim primarily at some kind of equality of outcome between women and men. Whereas gender neutral policies aim at securing the same formal citizen rights for women and men, gender recognition and gender reconstruction policies aim at removing hindrances to women in using these rights.

The fourth approach, the *gender reinforcement* approach, differs from the former three by highlighting differentiation between the sexes. While the gender reconstruction approach views changes of both male and female roles in society as a precondition for gender equalisation, supporters of the gender reinforcement approach advocate the continuation of traditional, complementary gender roles. The main aim is to reinforce and promote traditional female values, rewarding all kinds of home-care and domestic work. It is worth mentioning that although the gender reinforcement approach emphasises the preservation of differentiated gender roles, it does not necessarily imply a preservation of gender unequal *outcome*. Preventing a systematically unequal economic distribution among women and men in a political system dominated by a gender reinforcement approach, however, presupposes that work in the domestic and work in the public spheres are both equally rewarded.

Although Chamberlayne's typology represents a useful frame for analysing differences in the gender equalising process across countries and time, the gender-related policies of one country, or at one point in time, cannot be described by only one of the four approaches. I will argue that some elements of each and every one of Chamberlayne's four gender approaches may be found in all the countries compared in this chapter. I will also argue that the chronological development and shifts in gender policies have many similar traits in the actual countries. Nevertheless, there are reasons to believe that each country can be characterised by one or two predominant approaches during recent years. The predominant gender equality policy approach of each country may in turn explain the various levels of gender equality in their different social arenas. In the following I shall draw a rough sketch of some relevant policy areas and some important policy differences between the six countries, based on Chamberlayne's typology.

Policy approaches and the process towards gender equality

'First wave and early second wave feminism': mainly gender neutral approaches

The first steps towards national gender equalising processes, often called 'first wave feminism', were in most countries characterised by movements and questions of equal rights and equal opportunities between women and men, i.e. a gender neutral approach in Chamberlayne's terminology. The main areas of concern were basic political rights, such as the right to vote and to be elected in national local elections.

'Second wave feminism' is usually dated back to the early 1960s, when access to education, the labour market and to political and other influential positions on equal gender terms, together with equal pay for equal work, were put on the agenda.[4] Partly made possible by, and partly accompanied by, legislation and national machinery established to promote women's access to public arenas, the educational systems and labour markets were gradually invaded by women. However, the 'women's revolution' in the labour market (Skrede and Tornes 1994a,b) came later in some countries than others. Of the Nordic countries, Finland has the longest history of significant female labour force participation. Whereas in Sweden and Denmark the post-war female employment increase gathered pace during the 1960s, the corresponding increase in Norway did not commence until the beginning of the 1970s (Nordic Council of Ministers 1994; Ljones 1979). During the period 1975 to 1985, however, although still ranking at the bottom, Norway caught up with the other Nordic countries somewhat. To the extent that one can talk about a women's revolution in the Dutch labour market, it did not commence for some years yet; until 1980 less than one-third of Dutch women were employed (Keuzenkamp 1998). Relatively high and slowly increasing labour activity among British women during the 1970s and 1980s indicate a relatively long and stable female labour market participation in the United Kingdom. Thus in the case of Britain and Finland, one can hardly speak of a women's labour market revolution in the same way as in Denmark, Sweden and Norway during the early and late 1970s, and the Netherlands a decade or two later.

The 1970s was the decade where the first serious steps were made towards 'mainstreaming' gender equality perspectives in politics. By 1979 both the United Kingdom and the Netherlands had, as members of the European Union, adopted several directives on gender equality issues. The most important directives concerned equal pay, equal treatment in job engagement, on-the-job-training and work environment, and in social security. At the same time all the Nordic countries except Finland (where a gender equality and a Gender Commission Act were passed in 1986), had legislated on equal opportunities and/ or established state bodies to promote gender equality in all areas of society. The approach was mainly gender neutral, although a gender recognition approach was often also present. One purpose of the Norwegian Gender Equality Act of 1978 is to promote gender equality by eliminating discrimination in general, *and* to improve the status of women in particular. The Act applies to all areas of society, with the exception of internal affairs of religious committees. As the gender equality laws of the other Nordic countries are mainly focused on the labour market and on public positions, the Norwegian law is probably more comprehensive than the legislation in other countries (Nordic Council of Ministers 1994; Ministry of Children and Family Affairs 1994).

Gender recognition approach: gradually grasped by the Nordic countries, with Dutch and British reluctance

By late 1970s and throughout the 1980s the gender-related political agendas of several countries gradually shifted towards a greater focus on the many hindrances, both in the family and in public life, to women's access and participation in public arenas. Gender recognition approaches in most countries included political measures to relieve some of women's care responsibilities in the household through establishing and expanding public institutions for child and elderly care (for a more detailed analysis of care services, see Chapter 7). During this period there was a tremendous expansion of publicly financed day care institutions in the Nordic countries. Such coverage was doubled on the average within fifteen years (Nordic Council of Ministers 1994). Several gender recognition initiatives were pioneered by Sweden. Already by the end of the 1970s, 60 per cent of Swedish children aged 3–6 were enrolled in publicly financed day care. Sweden was also the first country to introduce a public day care guarantee to all pre-school children. The Swedish law was passed in 1985, and similar guarantees followed in Finland and Denmark a few years later. The fact that the expansion of day care came later in Norway may partly explain why Norway fell behind in women's employment development during the 1960s and 1970s. By 1997, however, it had achieved about the same coverage as the other Nordic countries, and even passed the Finnish level. Unlike in the other Nordic countries, however, Norwegian pre-school children have no statutory right to public day care.

The Dutch government's response to demands by the Women's Movement to expand public day care in the 1970s was to introduce a 12-week maternity leave with full wage compensation in 1977 (Rostgaard and Fridberg 1998). Dutch advocates of public day care have traditionally met strong opposition. While public child care has been accepted as a support for lower income groups, most children have been expected to be cared for in their families. In 1990 and the three following years, however, the Dutch government provided partial funding for new municipal day care places for children under the age of five. This led to a significant increase in day care institutions. But by the late 1990s the number of places was still so low that a woman's job position was in most cases the determining factor for obtaining a place (*ibid.*). Support for public day care in the United Kingdom has also been low. Except in war time, when women were needed in the labour market, children have been regarded as better off when cared for in the family. Still today, care for pre-school children is provided exclusively for families in need, although parents of children aged four years have recently been guaranteed places for their pre-school children in the education system (*ibid.*, see also Chapter 7).

As with day care expansion, Sweden was a world pioneer in introducing a generous system of parental leave connected to the birth and care of small children. Finland followed, and by the beginning of the 1990s Swedish and Finnish parents had the right to twelve and eleven months paid birth leave with 90 per cent and 80 per cent wage compensation, respectively. Danish parents were entitled to seven months and Norwegian parents (in 1991) to ten months leave, with 90 per cent and 80 per cent wage compensation, respectively. Throughout the 1990s, however, there were relatively modest improvements in child care cash benefits in the Nordic countries. In Sweden the wage compensation during parental leave was actually lowered for a period, whereas in Norway the parental leave period was extended (to 52 weeks in 1993).

When the EU Commission passed a directive granting a minimum of 14 weeks maternity leave with wage compensation at the level of the respective countries' sick leaves in 1992, 'protecting pregnant women and women after childbirth', the United Kingdom had already extended paid leave to 18 weeks. In the Netherlands, however, the directive brought about an extension of paid maternity leave. During the late 1990s the United Kingdom and the Netherlands extended the rights to parental leave somewhat, although these applied only to *unpaid* leave. By 1999 and in both countries, mothers (and partly fathers) were entitled to an additional three months unpaid leave after birth as a consequence of an EU directive. Accordingly, and following collective agreements, fathers have obtained some leave rights, albeit restricted compared to the Nordic countries. Thus in most European countries, the care of newly born children is today viewed as something both parents should be able to choose at least for some weeks after the birth. Imposing on, or mildly forcing, fathers to take part in post-natal child care, however, is a *reconstruction* rather than a *recognition* initiative in gender equality terms, and has so far been adopted in very few countries (see later in this chapter).

In many countries, the gender recognition approach of the 1980s and early 1990s drew attention to the male-dominant structures in work places and the corridors of power. In some countries legal measures were initiated against structural hindrances to women's participation in public arenas, and in the Nordic countries the need for special actions to integrate women in the public sphere became identified. The legal position of pregnant women was strengthened, and employers were prohibited from attaching importance to the pregnancy of a job-seeker. In the Nordic countries there was increasing concern about the segregated labour market as an important obstacle to gender equality in society. Since it was presumed to reinforce gender stereotyping and exert a negative impact on women's career opportunities and the valuation of women's work, the gender-segregated labour market was seen as a major determinant of male–female wage differentials (Ministry of Children and Family Affairs 1992; Nordic Council of Ministers 1995; Anker 1998; Melkas and Anker 1998). Some Nordic countries introduced quota systems to secure approximately equal representation of both sexes in strategic educational institutions and occupations. Employers were instructed to practise positive discrimination towards women, and public subsidies were granted to male-dominated businesses engaging women (Skjeie *et al.* 1989). The objective was to reduce the tendency for women and men to be in different occupations and sectors of the labour market (horizontal segregation) *and* in different positions within the same occupational groups or sectors (vertical segregation or segmentation).

At the same time there was growing concern about the large gender gap in access to and influence in political institutions. By the early 1970s it was acknowledged in most Nordic countries that the right to vote was not enough to assure women real political influence; they must also be nominated and elected to political bodies in sufficiently large numbers. It was argued that the proportion of women must exceed a certain level to ensure that their views had political impact. According to the Norwegian Ministry of Children and Family Affairs (1994), a 30 per cent proportion of women was seen to be a critical minimum. The means to this goal have partly been campaigns to increase women's political awareness and their numbers in political posts, and partly resolutions on minimum quotas of women in political bodies and parties. However, attitudes have differed across the Nordic countries on the merits of quota systems as the best instrument to achieve gender equality in this field. Such strategies, therefore, have been applied in slightly different ways among the Nordic countries (Nordic Council of Ministers 1995). Except for Denmark, where mobilisation strategies have been relatively sporadic, various quotation practices have been used in all the Nordic countries. The deployment of minimum quota systems within political bodies has proved most effective in Norway, however (Christensen 1999).

Owing to the prevailing liberal political traditions *and* to the predominantly gender neutral legal principles of the EU, positive discrimination has been seen as an alien element in British and Dutch policies. Compared to the Nordic countries, there is a general reluctance towards state interference in social recruitment processes. Quota systems, therefore, are generally unwelcome in these two countries, although both governments do aim at greater public participation of woman and a more equal distribution of public positions. This has been especially true since 1992, when both countries launched plans including quantitative targets for women's participation in political and public life. In recent government documents, political bodies are invited to take measures to promote gender equality (Minister for Women 1999 and SZW undated). To the extent concrete target figures are put forward, however, they are recommendations rather than instructions.

Gender reconstruction policies: rhetoric and actions

By the end of the 1980s and throughout the 1990s attention was gradually drawn towards women's and men's roles within the family as partners and parents. This policy shift is particularly evident in the Nordic countries, where several initiatives were taken to encourage the active involvement of men in the care of children. At the Nordic level, The Nordic Council of Ministers in 1995 agreed on a gender equality platform for action stating that 'the active involvement of men is necessary in order to achieve equality between women and men'. To achieve this, the platform states that 'the distribution of the workload between women and men in the family and in society must be changed' (Nordic Council of Ministers 1995: 12). While Norway was the most reluctant of the Nordic countries to introduce gender recognition measures on a large scale, it was among the first to introduce gender reconstruction policies. In 1986 a Government Commission on the Role of Men was appointed, and its work had considerable influence on public opinion and on policies in the early 1990s. The role of men as *fathers* was particularly debated, focusing not only on fathers' duties, but also on their *rights* to be with, and to care for, their children. As a result of the commission's work a father's quota, i.e. part of the parental leave reserved for the father, was introduced in 1993. Norway was the first country to give fathers a statutory right to four weeks of paid leave from work connected to childbirth.

Sweden was close behind, introducing the same regulations in 1995, and by 1997 fathers of newly born children in all four Nordic countries had an exclusive right to paid leave for two, three or four weeks (NOSOSCO 1999).

In contrast to the former regulations, where parental leave was partly reserved for the mother and could be partly split between the parents on an optional basis, the father's quota system represents a 'forced' father care period. That is, if the father neglects to take the leave it cannot be transferred to the mother or someone else, leaving the family without the right to a full parental leave period. This mild forcing of fathers to take part in post-natal child care has proved very successful. While only a few per cent of Norwegian fathers shared parental leave with their partners earlier, almost 80 per cent use the father's quota today (Branth and Øverli 1998). According to Branth and Øverli (*ibid.*), fathers using their quota report a strengthened relationship with the new born child and a more equal sharing of child care and housework with their partner than non-users. Although one should be aware of possible selection effects, Branth and Øverli maintain that their analysis of Norwegian fathers' use of the father's quota indicates that dividing parental leave forms an important basis for increased equality between women and men in the family.

Other Nordic examples of legal measures aimed at a more equal share of paid and unpaid work among partners are restrictions of the rights to work extra long hours in the public sector. As men and fathers are the ones who have traditionally worked the longest hours, these regulations may impose upon fathers more 'family-friendly' hours, enabling them to take a greater share of child care and household duties. Otherwise, however, very few concrete measures have been introduced to alter the roles of men and fathers. Actually, at the state level, gender reconstruction policies have so far been more visible through rhetoric than actions. Moreover, when gender reconstruction policies are stated as a political objective, the aim is very often to *encourage* rather than enforce behavioural changes. This applies to most Western countries, although more so to the Netherlands and United Kingdom than to the Nordic nations. Thus the element of gender reconstruction policies has played a much more superficial role in practical politics in the former two countries than in the latter. Nevertheless, both the Dutch and the British governments have established strategies to ease the co-ordination of paid work and unpaid care for parents of small children. In the Netherlands 'The Daily Routine Committee' appointed by the Dutch government in 1996 has proposed several ways of encouraging more flexible everyday routines in the labour market and the school system. At the same time, the Working Hours Act and the Equal Treatment Act provide certain rights to flexible working hours and protection against discrimination on the basis of working hours. The aim is to increase part-time work among parents – fathers included. Unlike the Nordic policies of mildly enforcing behavioural changes among men (and employers), however, Dutch emancipation policies are mainly confined to policies and programmes to change stereotyped attitudes and perceptions in society. The measures are restricted to media programmes, advertising and brochures rather than economic incentives and pressure, and political priority is not given to concrete initiatives to reconstruct the mutual rights and duties of women and men (SZW undated).

Since the Labour government was installed in the United Kingdom in 1997, British welfare policies have shown some new signs of gender recognition and reconstruction objectives. As part of the new 'Family-Friendly Employment Policies' the government will be providing 'a package of family-friendly policies'. The package includes prohibition against the discrimination of part-time workers, and parental leave in addition to the established maternity leave. During the 1980s similar initiatives were halted as Britain blocked EC attempts to standardise protection for part-time workers and vetoed an EC parental leave directive on the sharing of parental leave between partners (Chamberlayne 1993). The new reforms signal a certain shift in the British approach to gender equality, although changing the roles of men is still not a pronounced objective of British policies (Minister for Women 1999).

Converging gender policies?

When related to the general historical process towards increased gender equality in Western societies, the three gender equality approaches described in this section correspond fairly well to the notion of the 'three stages of the gender equality process' developed by Jonung (1979; see also Skrede 1998), which describe the milestones in Nordic gender equality history. *The first stage*, where equal formal and societal rights of women and men are established to secure basic democratic and economic rights, such as the right to vote and the right to earn a living, may be seen as an historic period dominated by a gender neutral approach. *The second stage*, characterised by women gaining access to the same arenas as men in society, such as the labour market and important influential positions in the public sphere, may also to a certain degree be regarded in a gender neutral perspective. However, to reach full 'maturity', it to a large degree presupposes political measures of the gender recognition type. Finally, *the third stage*, implying full integration of women and men at all levels of the labour market and in the private sphere, i.e. women and men sharing both economic and care responsibilities of the family, may be seen as a phase dominated by a gender reconstruction approach and gender reconstructive political measures.

Throughout recent history, where, albeit at somewhat different points in time, the three approaches successively have influenced state policies in the Nordic countries, Nordic gender equality policies *and* gender equality have gradually converged. Today it appears relevant to speak of a 'Nordic model of gender equality'. Still, as has been shown earlier in this chapter, minor, though important, national differences exist. While from a welfare state perspective Denmark is often seen as somewhat different from the other Nordic countries, several feminist analyses find that Norway appears somewhat different among the Nordic gender equality 'regimes' (see also Sainsbury 1998). A striking example is the influence of a certain gender reinforcement element in the new 'pro-familism' during recent years, which has led to some very controversial changes in welfare and family policies, especially in Norway. Most striking is the introduction of the child care cash benefit with the intention of encouraging parents to spend more time caring for their children. The reform has led to a new debate of the core feminist questions concerning the policies of caring. Some feminists argue that the benefits contribute to a setback of the gender equality process because they discourage mothers of small children from taking employment. Some applaud the benefits for securing mothers the opportunity to care for children at home on a certain income (Andenæs 1998; Leira 1998; Likestillingssenteret 1998; Wærness 1998). Thus the problem of social distribution vs. gender equality has been put back on the agenda.

It seems as if the gender reinforcement approach has not had the same political impact in Sweden, Finland and Denmark as in Norway. To be sure, Finland and Denmark introduced a child care cash benefit several years before Norway. But the anticipated impact on gender equality was less dramatic than in Norway, as all Finnish and Danish parents of pre-school children have a statutory *right* to choose public child care, which is not the case for Norwegian parents (see earlier in this chapter and Chapter 7 in this book).[5] However, it should be admitted (which Chamberlayne does), that policies on caring are not always easily categorised in terms of Chamberlayne's typology. The problem may be illustrated by the question of parental leave vs. child care cash benefits. According to the typology, generous parental leave would most probably be seen as an example of gender recognition or reconstruction policies, while child care cash benefits would most likely be regarded as an example of gender reinforcement policies. Still, as a matter of fact, the two examples may very well be two names for the same phenomenon.

Whereas the *gender reinforcement* approach has generally been of little influence in the Nordic political gender equality process, it has a fairly long historical tradition in the Netherlands. According to Knijn, in the 1970s motherhood was still a very strong institution with deep ideological roots in Dutch society (Knijn 1994). Although the problems of the traditional mother role were a main target of the women's movement in the following years, the assumption that there is (or should be) a strong relationship between mother and children was never challenged. Even today, the Netherlands has a relatively gender-differentiated social policy, and the position of mothers as caregivers has been a more important gender equality issue in the Netherlands than in the Nordic countries. Accordingly, recognising the obstacles to women's participation in social arenas, and reconstructing gender relations to promote the integration of women and men in both family and public life, have been given lower priority in practical politics. During recent years, however, the increasing demand for women in the labour market has necessitated public day care expansion, and today the former notion that public day care is immoral has been replaced by a notion of day care as a means to combat the waste of women's human capital (Bussemaker 1998). Not unlike Norway in the 1980s, the Dutch government taking this new responsibility is inspired by economic, rather than emancipatory arguments (Knijn 1998). The Dutch public engagement, however, has gradually been handed over to parents and employers, and the general coverage is still low, both in numbers of places and hours per week (*ibid.*). Although the 1990s have entailed a shift in the attitudes to women as workers *and* certain policy changes, the gender reinforcement elements remain substantial in Dutch policies. In relation to Chamberlayne's typology, today's Dutch gender equality approach is mainly gender reinforcement with certain gender recognition elements. To be sure, official statements call attention to the importance of attitudinal and structural changes to ensure equal shares of rights and duties between women and men (see earlier in this chapter). However, as few active steps have been taken to change the role of men, gender reconstruction elements play a very minor role. As Knijn (1998) sees it, the role of fathers is not *really* taken up for discussion in Dutch politics.

Among Chamberlayne's categories, the one best suited to characterise the gender impact of British state policies is the *gender neutral approach*. This approach appears to have been fairly persistent during recent history and, despite several changes of governments, is based predominantly on a liberal reformist political approach to gender equality. Chamberlayne argues, however, that there have been signs of gender recognition within labour market policies in the United Kingdom during recent decades, and a certain movement towards gender reinforcement during the Thatcher years. During the early 1990s some gender recognition initiatives were taken by employers, including introducing workplace nurseries and children's holiday schemes. Until the late 1990s, however, when the 'Package of family-friendly policies' was introduced, such initiatives were not followed up by state policies. But the gender recognition elements of the new family policies remain dubious, and the impact on gender equality uncertain. For instance, the state funding for free nursery education for 4-year-olds in 1997 (and 3-year-olds in 2002) (Minister for Women 1999) was introduced mainly for pedagogical purposes. As the school hours of small children are usually short, this reform may contribute to a more gender equal sharing of paid and unpaid work only if supplemented by additional arrangements.

Compared to the United Kingdom and the Netherlands, the similarities of the gender equality process among the Nordic countries are striking. While during the last two or three decades the United Kingdom and the Netherlands may be characterised more or less by *one* predominant gender policy approach, the nature of Nordic gender equality policies is of changing approaches. Another Nordic similarity which distinguishes the Nordic 'gender equality model' from those of the Netherlands and the United Kingdom is the role of the state. The Nordic shifts of gender equality approaches have predominantly been carried through as a consequence of state involvement, either initiated or supported by political and administrative bodies. In the Netherlands and the United Kingdom radical gender equality initiatives have to a larger degree been confined to local or organisational levels without state support.

Summing up so far, there are certain signs that approaches to gender equality within the countries discussed have converged towards stronger elements of gender recognition and gender reconstruction policies. This is the case among the Nordic countries during the last two or three decades, and to some extent among all the countries during the 1990s. But the differences are still significant. Today there are three main dividing lines: between the Nordic countries characterised by a relatively strong weft of gender recognition and gender reconstruction policies, the Netherlands still characterised by a stronger element of gender reinforcement policies than the other countries, and the United Kingdom mainly characterised by a gender neutral policy approach.

Gender equality in the 1990s: women's access and integration in public arenas

In the following I shall discuss some of the implications of differences in gender-related policies by confronting the framework of national variations in gender equality approaches with recent statistics. Ideally, a comparative analysis of women's relative position in society should take into consideration both the 'contributory' and the 'remunerative' sides of life, i.e. both the extent to which women participate in various social arenas *and* the outcome in the form of salaries, benefits, services, influence, etc. Here, the focus is on employment and political participation, so the discussion will mainly concentrate on 'contributory' aspects. Although far from being a complete gender equality status report, I believe that a statistical overview of women's positions in public arenas may serve as a fruitful illustration of national variations in gender policies and processes. 'Remunerative' aspects in turn are examined in more detail in Chapter 5.

Labour market participation

The different labour market participation profiles of the Nordic countries as compared to the Netherlands and the United Kingdom (Table 4.1) should of course to some degree be related to different national economic developments. The same is true regarding differences *among* the Nordic countries. As mentioned earlier, recent Nordic history covers important cultural variations. Economic and industrial variations have also been significant, as economic slowdowns and upswings have not occurred at the same time in the four countries. Norway, for instance, experienced less unemployment than the other Nordic countries during the 1990s. In all the Nordic countries, however, despite different timing and dimensioning, the evolution of the welfare state has been of significant importance to female employment. Finland represents somewhat of an exception to this rule, as many Finnish women were integrated into the labour market before the

Table 4.1 Labour force participation rates for women and men, and women to men ratio. Population 15–64 years: 1980 (1981), 1986, 1990 and 1998 (1997). Population 25–49 years: 1986, 1990 and 1997, per cent

		Population 15–64 years			*Population 25–49 years*		
		Women	*Men*	*Ratio*	*Women*	*Men*	*Ratio*
Denmark	1981	72	88	82	–	–	–
	1986	77	88	88	88	94	94
	1990	79	90	88	89	95	94
	1998[a]	75	85	88	84	93	90
Finland	1980	70	83	84	–	–	–
	1986	74	82	90	88	94	94
	1990	73	81	90	87	94	93
	1998[a]	70	77	91	85	91	93
Norway	1980	62	88	70	–	–	–
	1986	71	87	82	79	95	83
	1990	71	85	84	80	93	86
	1998[a]	76	86	88	82	92	89
Sweden	1980	74	88	84	–	–	–
	1986	78	84	93	90	95	95
	1990	80	85	94	91	95	96
	1998[a]	73	78	94	86	91	95
Netherlands	1980	36	79	46	–	–	–
	1986	41	75	55	56[b]	95[b]	59[b]
	1990	53	80	66	61	95	64
	1997	62	83	75	73	94	78
UK	1980	58	91	64	–	–	–
	1986	61	88	69	69	96	72
	1990	66	86	77	74	96	77
	1998[a]	67	83	81	76	93	82

Sources: Population 15–64 years: OECD Labour Force Statistics; Population 25–49 years: Eurostat Yearbook 1997 and 1998/99.

Notes:

a 1997–figures for age groups 25–49 years (Norway: 1996)

b 1987

Note that due to different sources, total and age-specific rates are not directly comparable.

development of the welfare state. This was mainly due to prevailing general economic hardship and low wages, making it necessary for both women and men to contribute to family maintenance. Thus the distinct 'housewife' phase between the agrarian and post-industrial society which characterised the other Nordic and most other Western countries was less pronounced in Finland (Melkas and Anker 1998).

Through the expansion of public health services and care services for children and the aged, considerable parts of women's traditional work at home has been monetised. This development has been more comprehensive in the Nordic area than in most other European countries. The process, which Hernes has called 'reproduction going public' (Hernes 1987a), was pioneered by Sweden and Denmark, which were the first countries to expand public day care for pre-school children and public services for the elderly (see earlier this chapter and Chapter 7), recruiting almost exclusively women to the new jobs. By the early 1980s, more than half of employed Swedish and Danish women were working in the public sector (Table 4.2). The lower proportion in Finland and Norway at the time illustrates on one hand the long tradition of female employment in the private sector in Finland, and on the other hand the somewhat delayed public expansion in Norway as compared to the other Nordic countries.

By the mid-1980s all the Nordic countries had high female activity rates, Sweden at the top (Table 4.1). The ratio of women to men was highest in Sweden and Finland, and this persisted throughout the 1990s. Due to the economic recession the activity *rate,* however, decreased for both Swedish and Finnish women and men, leaving Norway at the top in 1998. The Swedish and Finnish economic recessions during the 1990s had significant effects on welfare expenditure. One result was decreased labour demand in the public sector. In Norway and Denmark, however, public employment continued to increase (Table 4.2).

The Netherlands has had clearly the strongest female labour force participation increase since 1980. From a level corresponding to approximately half of the Nordic level and half of the level of Dutch men by the mid-1980s, the difference in activity rate between Dutch and Nordic women has been reduced to approximately 10 per cent within a period of 10–15 years, and to approximately three-quarters of the level of Dutch men. The increase among British women has been more moderate. But the women to men ratio has still risen, and by 1998 the British ratio was close to the Danish and Norwegian ratios (Table 4.1). However, the British and Dutch female activity increase has been less attached to welfare state development than in

Table 4.2 Public sector employment among women and men, and women to men ratio in 1980, 1991 and 1998, per cent

	1980			*1991*			*1998*		
	Women	*Men*	*Ratio*	*Women*	*Men*	*Ratio*	*Women*	*Men*	*Ratio*
Denmark	54[a]	20[a]	270	50	24	208	53	26	204
Finland	41[b]	24[b]	171	45	26	173	41	18	228
Norway	37	19	195	43	22	195	46	21	219
Sweden	55	25	220	57	25	228	50	17	294
Netherlands	–	–	–	23	20	115	–	–	–
UK	–	–	–	21	14	150	–	–	–

Sources: Gornick and Jacobs 1997; Nordic Council of Ministers 1994 and 1999.
Notes: a 1981; b 1985

the case of the Nordic countries. Due to a lack of comparable gender statistics on public employment in the 1980s and late 1990s, we cannot draw very strong conclusions on this issue. The numbers presented in Table 4.2, however, show that despite women being more often publicly employed than men in the Netherlands and the United Kingdom, the public sector plays a significantly less important role as employer, and as employer of women, in these countries than in the Nordic countries. The role of the Dutch and British welfare states has accordingly been significantly less important in the process of increasing female employment. An extensive public sector is, however, no prerequisite for a certain female employment level. Quite differently from the situation in the Nordic countries, broad comparative studies of other Western countries show only a modest relationship between the size of the public sector and women's share of total employment (Gornick and Jacobs 1997). Unlike the Nordic countries, the employment increase of Dutch and British women is mainly due to increased labour demand in the private sector.

Employment and policies

Along with welfare states being unequally important as an employer of women, welfare policies and arrangements in various countries constitute different terms for women's labour market participation. As Esping-Andersen argues, some countries exhibit high women's employment rates by pulling women into the labour market, while other countries with minimalist welfare states tend, at least to some extent, to push women into employment by restricting income options outside paid work (cited in Gornick and Jacobs 1997: 24). One characteristic of recognition and reconstruction policies is the arranging for mothers (and fathers) of dependent children to participate in paid labour without having to sacrifice their role as mothers (fathers) and carers. During recent decades child care and care leave arrangements have gradually relieved Nordic women of having to choose between children and work, and have made motherhood compatible with a work career. Quite uniquely, therefore, the female employment increase of the 1980s was accompanied by a strong fertility increase in all the Nordic countries, while in the Netherlands and the United Kingdom it was accompanied by stable and decreased fertility. However, the more or less universal fertility decrease in the Nordic countries (as well as in the Netherlands and the UK) during the 1990s should warn against interpreting the relationship between policies and fertility as unambiguous. In Norway, expanding parental services and benefits did

Table 4.3 Part-time employment among women and men, and women to men ratio in 1983, 1990 and 1998, per cent

		1983[a]			*1990*			*1998*	
	Women	*Men*	*Ratio*	*Women*	*Men*	*Ratio*	*Women*	*Men*	*Ratio*
Denmark	37	7	529	30	10	300	25	10	250
Finland	11	3	367	11	5	220	13	7	186
Norway	–	–	–	39	7	557	36	8	450
Sweden	30	5	600	25	5	500	22	6	367
Netherlands	45	6	750	53	13	408	55	12	458
UK	40	3	1333	39	5	780	41	8	513

Source: OECD Labour Force Statistics.

Notes:

Part-time employment refers to persons who usually work less than 30 hours per week in their main job.

a Finland: 1980, Sweden: 1987.

not prevent a slight fertility decline. The relation between economic slowdown and declining fertility is noticeable in Sweden, which experienced by far the strongest fertility decline of the six countries during the 1990s. According to Hoem (SOU 2000), the Swedish fertility decline has mainly occurred among low educated and non- and unemployed women. This indicates increasing uncertainty concerning the possibilities of combining motherhood and a work career, especially among the least privileged.

The impact of policies on the increase in mothers' employment is less ambiguous. Because Sweden, Finland and Denmark were very early to make arrangements for combining employment with child care, female activity rates during the childbearing years were already high in the 1980s; by the mid-1980s women's labour market participation was almost as high as men's in the 25–49 year age group (Table 4.1). The equality of Swedish and Finnish gender ratios among the '25–49s' remained stable throughout the general employment decline of the 1990s. In Denmark, however, the activity rate declined more strongly among women. Notwithstanding some inter-country variations, these changing (or rather *lack of* changing) activity figures underline the well-established position of Nordic women in the labour market. Despite periods of economic slowdown and general employment backlash, women have stayed in the labour force even during childbearing and child caring phases.

Norway's role as a latecomer among the Nordic countries applies particularly to women of childbearing age. However, the expansion of child care and leave arrangements made it possible for mothers of small children to keep pace with the general female employment increase of the 1990s. The somewhat stronger British and much stronger Dutch activity increases among women in this age range are not so easily explained by welfare and gender equality policies. To be sure, child care services have increased in these countries too. But as the public child care increase has not been targeted towards improving gender equality, the arrangements are often incompatible with employment of both parents (see earlier in this chapter). Thus the British and Dutch female employment increase has been made possible mainly by means of private and individual child care arrangements, *and* by part-time employment. Whereas female part-time work has been decreasing in the Nordic countries during the last two decades, it has remained at a high level or increased in the United Kingdom and the Netherlands (Table 4.3).[6] Thus directing their political efforts towards increased part-time work has been successful in these countries, especially in the Netherlands. The Nordic countries, on the other hand, have encouraged full-time work of both women and men. The reduction of part-time work during the 1990s was however caused by somewhat different labour market processes. Whereas in Norway the decreased part-time proportion was mainly a result of more and more women and mothers taking full-time employment, in Denmark and Sweden it was largely a consequence of a reduced employment rate among women and mothers formerly part-time employed. There are also national variations distorting the universal picture of women being by far the main 'part-timers'. In Finland and Denmark the women to men ratio indicates somewhat less gender-segregated working time 'regimes' than in the other countries. The declining women to men ratio in all the countries since the early 1980s does, however, reveal a long-term trend towards generally less gender-segregated time regimes. In the Netherlands the slightly increasing time segregation among the employed during the 1990s was caused by formerly non-economically active women taking part-time work. Thus the increased registered time segregation actually reflects a general reduction of gendered time use in the Netherlands, too. Since 1990, however, little effect can be seen from the political encouragement of male part-time work in that country.

Women's labour force participation and working hours, measured in absolute terms and relative to men during the last two decades, reveal a clear converging trend among the six countries. This is mainly a result of those formerly characterised by low female labour market participation catching up with the pioneering countries. The former category includes the Netherlands and to a certain degree the United Kingdom and Norway. The latter category includes Sweden, Denmark and Finland. The fact that Norwegian mothers caught up with the other Nordic mothers during the 1990s is usually interpreted as a consequence of Norway's somewhat delayed adoption and implementation of the 'Nordic model' of welfare and gender equality policies. The line of thought was that 'politics matter'. But it is important to bear in mind that, with the partial exception of Sweden and Denmark, in all the countries discussed here the onset of the female employment increase came before second wave feminism had gained a proper foothold, *and* before the advancement of gender equality policies. Thus one should be cautious in giving politics *all* the 'credit'.

At the same time, the fact that women of childbearing age in the Netherlands – where approaches to gender equality have traditionally been quite different from Nordic policies – are rapidly catching up is poorly explained by a single, exclusive policy approach. The same 'problem' applies to the United Kingdom. The differences in employment patterns and development between Norway and the United Kingdom are actually much smaller than should be expected from the different gender equality approaches of the two countries. As a matter of fact, in general, female employment seems to have increased rather independently of national welfare and gender equality policies. This also applies to women with pre-school children. However, there is reason to believe that policies *do* matter in terms of the ways women and men are able to combine and practise their roles as parents and workers. One question is whether absence of gender recognition and gender reconstruction measures – and thereby neglect of society's and fathers' share of the caring responsibilities – may lead to female employment increase at the expense of children being born. Such an effect might be increasing inequality among women – between women choosing not to have children to pursue a work career, and mothers mainly preoccupied by family care at home. In the long run the former might end up outnumbering the latter (Lappegård 1998, 1999).

Labour market segregation

Different policy approaches most probably also have different effects on the way women are integrated in national labour markets. The vast female majority in public sector jobs in the Nordic countries (Table 4.2) illustrates this argument, as Nordic welfare state development has largely been based upon the monetising of women's traditionally unpaid work. To some degree one may say that the more comprehensive the welfare state, the stronger the female majority in the public sector. Whereas the gender composition in the public sector is almost even in the Netherlands and the United Kingdom, the proportion of publicly employed women is approximately twice that of men in the Nordic countries.

Comparing gendered occupational structures between countries is a difficult task, and the information on the subject is not always easily interpreted. In a large international study mainly based on census data, Anker and Melkas (Anker 1998; Melkas and Anker 1998) analysed occupational sex segregation in a great number of countries during the period 1970–90. They found that the level of segregation by sex is on the average higher in the Nordic nations than in the other OECD countries. This is mainly explained by the greater extent to which Nordic women work in 'female' occupations, i.e. in occupations where at least 80 per cent of workers are women. Again, Norway represents a certain deviation from the Nordic pattern. With approximately one-third of women in these occupations, Norway resembles the Netherlands more than Sweden and Finland. Out of the six countries, however, the United Kingdom differs the most, as only 14 per cent of British women are employed in female-dominated occupations. On the other hand, the typical male-dominated occupations are somewhat more gender-integrated in the Nordic nations than in most other OECD countries, including the Netherlands and the United Kingdom. Whereas Melkas and Anker reveal relatively small differences among the Nordic countries, such differences appear somewhat more significant in a recent analysis by Nermo (1999), who concludes that the overall association between occupation and sex is stronger in Finland, Norway and the United Kingdom than in Sweden (also in Spain, the United States and Austria). At a general level, however, he finds that the size and characteristics of the service sector in the analysed countries are important in explaining national variations in sex segregation. According to Nermo, the Nordic female employment increase caused by the demands of a large public sector has had less positive effects on gender equality in terms of integration than the market-driven female employment increase in countries like the United Kingdom and the United States (*ibid.*). It may be seen as a Nordic paradox that welfare state policies, involving a broad recruitment of women to public sector service jobs, most probably contribute to gender-segregated job structures, whereas one main objective of gender equality policies is to integrate women and men on equal terms in the labour market.

It might, however, be argued that a high percentage of women in female-dominated occupations does not necessarily represent a disadvantage to women as long as 'male' and 'female' occupations are similar in terms of pay, status and promotion possibilities. Accordingly, as pay differentials are relatively low in the Nordic countries (see Chapter 5), one might argue that the Nordic sex-segregated labour market does not represent an important impediment to gender equality. In addition, for the time being the Nordic situation offers women a relatively large segment of the labour market with little or no competition from male workers (Melkas and Anker 1998). Moreover, the fact that a large number of these jobs are public sector jobs also implies in practice a certain protection in periods of labour market slowdown and unemployment. In any case, whether or not the Nordic version of horizontal occupational segregation actually tends to hamper the process towards gender equality, the above analyses show that in this field the Nordic gender recognition policies of the 1980s and early 1990s brought few visible results. To be sure, the analyses conclude that occupational segregation by sex has fallen over the past two decades in the Nordic countries. But the same is true in the United States, Canada and most of Western Europe, including the United Kingdom and to a lesser extent the Netherlands. Even though the authors conclude that government-supported facilitating policies have probably contributed to decreased gender segregation in the Nordic countries, their findings give no reason to conclude that Nordic policies have had greater effects than those in, for instance, the United Kingdom. Thus (with Sweden as a possible exception) the Nordic gender recognition policy tradition of seeking to control certain labour market segregating processes has not proved more successful than traditional non-interference or, at the most, the persuasive policies of the United Kingdom, for example.

Gendered social hierarchies

Similarly, the effects of various policies and policy approaches concerning *vertical* gender segregation appear rather ambiguous. Nordic gender recognition policies, including affirmative action, quota systems and positive discrimination of women in influential public positions, would lead one to expect a high proportion of women in leading positions as compared to most other countries. Gender reconstruction policies aimed at easing women's care burden should have similar effects. In addition, the fairly long female employment tradition should make Nordic women more inclined to seek and get higher level jobs than women in other countries. In any case the latter should imply a relatively good basis for recruitment of women, simply because the number of employed women almost equals the number of employed men in these countries.

Table 4.4 presents a scattered picture of national variations of gender hierarchies in the labour market and political system. The five occupational groups presented are presumed to represent relatively high status occupations in each country, based on educational level, earnings and relative authority. Table 4.4 reveals no unique 'Nordic model' of labour market segmentation. Finland has the highest female proportion of employers and own account workers, Britain, Sweden and Norway the lowest. Sweden has the highest female proportion among managerial administration workers and teachers in tertiary education, Denmark and the Netherlands the lowest. Comparable figures on managers and managing directors in private sector businesses do not exist for all the countries considered here. The very low proportion of female managing directors in the largest private enterprises of the

Table 4.4 Female proportion in influential positions in early to mid-1990s, per cent

	Employers and own account workers 1995	*Admin. and managerial workers 1995*	*Teachers in tertiary education 1995*	*Managers in private sector 1990*	*Managing directors in 100 largest enterprises 1992/1993*	*Parliament 1995*	*Government ministerial positions 1995*	*Municipal Councils 1994/1995*
Denmark	29	19	30	–	0	33	30	26
Finland	38[a]	21	36[c]	25	2	33	39	30
Norway	27	31	33	17	0	39	41	33
Sweden	26	40	47	–	2	40	50	34
Netherlands	30[b]	23	24[d]	13	–	31	26	22
UK	25[a]	32[a]	30	–	–	9	9	–

Sources: Economic Commission for Europe 1995; Nordic Council of Ministers 1994; Eurostat 1995; Statistics Norway 1998b; Anker 1998.

Notes:

a 1994
b 1990
c 1992/93
d 1993/94

Nordic countries does, however, reveal a severe shortcoming of Nordic gender equality polices in this area. Accordingly, among the many challenges to gender equality policies, the corridors of labour market power seem to be the most difficult to change. This applies of course to most countries. Still, the Nordic situation is particularly striking in the sense that these countries have for many years practised radical political measures to alter the male-dominant recruitment and career structures of the labour market. But gender recognition policies have had somewhat greater impact on Nordic women's career prospects in the public than private sector. Although still strongly underrepresented among public sector leaders, women increased their proportion considerably during the late 1980s and 1990s, albeit more at lower management levels (Kjeldstad and Lyngstad 1993; Statistics Sweden 1997; Veikkola 1999).

The Nordic gender recognition policies have proved far more successful in the political system. Although measures and practices have not been identical, in all the Nordic countries during the 1980s and 1990s there was an active engagement, both at state and grass-roots levels, to boost the nominations, elections and appointments of women. Grass-roots mobilisation during the 1970s initiated a more or less steady increase in female Nordic members of parliament. But it was not until a decade or so later that women became integrated into political leadership (Nordic Council of Ministers 1994, 1999; Raaum 1995, 1999). The relatively successful integration of Nordic women in top political positions owes much to the systematic implementation of gender recognition measures in party organisations and political bodies at all levels. Denmark, however, deviates from the other Nordic countries in this area, having only to a limited degree practised institutional integration strategies (Christensen 1999). The difference in the female proportions in government and municipal positions in Denmark compared to Sweden, Finland and Norway (Table 4.4) should therefore most probably be interpreted as an effect of differences in imposing gender recognition practices in political life. The same argument goes for the even lower Dutch and British female proportions, although quantitative targets formulated by the Dutch government contributed to a certain increase of women ministers during the 1990s (SZW undated). At the same time, in the United Kingdom the Labour party landslide and new cabinet of 1997 more than doubled the female parliament and cabinet proportions at a stroke to respectively 28 and 23 per cent in 1998 (Minister for Women 1999). This change, however, is largely a reflection of party specific priorities, and there is no guarantee that British women's newly won political influence is the beginning of a lasting or expanding process. This is of course in accordance with a predominantly gender neutral policy tradition at national level. In comparison, the Nordic political tradition renders a stronger injunction to avoid regression of the process. As part of this tradition all Nordic political parties, with a few exceptions, have adopted the objective of approximately even sex distribution of political positions.

Conclusion

From the commencement of second wave feminism some decades ago and until today, there has been, albeit slight and uneven, a gradually converging process of gender policies and gender equality among the six countries compared in this chapter. This process has been longer and more extensive among the Nordic group of countries. During the 1990s, however, certain general converging trends appeared, which included the Netherlands and the United Kingdom. The most striking example at the behavioural level is the increasing labour market participation and integration of women. At the political level one of the most important characteristics is the growing tendency to recognise a certain public responsibility for the care of small children. Even though the political processes in some countries have often preceded new social adjustment processes, this has far from always been the case. In some countries, and in some periods, the gender equality process has developed in spite of absent gender-sensitive policies. In such cases policies have usually followed within a relatively short time period. The impact of policies varies, however, depending on which aspect and which area of gender equality is studied. Whereas the rise of women's employment appears largely to have evolved independently of deliberate gender equality measures, the integration of women on equal terms with men in the labour market as well as in politics seems to presuppose certain policy measures at state and institutional level. This is particularly true concerning the integration of women during child caring phases. As shown in this chapter, however, Nordic experiences from implementing such policy measures have not always proved successful.

The question of whether the notion of a 'Nordic model' is fruitful in a comparative analysis of the gender equality process is answered positively in this article. This is mainly based on the fact that the Nordic countries in general have had a longer and stronger tradition of institutional arrangements for the integration of women in politics and the labour market. This does not mean that I disagree with analysts who draw attention to important differences in gender equality policies and development between the Nordic countries. Compared to most other countries, including the Netherlands and the United Kingdom, however, the similarities between the Nordic countries appear more important than the differences.

Notes

1 Many thanks to Jane Millar, Prue Chamberlayne, Saskia Keuzenkamp and Joyce Outshoorn for welcoming me so kindly during my trip to England and the Netherlands in April 1999, and discussing with me the very first outline of this chapter. They gave me lots of ideas and information. The final result is, however, my responsibility alone.

2 The UN Human Development Report publishes two gender equality indexes showing the inequalities in achievement between women and men of the world. One of these (the Gender Disparity Index) measures the gender disparity in life expectancy, literacy, education and income, and the other (the Gender Empowerment Measure) measures gender differences in participation in economic and political life. The first measure ranks Norway, Sweden, Finland and Denmark as numbers 2, 3, 5 and 10, respectively, and Britain and Netherlands as 11 and 12, while the other measure ranks the four Nordic countries among the top five, and Netherlands and Britain as ninth and twentieth, respectively (1998).

3 The quote is roughly written out from memory of my discussion with Joyce Outshoorn, April 1999.

4 The struggle for reproductive rights, particularly the liberation of abortion laws, was an important part of early second wave feminism in many countries. This and other related topics will not be discussed here as they lie outside the main focus of this article.

5 For a very short period in 1994, a similar child care cash benefit was instituted in Sweden, but was eliminated in 1995 on the grounds that the scheme was a threat to publicly-funded day care.

6 The part-time rate has actually been fairly stable in Finland, albeit at a very low level. Norwegian data from early 1980s are not internationally comparable, although separate Norwegian analyses show a slow decline of female part-time work during the 1980s (Kjeldstad and Lyngstad 1993).

5 Gender equality in earnings at work and at home

Annemette Sørensen

Introduction[1]

One of the defining characteristics of gender relations in modern society is that women earn clearly less money than men on average, and most earn less than the man they live with. This economic dependence of women on men has been seen as the major bulwark of systems of gender inequality (Chafetz 1990), and as a central mechanism by which women's subordinate position in society is maintained. Economic dependence on men is an important means of support for the majority of women, but it entails a lack of control, a lack of rights and a sense of obligation (Lister 1990). By contrast, income from earnings brings not just money but control, independence and self-esteem. During the twentieth century, women's labour force participation increased, entry barriers to occupations were lowered and wages improved (Reskin and Padavic 1994). The sexual division of labour has changed, and a convergence of women's life course towards men's has been observed in all the rich industrialised countries, although to varying degrees. The Nordic countries of Denmark, Finland, Norway and Sweden, enjoy the reputation of having approached gender equality much more closely than the three other countries discussed in this chapter, namely Germany, the Netherlands and the United Kingdom. There is good evidence that this is indeed the case with respect to labour force participation and wages (Blau and Kahn 1992; Asplund *et al.* 1996; Blossfeld and Hakim 1997; see also Chapter 4). However, it is less clear how distinct the Nordic countries are from the other three in terms of gender earnings inequality, which is the focus of this chapter.

As women's life course has become more like men's, gender inequality in earnings has narrowed and gender relations have changed. Many women have gained financial independence, and men are less likely to shoulder the responsibility of being the sole supporter of the family.

Such changes have been celebrated by feminists as emancipatory and liberating for both women and men, and as strengthening the foundation for true love between partners. Other commentators have taken them to mean that marriage (or partnerships) stand to be undermined; women will lose interest in marriage because they can support themselves, and both men and women will be more likely to leave unsatisfactory marriages. This independence thesis finds proponents both in sociology (from Parsons 1949 onwards) and economics (Becker 1981). Central to this argument is that as women become more economically independent of men, the gain to marriage is reduced for both sexes. The complementarity and interdependence that exist in partnerships where one spouse specialises in market production and the other in domestic activities dissolves if both spouses are employed full time and share housework (Becker 1981).

This view has been challenged by Oppenheimer (1997), among others, who suggests that while women's earnings provide financial independence, they also raise the family income and the standard of living. An increase in both spouses' gain to marriage is thereby possible. As more married women make substantial contributions to family income, men may become more interested in marriage because they are no longer expected to be the sole provider for the family and because they have an opportunity to share in their wife's earnings. It has been shown, for example, that in countries where married women are not heavily penalised in the labour market, highly educated women are more likely to marry than those with less education (Blossfeld 1995; Oppenheimer and Lew 1995). Men also become more dependent on women's earnings for maintaining a satisfactory standard of living and they share more equally in the financial risks associated with a loss of one income due to a breakdown of the marriage. This suggests that as a society moves towards more earnings equality between spouses, both husband and wife will have some financial independence, yet at the same time remain quite dependent on each other. Independence for women may then *not* undermine interdependence between spouses, but rather strengthen it. In this chapter, I show that gender equality in earnings between spouses does in fact increase men's dependence on their partner's income, and that more equality in earnings means more equal sharing of the economic risks associated with divorce.

An increase in women's earnings will of itself reduce gender inequality in earnings, unless men's earnings increase at the same rate. However, the equalising process might be accelerated if men saw this as an opportunity for working less and making less money, and instead taking more responsibility for the domestic sphere. If this were the case, we might see men less likely to have very high earnings and women more so, and there may be an increase in the proportion of couples contributing fairly equally to family income. Another possible outcome of women's greater earnings is a *qualitative* change in the sexual division of labour. If more men took on a greater share of domestic responsibilities so that both parents were about as likely to take primary responsibility for children and family and to be the secondary earner, men would become equally likely to have low earnings and be financially dependent on their spouse. Under this scenario there would also be more earnings equality between men and women, but it would be equality only on the aggregate level; on average, men and women would earn about the same, but inequality between spouses would be fairly large with one dependent on the other for financial support. The difference between this scenario and the more familiar situation is that economic dependence in marriage would be unrelated to gender; men would be as likely as women to earn less than their spouse. It remains an empirical question whether the increase in women's earnings, in addition to reducing the gender gap in earnings, has also resulted in the more fundamental shifts in gender relations that these two scenarios depict.

In this chapter I examine how far Denmark, Finland, Norway and Sweden have achieved gender equality in earnings. I contrast these Nordic countries with Germany, the Netherlands and the United Kingdom in the mid-1990s, and include some comparisons with the situation in the 1980s. While all these countries have experienced the same general changes in women's roles and positions, when these began and how fast they have progressed vary greatly. There is every reason to expect substantial country differences at the end of the twentieth century, and that the four Nordic countries as a group have moved closer to realising the political goals of gender equality in the labour market and a lessening of women's economic dependence on men. The reason for examining change between the 1980s and the 1990s is to see if there are indications that the non-Nordic countries have caught up with the others, either because the Nordic countries have reached a saturation point or because there has been a backlash there, especially in Sweden and Finland, due to the economic depression of the early 1990s.

There are three parts to the empirical analysis. The first is an examination of the gender differences in earnings for adults aged between 18 and 60. The second part concerns women's economic dependence on the men they live with and how much having small children increases that dependence. The third part of the analysis takes up the question of how more equality between spouses affects their dependence on each other and the inequality of economic risks.

Data and measures

The Luxembourg Income Study (*http://www.lis.ceps.lu*) provides data for all seven countries. Most of these analyses are based on data from the late 1980s and early to mid-1990s, depending on availability. The LIS data are relatively well suited to the study of gender equality in earnings because each survey provides information on individual earnings for all adult household members, as well as relatively good data on total household income and transfer income. Earnings are defined as a person's income from salary, wages or self-employment. Self-employment income is reported only at the household level. To assign self-employment income to individual members of a household, data on employment status and occupation were used to determine who in a given household was self-employed. If both the head and the spouse were self-employed, they were each assigned half of the reported self-employment income. This probably means that men's self-employment income is underestimated, resulting in a conservative estimate of the gender disparity in earnings. Pre-tax earnings were used throughout the analyses and only respondents between 18 and 60 years of age were included. This means that I am not describing gender inequalities in take-home pay or standard of living but in incomes generated from the labour market.[2]

Gender equality in earnings is measured in two ways. The gender gap in earnings is simply the ratio of women's to men's mean earnings, including individuals with no income from earnings. The other measure examines the position of men and women in the earnings distribution for those aged 18 to 60, again including those without income from earnings. The percentages of male and female earnings at different deciles in the earnings distribution provides a more sensitive measure of inequality between the sexes than the gender gap measure because it is insensitive to the overall level of earnings inequality. In the Nordic countries, earnings inequality is low compared to Germany, the Netherlands and the UK (see Chapter 2). For this reason, the gender gap in wages may emerge as considerably smaller in the Nordic countries, while measures that look at the position of men and women in the earnings distribution tend to show considerable gender differences also (Blau and Kahn 1992; Asplund *et al.* 1996).

A woman's economic dependence on her partner is measured by her contribution to the couple's income from earnings (Sørensen and McLanahan 1987). Couples are assumed to pool their earnings and share them equally. The economic dependence of the woman is then measured as the difference between the man's and woman's relative contribution to the family earnings:

$$\text{DEP} = (\text{his earnings} - \text{her earnings})/(\text{his earnings} + \text{her earnings})$$

The measure, DEP, varies between +1 and −1. If the woman is completely dependent on her partner, DEP is 1; if they contribute equally it is zero, and if he is completely dependent on her, DEP is −1. There is a direct relationship between this measure of dependence and the wife's relative contribution to the couple's earnings (REL = (1 − DEP)/2).

The measure of dependence employed here is somewhat limited because it does not take into account income from earnings-determined transfer income, the most important sources of which are unemployment insurance, disability insurance and parental leave schemes. By excluding such sources of income, I clearly underestimate earnings-related income for some people. Take the case of a Norwegian woman who takes parental leave for a year. She will have no earnings, but she will receive income from the parental leave insurance, which may be almost as high as her regular earnings. With the measure I employ here this woman will be completely dependent on her partner, which is not the case in reality. Another example is of an unemployed husband who while searching for a job receives unemployment compensation. One could argue that income from parental leave schemes or unemployment insurance is a less valued currency than earnings, but that seems difficult to defend since both are dependent on being in the labour force and thus normally having earnings. It is thus likely that the validity of my measure of income dependence is somewhat problematic because it will systematically overestimate the dependence of some people. Since the main interest here is to compare seven countries, the most important question is how the comparisons may be affected by this weakness in the dependence measure. I predict that I will somewhat overestimate women's economic dependence in the Nordic countries and thus underestimate the extent to which those societies have actually moved towards equality between partners. Women in all seven countries are more likely to have reduced earnings due to family responsibilities, but it is in the Nordic countries that the shortfalls are most likely to be made up by transfers from the government or an insurance programme. In other words, it is likely that the results presented below give a conservative picture of the true differences between the Nordic countries and the rest with respect to income equality between partners.

Based on the continuous measure of income dependency, a variable is constructed classifying people according to the level of equality in earnings between partners. The variable has five categories: respondent provides all earnings; respondent has the higher earnings; equal contribution, meaning respondent provides 40 to 60 per cent of earnings; respondent has the lower earnings; respondent has no earnings.

I use a very simple measure to gauge the extent to which men and women share the financial risks associated with a divorce and thus the degree to which men, even when earning more than their spouse, depend on their wife's earnings. Couples' gross income from earnings and transfers is compared with what the gross income would be in the absence of one partner's earnings.

The gender gap in earnings

If women and men work the same number of hours and are paid equal wages, there will be earnings equality. If women work fewer hours but are paid equal wages, there will be earnings inequality between the sexes, and if women not only work fewer hours but are paid less than men per hour, earnings inequality will be substantial. In this analysis, I am only interested in the joint outcome of labour supply and wages. The average woman's earnings is compared to the average man's. This provides a simple indicator of the degree to which there is gender equality in earnings in a society. Individuals without earnings are included in the calculations, since the interest is in forming a global picture of women's income from earnings compared to men's, not to gain insight into gender differences in wage rates, discrimination and the like.

Table 5.1 shows the ratio of women's average earnings to men's in the mid- to late 1980s and the early to mid-1990s. In the 1990s the Scandinavian countries as a group had the lowest gender gap in earnings, with ratios ranging from 0.54 in Norway to 0.72 in Finland. German and British women earned about 45 per cent of what men earned, and Dutch women 40 per cent. Clearly, there was more equality by this measure in the Nordic countries, and it resulted from relatively low gender differences in wages (Asplund *et al.* 1996) and labour supply (Blossfeld and Hakim 1997). However, despite decades of efforts to

Table 5.1 The gender gap in earnings, all women and men 18–60 years old

Country	*1980s*	*1990s*
Denmark (1987, 1992)	0.63	0.66
Finland (1987, 1995)	0.68	0.72
Norway (1986, 1995)	0.49	0.54
Sweden (1987, 1995)	0.64	0.66
Germany (1984, 1994)	0.38	0.44
Netherlands (1987, 1994)	0.31	0.40
UK (1987, 1995)	0.37[a]	0.45

Note:
a excluding income from self-employment.

achieve equality in both labour supply and wages, Nordic women continue to earn considerably less on average than men.

Compared to the 1980s, all seven countries have narrowed the gender gap in earnings. In Germany, the Netherlands and the UK the greatest changes took place, but the gender gap in these countries in the 1990s remained larger than it was in the Nordic countries in the 1980s. It is interesting to note that the sharp economic downturn in Finland and Sweden early in the 1990s does not seem to have resulted in a widening of the earnings gap between men and women.

The gender gap in earnings is a rather crude measure. Table 5.2 therefore takes another look at the gender differences in earnings by comparing the relative position of men and women in the pre-tax earnings distribution for all 18 to 60 year olds in the early to mid-1990s. Men and women without earnings are again included in the analysis, so that what we are looking at is the overall similarity or difference between men and women.

Women in all countries were more likely to have very low earnings compared to men. For example, while 17 per cent of men in Denmark had earnings at or below the second decile, 23 per cent of women did; the respective figures for the other Nordic countries are fairly similar, although in Norway the disparity is somewhat less. In Germany, almost a third of women had no earnings, compared to 12.8 per cent of men. In both the Netherlands and the UK high percentages of the sample had zero earnings. In the Netherlands 20 per cent of men and almost 40 per cent of women were in this situation in 1994. In Britain, 24 per cent of men and 38 per cent of women had no income from earnings. Overall, women in the Nordic countries were somewhat less concentrated in the lowest deciles of the earnings distribution

Table 5.2 The gender gap in earnings, and the percentage of women and men with very low and very high earnings in Denmark, Finland, Norway, Sweden, Germany, the Netherlands and the United Kingdom in the 1990s, all women and men 18–60 years old

Country		*Earnings 2nd decile*	*Earnings in 3rd, 4th and 5th decile*	*Earnings in 6th and 7th decile*	*Earnings in 9th and 10th decile*
DK 92	Men	17.0	22.9	17.5	30.8
	Women	23.0	37.3	22.5	9.0
FIN 95	Men	18.7	26.8	15.3	28.5
	Women	21.3	33.3	24.7	11.4
N 95	Men	13.7	21.9	18.1	33.0
	Women	26.4	38.1	21.9	6.9
S 95	Men	17.8	21.9	16.7	30.7
	Women	22.2	38.3	23.2	8.9
D 94	Men	10.6% No	19.8[a]	22.9	32.5
	Women	31.5% earnings	38.1[a]	17.0	7.7
NL 94	Men	19.7% No	11.7[a]	18.7	35.2
	Women	39.8% earnings	28.4[a]	21.3	4.9
UK 95	Men	24.3% No	8.3[a]	21.2	32.4
	Women	37.7% earnings	28.0[a]	18.9	8.6

Note:
a Percentage with earnings below the median.

than in the other three countries, but were still more likely to be there than men.

If we turn our gaze to the upper part of the earnings distribution, it becomes quite clear that the Nordic countries differ little from the Netherlands, Germany and the UK in terms of women's chances of having very high earnings. The percentage of women with earnings in the 9th or 10th decile ranges from a high of 11 per cent in Finland to a low of 5 per cent in the Netherlands, with the other countries varying between 7 and 9 per cent. In contrast, it is quite common for men to have earnings this high. In the non-Nordic countries and Norway, fully one out of every three men falls into this category. The respective figure in Denmark, Finland and Sweden is about 30 per cent, which means that the *gap* between men and women's chances of being high earners is slightly lower in these three countries than in the other four. However, the overwhelming impression from the figures in Table 5.2 is that the Nordic countries do not distinguish themselves as societies where women and men have equal chances of having high earnings. This is quite remarkable given the claims of gender equality made in all the Nordic countries. While there is an element of truth in these claims, the hard fact remains that women in Denmark, Finland, Norway and Sweden are no more likely than their sisters in the other countries to have earnings that place them in the upper two deciles of the earnings distribution.[3]

Thus the achievement in the Nordic countries seems to have been to pull the majority of women out of the bottom part of the earnings distribution, both by encouraging employment and by having relatively high minimum wages. The modal category for women in all the Nordic countries is the 3rd to 5th decile, and a substantial percentage have earnings that place them above the median in the 6th to 7th decile. Compare this to the modal category for Nordic men, which is the 9th to 10th decile, and we see how far these countries are from having achieved gender equality in earnings.

The figures in Table 5.2 do show an increase between the 1980s and 1990s in the percentage of women with earnings above the lowest earnings category in all seven countries. There was also a small increase in the percentage of women with very high earnings (figures not shown). Typical of change in the high earnings category is that whereas 9 per cent of Danish women in 1992 had very high earnings, 7 per cent did so in 1987. In Sweden, the percentage increased from 8 to 9 over a seven-year period (1987 to 1995). Glacial change indeed.

Summary

This picture of gender equality in earnings shows three important things: 1) despite great increases in women's labour force participation and a narrowing of the gender gap in wages, there remained substantial inequality in earnings between the sexes towards the end of the twentieth century. 2) The Nordic countries do appear to have moved further than others in the direction of equality in earnings between the sexes. This is evident both in the smaller gender gap in earnings and in the somewhat better position of women in the earnings distribution. 3) The important achievement in Denmark, Finland, Norway and Sweden has been to provide the vast majority of women with the opportunity to have income from earnings that provide some financial independence. But the achievement is considerably more modest in terms of high earnings: Nordic women are unlikely to have very high earnings and are only marginally more likely to be high earners than women in other European countries. 4) Taken together this means that greater gender equality in earnings in the Nordic countries has been achieved because most women have some earnings, not because of a fundamental change in gender relations. We do not see evidence of large numbers of Nordic men earning modest incomes or no incomes at all. Put differently, women's economic roles have become more like men's, whereas there is little indication that men have responded to this change by reducing their earnings or labour supply.

Women's economic dependence on men

Inequality in earnings between men and women translates into inequality in earnings between men and women living together, so that many women contribute less to household income than their partners. If we assume that couples pool and share resources, this means that many women are financially dependent on their spouse (Sørensen and McLanahan 1987; Ward *et al.* 1996). As a society moves towards greater earnings equality between the sexes in the labour market, women's economic dependence should decline, although it is impossible to say by how much without knowing whether there are changes in the pattern of mate selection. The figures presented in Tables 5.3 and 5.4 show how much women depend on their spouse in each of the seven countries considered here. The results in Table 5.3 are for men and women living with a partner where at least one has income from earnings. Table 5.4 reports results for couples with at least one child under seven years of age. As discussed above, the limitation of the dependence measure to income from earnings probably means that women's economic dependence is overestimated, especially in the four Nordic countries.

It is clear that women in the four Nordic countries are far less dependent on their partner than women in the other three countries. The differences are all the more surprising given that I have probably overestimated women's economic dependence in the former (see earlier). Finnish women's average dependence is 0.15, meaning that they rely on their spouse for 15 per cent of their share of the couple's combined earnings. In Denmark, Norway and Sweden the corresponding figures are about 22 per cent. These low dependency scores are in stark contrast to what we see for the Netherlands, where married women in 1994 relied on their spouse for 53 per cent of their share of the couple's earnings. In Germany and the UK, the figures are 39 per cent and 36 per cent, respectively. Put differently, Finnish women contribute about 42 per cent of the couple's earnings, compared to only 23 per cent in the Netherlands.

There was a decline in women's economic dependence from the 1980s to the 1990s (figures not shown). This was most pronounced in

Table 5.3 Women's economic dependence on their partner, couples with income from earnings

Country and year	*Mean dependence, %*	*Woman has no earnings, %*	*Woman earns less than man, %*	*Equality in earnings[a], %*	*Woman earns more than man, %*	*Woman sole earner, %*
Denmark 1992	0.22	12.2	50.4	21.3	10.5	5.6
Finland 1995	0.15	12.1	44.5	17.6	16.7	9.1
Norway 1995	0.22	13.4	53.4	14.0	10.1	9.1
Sweden 1995	0.23	8.7	57.9	15.5	12.3	5.5
Germany 1994	0.39	33.5	39.2	9.6	6.3	11.5
Netherlands 1994	0.53	39.8	41.2	7.6	2.5	7.8
UK 1995	.36	25.8	46.3	12.5	5.0	10.3

Notes:
Dependency = (man's earnings − woman's earnings)/(couple's earnings)
a Equality in earnings is defined as each partner contributing between 40 per cent and 60 per cent to the combined earnings.

Norway, where the mean dependence for married women was almost halved in nine years. Germany also saw a substantial decline, from 0.58 in 1984 to 0.39 in 1994.[4] However, it is interesting to note that Germany, the Netherlands and the UK by the mid-1990s still had dependence scores that were higher than those for the 1980s for Denmark, Finland and Sweden.

The low economic dependence of women in the Nordic countries does not mean that the majority of couples are equal with respect to earnings, nor that a major shift in the sexual division of labour has taken place, with men as likely as women to be the dependent partner. This is clear from the results in Table 5.3, and of course consistent with the findings on gender inequality in earnings. We see in Table 5.3 that the modal category in all seven countries is the couple where the woman earns less than her partner. This group constitutes 58 per cent of all Swedish couples, half of all Danish couples, and almost half of British couples. The Nordic countries stand out in three respects from Germany, the Netherlands and the UK. First, the percentage of married women without earnings in the former is considerably lower, ranging between 9 per cent and 13 per cent, while about a third of married women in the other countries have no earnings. Second, the percentage of couples where each partner earns about the same is a little higher, and third it is a little more common for Nordic women

Table 5.4 Women's economic dependence on their partner, couples with income from earnings and at least one child under 7 years old

Country and year	*Mean dependence, %*	*Woman has no earnings, %*	*Woman earns less than man, %*	*Equality in earnings*[a]*, %*	*Woman earns more than man, %*	*Woman sole earner, %*
Denmark 1992	0.27	12.7	56.3	18.1	8.9	4.0
Finland 1995	0.36	21.2	47.9	14.5	11.6	4.8
Norway 1995	0.34	16.0	57.7	13.4	7.1	5.8
Sweden 1995	0.41	13.1	66.7	9.4	7.9	2.9
Germany 1994	0.61	50.8	34.5	3.1	3.3	8.4
Netherlands 1994	0.61	44.8	41.0	5.7	3.6	5.0
UK 1995	0.56	41.4	41.4	7.9	3.2	6.1

Notes:
As for Table 5.3.

to earn more than their spouse. In Denmark one in five couples has equality in earnings, and in 16 per cent of couples the woman has the highest earnings. In Finland equality is a little less common, but the woman has the higher earnings in one of four couples. Norway and Sweden are somewhere between the Danish and Finnish cases. In contrast, we see that equality in earnings was found among only 10 per cent of couples in Germany, 8 per cent in the Netherlands and 12 per cent in the UK.

As shown in Chapter 4, a hallmark of family and gender equality policies in the Nordic countries has been to facilitate the employment of mothers with young children. The results presented in Table 5.4 show that these policies have worked in the sense that being the mother of a pre-school child has less of an impact on her economic dependence on her spouse than is the case in the other three countries. For example, in Denmark, married women with small children are as likely to have earnings as other employed women (87.3 per cent compared to 87.8 per cent). They do earn less, and are for that reason somewhat more dependent on their spouse, but the mean economic dependence remains low at 27 per cent. In the other three Nordic countries, having a small child has a slightly stronger effect on the mother's economic dependence, largely because a higher percentage of mothers have no income from earnings as in Denmark. In Germany and Britain married mothers with small children are considerably more dependent on their spouse for support than are other married women. There is less of a difference in the Netherlands because married women without small children are also highly dependent.

The results presented in Tables 5.3 and 5.4 show that while the Nordic countries have definitely made progress in earnings equality between spouses, the typical couple remains one where he earns more than she does, and where both spouses have earnings even when there is a pre-school age child in the household. It is perhaps in this way that the Nordic countries are most distinct from the other countries considered here. Both men and women expect and are expected to be employed and to help support the family, even when the children are small. The minor variations between the Nordic countries do not detract from the fact that more equality between spouses prevails than in Germany, the Netherlands and the UK. The Nordic countries also stand out as societies where a *substantial* minority of couples exemplify less traditional gender relations. More than one in four couples is not following the traditional pattern of female dependence in marriage. Perhaps this is among the first signals of deeper social changes in the ways men and women organise their lives in the Nordic countries.

Implications of equality between partners

While gender equality in the labour market and at home has not occurred in any known society, the present results reveal that the Nordic countries have arguably come closer to achieving this than others, and most certainly more so than the three other countries considered here. Gender equality would have numerous consequences for individual men and women, and for society in general. I shall here consider the argument presented earlier that equality between spouses means not only that women would become more independent but also that men would rely more on their spouse's income, and that both would share more equally the financial risks associated with a divorce (Oppenheimer 1997). This argument is important because it questions the common assumption that financial independence for women lowers the gain to marriage and undermines interdependence between men and women living as partners.

Having income from earnings provides the individual with a measure of financial independence, even if the earnings are low. As Valerie Oppenheimer notes: 'A relatively small amount of earnings may actually provide a married woman with the ability to act independently in the sense of making a variety of consumption decisions on her own and increasing her influence in joint consumption decisions'

(Oppenheimer 1997: 444). The twentieth century was when women gained such independence. How relations between men and women are affected by this independence has been the focus of much work on the family since the 1970s, the central concern being the decline in marriage and the increase in divorce that coincided with women entering the labour force in record numbers. Some of the earlier research on the effects of women's income on marriage and divorce emphasised that women's income had both income and independence effects (e.g. Hannan and Tuma 1978). Women's income (either from earnings or welfare benefits) increases family income and also provides women with a measure of financial independence. It remains unclear how women's income will affect the stability of a marriage. Better household income tends to have a stabilising effect; on the other hand, more economic independence may provide opportunities for leaving an unsatisfactory relationship. Since then, the literature in both economics and sociology has tended to favour the independence hypothesis, so that it is now virtually taken for granted that women's economic independence lowers the gain to marriage and thus poses a threat to both marriage formation and its stability. The aggregate trends in women's contribution to family income, and in marriage and divorce are consistent with this hypothesis, but at the individual level there is a surprising lack of empirical support for it (see Oppenheimer 1997 for details).

Women's greater financial independence clearly also has implications for men, one of which is that as women earn more money, men come to depend on that income.[5] They do so even if they are not economically dependent on their spouse in the sense that I have defined it earlier. The point made so forcefully by Oppenheimer (1997) is that when women begin to earn good money, albeit less than their husband, men enjoy the benefits of that income; they come to rely on it and will experience an economic hiatus if they lose it, either because the wife leaves the marriage or loses her job. This implies that the economic consequences of divorce for men should be worse in countries with more equality between spouses (Fritzell 1990). I agree with Oppenheimer that we need to take a careful look at the degree to which growing equality between partners, although providing financial independence to both, also creates economic interdependence and a sharing of economic risks which are absent in partnerships relying exclusively on male earnings.

The figures presented in Table 5.5 show in a very simple manner how Nordic men are more dependent on their partner's income than men in the other three countries with less equality. The mean decile positions for couples in the distribution of gross household income are examined

Table 5.5 Mean decile position in the distribution of gross household income based on the couple's earnings and transfer income and the respondent's earnings and transfer income, couples with income from earnings or transfers

Country and year		*Mean decile position. Couple's earnings + transfer income*	*Mean decile position if partner's earnings were zero*	*Mean decile decline (women/men ratio)*
DK 1992	Men	6.5	4.2	2.3
	Women	6.4	2.8	3.6 (1.5)
FIN 1995	Men	5.4	3.7	1.7
	Women	5.2	2.7	2.5 (1.5)
N 1995	Men	4.8	3.4	1.4
	Women	4.6	2.1	2.6 (1.8)
S 1995	Men	7.1	4.9	2.2
	Women	6.9	3.4	3.5 (1.6)
D 1994	Men	5.6	4.1	1.5
	Women	5.5	1.8	3.7 (2.5)
NL 1994	Men	6.1	4.9	1.2
	Women	6.1	1.8	4.3 (3.6)
UK 1995	Men	5.4	4.2	1.2
	Women	5.3	2.2	3.1 (2.6)

under two conditions: 1) counting their combined earnings and transfer income; and 2) subtracting the partner's earnings from the combined earnings. This provides a very crude measure of how much the couple's financial position would alter if one income were to disappear, all else remaining constant including the need for income.[6]

In societies with more equality between partners, we should find that men risk a greater decline in economic status if they lose their partner's income than men in less egalitarian societies. And for women the opposite should be the case: the more a woman earns compared to her partner, the less the slide down the economic ladder were his income to disappear. This implies, of course, that the discrepancy between men and women's economic decline will be less, so that in egalitarian societies men, too, would be likely to suffer economic decline following the loss of their partner's earnings. These expectations are well supported by the data. The three societies with most inequality between spouses are indeed characterised by relatively small decile declines by men and much larger ones by women, following the loss of spouse's earnings. In the Netherlands, for example, men would move 1.2 deciles down on average in the household income distribution, whereas women would drop a full 4.3 deciles if they lost their husband's earnings – more than a three-fold disparity. Although women in Germany and the UK are somewhat better off than in the Netherlands, the same pattern prevails with risks about 2.5 times those of men. Women in Finland and Norway would experience on average decline of 2.5 and 2.6 deciles, respectively, if they lost their husband's earnings. Men's risk in these countries is somewhat less, reflecting their higher earnings, with respective mean declines of 1.7 and 1.4 deciles. In Denmark and Sweden gender differences are also relatively small, with women's risk about 1.5 times greater, but the average decline for both sexes is somewhat higher than in Finland and Norway. In other words, Danish and Swedish partners are somewhat more dependent on each other's earnings for maintaining current economic status than is the case in Finland and Norway. Finally, the strong economic position of women in the Nordic countries is demonstrated by the fact that their decile category in the absence of their partner's earnings is above 2 in all four countries.

Conclusions

In the analysis presented here, I have shown that in some ways the Nordic countries do indeed live up to their reputation as societies where women have achieved equality with men. To be sure, gender equality in earnings has not been achieved, but compared to the Netherlands, Germany and the United Kingdom it is quite clear that the earnings of Nordic women and men are considerably closer. It is also obvious that the similarities between the Nordic countries far outweigh the differences. But the Nordic gender gap in earnings remains non-trivial, with women's incomes about two-thirds of men's. Perhaps the most striking finding was that while Nordic women have made it out of the bottom of the earnings distribution, they have most definitely not made it into the top. Not only that, women in Germany and the UK are as likely as Nordic women to have earnings that place them in the top 20 per cent of the earnings distribution. More than a third of men in all countries earn this much.

On the home front, too, it is clear that there is more equality in the Nordic countries. Although the economic dependence of women is quite low, men still tend to have the higher earnings, although women very often earn about the same or more than their partner. Finally, it was shown that increasing domestic equality between men and women does make men more dependent on women's income, so that their risk of economic dislocation upon losing spousal income becomes closer to the risk married women have always faced. While the simple analysis presented here is clearly only a first step, I believe it indicates that improved income equality between partners provides financial independence to both men and women, along with creating economic interdependence and a sharing of economic risks that is absent in partnerships relying exclusively on male earnings.

The four Nordic countries are approaching a situation where this type of economic interdependence is a fact of life for the vast majority of couples, and where gender inequality in earnings is low compared to other societies. It is tempting, of course, to attribute the distinctiveness of the Nordic countries in this way to the raft of gender and family policies assembled over the past four decades in the context of the Nordic welfare state (see Chapter 4). The welfare state did indeed at an early stage provide a framework in which it became easier and more acceptable for women to pursue employment without having to sacrifice a family. It is also likely that developments in the welfare state which tied benefits to labour force participation played a significant role in keeping many women in employment who would otherwise have preferred staying home with small children. The Nordic social democratic welfare state substantially increased the opportunity costs of being a housewife, and thereby doubtless played an important role in the emergence of greater gender equality at home and at work. At the same time, however, it also made it more difficult for parents to choose to have one of them stay at home with small children. Finally, it is probably fair to say that the family and gender policies we find in the Nordic countries at the end of the twentieth century are as much a *result* of the changes that women's employment and earnings have brought to men and to families as they are the *cause* of the transition towards more equality between women and men.

Notes

1 I have benefited from very helpful comments from Johan Fritzell during the preparation of this chapter.

2 Earnings after tax would provide a more valid picture of how much money people bring home. Several of the surveys used here do not, however, provide sufficient information at the individual level to calculate after-tax earnings for each member of a household. Since taxation tends to redistribute income between men and women, especially in the Nordic countries (Sørensen 1992), this means that I am somewhat overestimating gender inequality in take-home pay for these countries. In other words, the results

will tend to underestimate the difference between the Nordic and the other three countries.

3 The lack of Nordic distinctiveness is even more pronounced when comparing the percentage of men and women with earnings in the 10th decile. The similarity between the seven countries is striking: about 3 per cent of women (although only 2 per cent in the Netherlands) and 17 per cent of men (but only 15 per cent in Finland) have earnings this high.

4 Some of this decline should no doubt be attributed to the unification of the two Germanies in 1990. The data for 1984 are for West Germany only.

5 This is, of course, what people mean when they claim families today need two incomes to get by.

6 In case of divorce, children are more likely to live with the mother than the father. This means that the typical father's need for income will decrease substantially, while the mother's will change little. The gender disparities in the decile decline in the equivalent gross income distribution will thus be considerably larger than those shown for the gross income distribution.

6 Changing family patterns: A challenge to social security

Aksel Hatland

Introduction

Economic redistribution between families has traditionally been one of the most important objectives of social policy throughout Western Europe. When the initial social security schemes to pursue this goal were constructed during the first two-thirds of the twentieth century, they typically drew on certain assumptions about family structures and functions. Benefit schemes, for example, were founded on a common premise that adult partners were formally married; unmarried persons were looked upon as singles, and treated as such. In terms of family functions, important assumptions were made about the division of labour within the family. What Jane Lewis (1998a) states for Britain, is largely valid for all of Western Europe: 'Policy-makers followed William Beveridge in assuming that adult men would be fully employed, that women would be primarily homemakers and carers, and that marriages would be stable.' These assumptions had important consequences for what needs were recognised in social security schemes and what indicators were used to define the different need groups.

However, rapid changes in family patterns during the last three decades have seriously challenged these assumptions. Dual earner families have become the norm and one-earner families have become atypical in most European countries. Marriage has become a more unstable institution and to regard them as lifelong unions is less valid than before. New family forms have emerged as alternatives to marriage, and homosexual and lesbian couples are now widely recognised. More people are living as singles or single parents for periods of their lives, cohabitation among heterosexual partners has become a common alternative to marriage. There are signs that an institution which was traditionally looked upon as society's foundation, is crumbling. Legal marriage has lost its monopoly as the only socially recognised sexual union in Western societies.

For many years, studies of the family and of family policy were the domain of feminist researchers. During recent years, however, interest in the field has become more widespread, and at the turn of the millennium even the most prominent male researchers of the welfare state are focusing on family issues. Esping-Andersen, who admits that he is influenced by the 'feminist critique of "mainstream" male-centred welfare state theory' (1999: 48) thus writes: 'The problems that beset the welfare state are intimately connected with the malfunctioning of labour markets and families. Both function badly because they are in the throes of revolutionary change' (*ibid.*: 1). Anthony Giddens (1999: 51) expresses a similar view: 'Among all the changes going on in the world, none is more important than those happening in our personal lives – in sexuality, relationships, marriage and the family.'

That this challenge is recognised by the political authorities in Europe is clearly expressed in the EU's 'Convergence Recommendation' (EU 1992), the aim of which is to establish common objectives as a guide for national policies. The document stresses that

> social protection systems must endeavour to adapt to the development of behaviour and of family structures where this gives rise to the emergence of new social protection needs, related in particular to changes in the labour market and demographic changes.

It is part of conventional wisdom that the Nordic countries have spearheaded these 'revolutionary changes'. In this chapter I throw light on this assumption using comparative data, and analyse how policy makers in the seven countries compared in this book have responded to these new challenges in important fields of social policy. Yet it cannot be taken for granted that the causal process goes only in one direction – from changing needs and risks to policy responses. People should also be looked upon as actors who take social rights into consideration in their family decisions. Thus there is a complex interplay between social security and family behaviour or, which may be more important for our issue, between social security and policy makers' assumptions about changing behaviour. This chapter deals with both aspects of this interplay, but the main emphasis is on 'the challenge to social security' side of the relationship.

The responses to new family forms are analysed in terms of policies aimed at the most rapidly growing family type, i.e. cohabitation, and the responses to changing family functions are analysed by studying reforms in income maintenance for adult women.

Politicians may react to family changes in many ways. But to be able to understand these reactions, we should search for certain patterns. Relying partly on Jane Millar (1998), I would like to distinguish between three types of possible response patterns:

- Conservative responses see the new family patterns as negative trends and would use social policies as means to restore traditional family patterns, especially marriage. Social security legislation should thus be used to encourage people to marry and to stay married until separated by death.
- Pragmatic responses prefer to adapt to changing family patterns and needs by piece-meal reforms of social security systems. Such an approach takes a more neutral attitude to the new family practices, and accepts a more pluralistic society.
- Radical reactions would dismantle benefits derived from family status and advance further towards an individualised social security system. In this perspective, adults should have the same benefits irrespective of family status; justification of benefits lies in a person's labour market position, not in their family position.

Using this taxonomy as my starting point, I hypothesise that we find conservative responses in Germany and, although more hesitant, also in the Netherlands. In comparative welfare state research Germany is often classified as a familialist welfare state (i.e. Esping-Andersen 1999: 86). Social security there is traditionally based on the bread-winner model and the public responsibility for supporting people in need is subsidiary to the responsibility of the family. In the Netherlands familialist tradition is found to be strong when we study social services, but less so when we study benefits in cash.

I further hypothesise that we find pragmatic responses among the Nordic countries. There, the public obligation to provide universal economic support to all citizens is traditionally strong and the assumption that it is primarily the obligation of the family to care for people in need seems to be weaker.

The United Kingdom is a more open case. Mutual obligations within families are traditionally more limited in liberal states like Britain than in Central Europe, and the dominance of market ideology strengthens the drive towards individualised social rights. On the other hand, the widespread use of means-testing to limit public expenses promotes conservative responses to needs created by new family forms.

The relevance of family status in social security

In the history of social policy in Europe one line of development has been from discretionary poor relief given to households in need to rights-based social security benefits. Today, social security benefits are generally distributed as individual rights. But many of these rights depend on the individual's family status. Before I start to discuss changes in family patterns, it may be fruitful to describe benefits that are traditionally influenced by family status, although the pattern differs from country to country. Four groups of benefits may be distinguished.

a) Income maintenance due to lack of breadwinner

In this group is found the most traditional of all social insurance benefits, namely *survivors'* pensions. In the present context widows' pensions are of greatest interest. They have developed from a family model based on lifelong marriage, where the husband was responsible for the economic well-being of the family, and the wife was treated as an economic dependant of the husband. These benefits have come under pressure during recent years. Less stable families and increased labour participation by married women have weakened their legitimacy. On the other hand new risks have emerged due to new family patterns. Here it is in the interest of cohabitants to be treated as married couples.

Income maintenance to *single parents* has traditionally been justified on similar grounds as survivors' pensions, i.e. there is no father present to provide for his family. But the needs of single mothers have been less easily recognised than widows' economic needs. A major reason for this is that their needs have been perceived as a consequence of their own behaviour, and many policy makers have feared that generous benefits to single mothers would encourage irresponsible behaviour. The schemes are largely means-tested (see below) to prevent serious poverty among single parents. For poor parents who cohabit, it is usually advantageous to be treated as singles rather than married.

b) Compensation for extra costs to support a family

Family/child benefits both redistribute money from families without children to families with children and redistribute between different family types. In many schemes one-parent families are granted higher benefits than two-parent families. When this is the case, it is to the advantage of cohabitants to be treated as singles.

In many pension schemes *spousal supplements* are granted for invalidity and to old age pensioners who are supporting a spouse not receiving their own pension. If cohabitants are treated as married couples, they will be entitled to benefits of this kind.

c) Calculation of benefits according to economies of scale

Since two persons living together do not need twice the income of a one-person household to maintain the same standard of living, pensions and other benefits are often lower for married couples than for two single beneficiaries. In schemes where this is the case, it is in the interest of cohabiting couples to be defined as singles.

d) Means testing of benefits to people in need

Many social benefits are granted only when income/wealth falls below a prescribed limit, and social assistance is the most typical benefit in this category. But the income unit used to test the recipient's means differs between schemes. Sometimes only the individual income counts, sometimes the family income, sometimes the household income. It is in the interest of cohabitants not to be treated as one income unit when they apply for benefits that are subject to family means tests.

This overview shows that in social security there is no general rule for whether it is an advantage or a disadvantage for cohabiting couples to be treated as a married couple or as two singles. The answer will differ from scheme to scheme and accordingly from one type of need to another. If policy makers want to encourage marriage through social security legislation, it is not a viable method to treat cohabitants as *either* singles *or* married couples. If this is the policy goal, the most effective way would be to give cohabitants the worst of both worlds: to treat them as singles when this is to their disadvantage and as married couples when this is to their disadvantage. Whether any of the countries in this study has chosen this way is a question to which I will return.

Changing risk patterns

A well-functioning social security system must adapt to social changes that influence needs and risks. One of the most profound changes affecting family functions during recent decades has been women's increased labour market participation. The data presented by Randi Kjeldstad in Chapter 4 (see particularly Table 4.1) confirms and elaborates this well-known phenomenon. Women's economic activity outside the home has increased. The Nordic countries have held a leading position in this field, although Norway was a laggard for many years. The decreasing rates in Finland, Sweden and Denmark during the 1990s are mainly explained by a phase of high unemployment. The incentives to register in the labour force temporarily declined. But there are no signs that Nordic women have returned to housewifery. Since 1970 the differences between the Nordic countries and Germany, the Netherlands and the United Kingdom have gradually diminished, but the rates are still lower for the three latter countries.

These changes have important consequences. Women are ever less dependent on men to support them. Marriage is no longer an economic necessity for the majority of European women, since there are alternative ways of getting an income. And for women who do marry, the economic consequences of a loss of provider may be much less dramatic than, say, thirty years ago. In other words, European women's risk patterns have changed rapidly. Yesterday the main economic risk was to lose a provider, today it is to lose a job.

Another important driving force behind changing family patterns is the new reproduction technology (contraception and abortion) that has become available during the past 30–40 years. Women today control their own reproduction to a degree that earlier generations could not dream of. One of the consequences is that they do not need marriage as a frame around sexual life and as an economic safety net in case of pregnancy.

The facts in Figures 6.1 and 6.2 confirm the widely-held impression that marriage is in retreat in Northern Europe. Fewer marry and more divorce. Although 'serial monogamy' has become more widespread, i.e. more people marry for second and third times, this does not compensate for the general trend.

Figure 6.1 shows that marriage rates since 1970 have declined in all countries studied and that there has been a tendency towards convergence, especially in the early 1970s. The figure also confirms the popular belief that the Swedes are the pioneers in rejecting marriage. It may be more surprising that marriage rates have increased somewhat in Denmark since 1980 and that Danes are more likely to marry than the other nationalities studied here.

Figure 6.2 largely mirrors Figure 6.1. During the same period (1970–97) the general trend was an increasing divorce rate in all seven countries. In this respect, too, we see a weak tendency of convergence. But it may be worth noting that the curves flattened out during the last years of the period. One of the reasons may be that when fewer marry,

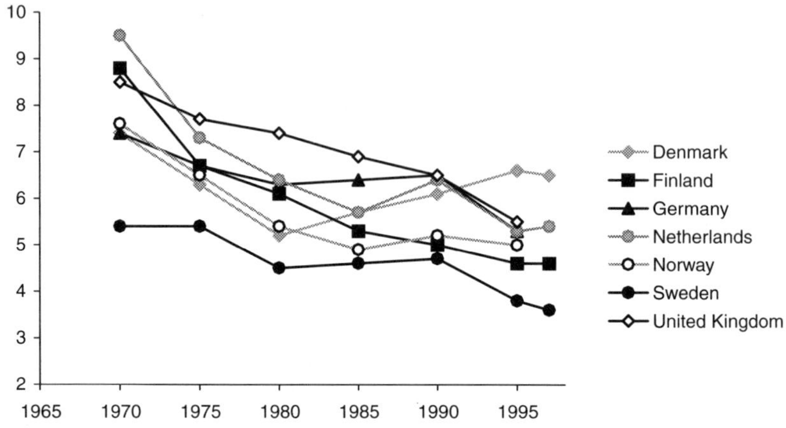

Source: Recent demographic developments in Europe 1998.
Note: Crude marriage rate refers to marriages per 1000 average population.

Figure 6.1 Crude marriage rates, 1970–97

there are necessarily fewer that can divorce. Another explanation is that the group of married people in Northern Europe today is more selective than before, and they may hold more traditional family values than those who choose to cohabit.

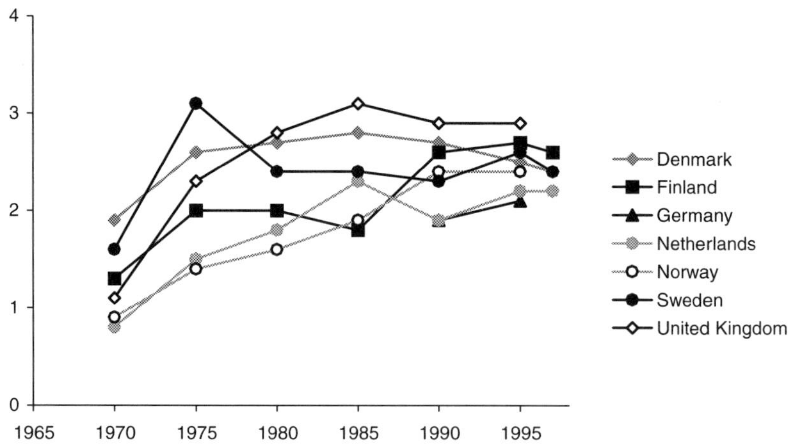

Source: Recent demographic developments in Europe 1998
Note: Crude divorce rate refers to divorces per 1000 average population.

Figure 6.2 Crude divorce rates, 1970–97

The growth in cohabitation[1]

This section discusses in more detail the growth in cohabitation. Modern cohabitation seems to have arisen throughout the Western world in the late 1960s, at a time when new lifestyles took root in many areas and traditional institutions were challenged. Studies from many countries show this. An indicator that widespread cohabitation is a relatively new phenomenon is the lack of statistical data; regularly collected comparative data on the growth and distribution of this family form do not exist. However, various sources give us a quite clear picture of the demographic tendencies. The most comprehensive effort to gather comparative data on cohabitation was by Kathleen Kiernan (1996). The data she collected from numerous sources on the development of cohabitation from the early 1970s to the late 1980s all point in the same direction: numbers of cohabitants have grown in all seven countries studied here, although at different rates. Denmark and Sweden show the highest levels of cohabitation, followed by Finland and Norway.

According to Manniche (1991) couples in *Denmark* started to opt out of marriage from the mid-1960s, instead preferring cohabitation, which was considered a deviant social behaviour at the time. By the end of the 1980s Manniche states that 'non-married cohabitation is an ancient phenomenon, but the current extent of it is new, at any rate in modern times, as is the general social acceptance of it in all social classes'. Another indicator of this trend was that in 1989 the non-marital birth rates reached 46 per cent.

As in Denmark, marriage rates in *Sweden* fell suddenly in the mid-1960s. The couples that started to cohabit at this stage did so 'mostly because they were against the social and religious institutions of marriage' (Trost 1996). 'Nowadays very few couples can be found who marry and start living together. Very few are against marriages, almost no-one actively chooses to cohabit, and no-one chooses to opt out of marriage' (*ibid.*). Trost suggests this means that people no longer *choose* to cohabit but just do it. It has become common social practice.

Compared to Denmark and Sweden, the phenomenon of cohabitation in Norway started later and developed much more slowly. The official Norwegian attitude towards living together outside marriage is illustrated by the Penal Code of 1902 (§ 379) which basically stated it was a crime to live in sexual unions without formal marriage. There was heavy opposition to the abolition of the paragraph in 1972, even though it had been a 'sleeping paragraph' for many years

(Bull 1990). By the end of the 1970s (in 1977 according to the *Family and Fertility Survey*) only 5 per cent of women in the age group 20–44 years cohabited, whereas this form of union had risen to 24 per cent in 1996 (Noack 1997). In an attempt to compare the forms of cohabitation cross-nationally, Noack suggests using number of children born to cohabiting parents. In Norway in 1996, 46 per cent of children were born out of wedlock, 39 per cent of these to cohabiting parents. In 1997, 49 per cent of children were born outside marriage in Norway (Statistics Norway 1998a).

In *Finland,* cohabiting couples constituted 2 per cent of all family unions (including single parent family units) in 1970. The rate increased steadily to 16 per cent in 1995 (Statistics Finland 1996). Cohabitation is often regarded as a trial marriage in Finland, since it is mainly young childless couples who cohabit and two in three will eventually marry.

The demographic discussion of cohabitation numbers in *Great Britain* is mainly based on the General Household Survey (GHS) starting from 1979, where cohabiting couples are defined as 'co-resident man and woman living together within a sexual union'. In 1979, only 3 per cent of all women aged 18–49 were cohabiting; a decade later there was an almost threefold rise to 8 per cent, but then a slower increase to 10 per cent in 1994. Seven out of ten first marriages were preceded by premarital cohabitation at the beginning of the 1990s. The average duration of a consensual union is about two years. There was a slight tendency for women with a university degree to cohabit more. In 1986, 4 per cent of children lived with cohabiting parents compared to 12 per cent with lone parents. In 1989, 26 per cent of all children were born outside marriage.

According to Blossfeld *et al.* (1994), consensual unions play an increasingly important role during the period of family formation in *Germany*. The average duration of such unions by the end of the 1980s was three years. In the 1980s more than 50 per cent of cohabitants either married or separated before they had lived together four years.

A rough indicator of the growth of cohabiting families with children is statistics on extra-marital births. As Figure 6.3 shows, the trend is the same in all seven countries, and there is little doubt that the rising numbers of such births are due to growth in the number of cohabiting parents. But the curves are diverging. The trend has been considerably stronger in the Nordic countries than in Germany and the Netherlands, with the United Kingdom in the middle. Today in Sweden, Denmark and Norway every second child is born to a mother who is not formally

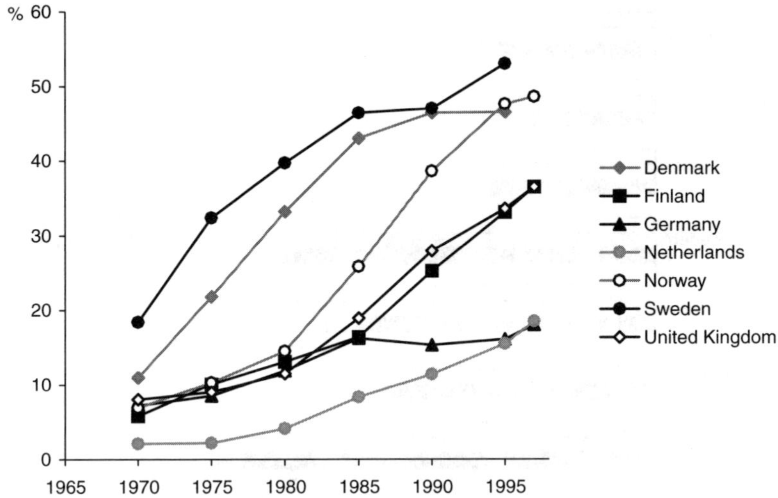

Source: Recent demographic developments in Europe 1998.

Figure 6.3 Extra-marital births as percentage of all births, 1970–97

married, while this is the case with every fifth child in Germany and the Netherlands.

Although there still are no comparable time series on the incidence of cohabitation, surveys during recent years show how many persons define themselves as cohabitants. Figure 6.4 presents Eurobarometer data from 1996 analysed by Kiernan (1999), supplemented with data from Statistics Norway. The figure confirms a picture that has now become familiar to us. The Nordic countries are leading the spread of cohabitation and all over Northern Europe cohabitation has become commonplace. We also see that this family form is most popular among young people, and that the numbers decline after the age of thirty.

A common interpretation, which is supported unanimously by empirical studies, is that cohabitation should basically be regarded as 'test marriages'. But there are indications that cohabitation is also gradually becoming a permanent alternative to marriage. And there seem to be pockets of cohabitants in the middle-aged and elderly population, especially among divorced and widow/widowers. However, the statistical evidence to support these impressions is weak.

As pointed out by Manting (1996), there is little consensus among scholars on the social importance of the growth in cohabitation. 'Some

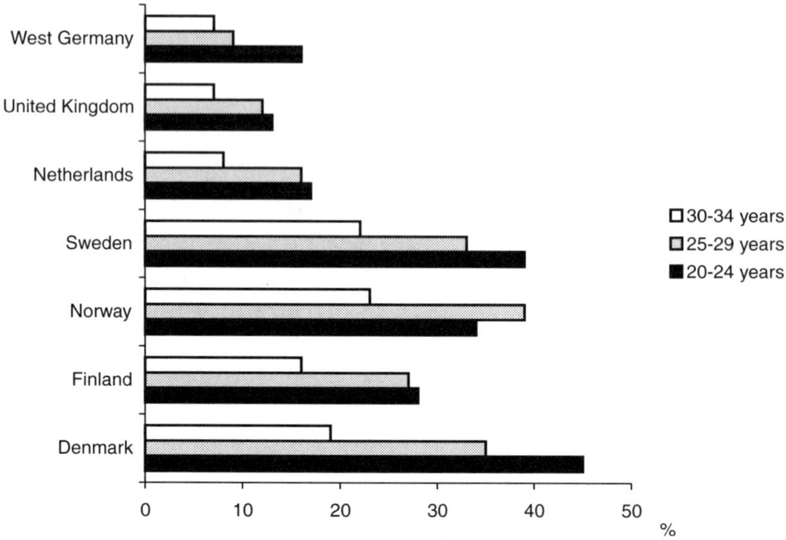

Sources: Population Trends 1999 and Statistics Norway 1999

Figure 6.4 Women cohabiting in 1996

argue that marriage and cohabitation are more or less the same . . . others are convinced that cohabitation is something completely different while others suggest that cohabitation serves different functions' (Manting 1996: 53). These different attitudes are also reflected in the political debates on social policies towards cohabitants.

Policy responses[2]

Derived pension benefits

We now return to the question of how policy makers have reacted to these changes we have described. We will focus mainly on changes in widows' and old age pensions. Widows' or survivors' pensions have traditionally been the most important derived benefit (as opposed to individual benefits), and the legitimacy of this benefit is under intense pressure from the demise of the traditional life-long marriage and increasing labour market participation. Old age pensions are the most important of social security benefits. In most countries they have been constructed as a mixture of derived and individual elements. These two benefits should therefore be suitable candidates to illustrate the pressure on social security systems.

Let us start with *Sweden*, which has been a pioneer in the field of family changes. Major reforms of survivor pensions took place in 1990. Before then, widows' pensions could be paid until the widow reached retirement age (65 years), but the reform introduced a time limit. An adjustment pension is now payable for six months for both men and women. For survivors with a child under the age of twelve the pension can be paid for a longer period, but not beyond the child's twelfth birthday. A survivor who cannot support herself (or himself) by working when the adjustment pension terminates may be entitled to a special survivor's pension. In other words, the norm is now that widows are expected to support themselves by participating in the labour market after a relatively short transitional period. The new system will be phased in gradually. Women born in 1944 or earlier will keep their right to the widow's pension.

During the period 1962–99 obligatory pensions in Sweden consisted of two tiers. Basic pensions were universal, but were somewhat lower for couples than singles. The spousal supplement has been phased out of the system since 1995; it is now only payable to women born before 1934 and is of little practical importance.

In 1999 a new old age pension system was introduced in Sweden, and represented a further step towards the individualisation of social security. Pension rights as a rule are calculated on the basis of individual contributions, and family situation does not influence these rights. But people with little or no previous income are granted a 'guarantee pension'. This pension is about 11 per cent lower for married pensioners than for singles. Spousal supplements are not granted under this new scheme.

Denmark carried through a major pension reform in 1984. Widows' pension was abolished, but widows with difficulties in finding suitable work may qualify for a social pension, a benefit also payable to people with disabilities and other groups with difficulties in the labour market. The justification for paying a pension to a woman who has lost her husband is not her widowhood but her position in the labour market. Spousal supplements were also removed in 1984. The only important consequence of family status in the Danish pension system today is the calculation of pensions. A married couple gets a lower pension than two singles. Denmark today is very close to operating a fully individualised pension system.

Finland has also had a dual system of basic pensions and employment pensions for all economically active persons. Until 1996 supplements for dependent spouses were paid as a part of the basic pension, but since 1 January 1996 no new supplements have been available.

Survivors' pensions were reformed in Finland in 1990. While equal rights for widows and widowers were introduced, qualification for a pension became more limited. Before 1990 a childless widow qualified for a pension if she had reached forty years of age when her husband died. Since 1990 the age limit has been fifty.

In *Norway* there have been only minor changes in family-related pension rights since 1980. Norway has, like Finland and Sweden, a dual obligatory pension system with basic pensions (or guaranteed minimum pensions) and earnings-related pensions. Supplements to spouses were paid as a universal benefit until 1990, when income testing was introduced, after which the benefit was gradually reduced if the pensioner's income exceeded a certain level. It is no longer looked upon as a universal norm that a pensioner maintains his wife. Survivor pensions to widows and widowers were integrated in the National Insurance Scheme in 1967, and the system still has the same characteristics. A reason for the system's ability to survive may be the flexible use of income testing. The pension is reduced if the surviving spouse has, or may be expected to get, income from work exceeding a certain level. The system seems somewhat adaptable to changing norms of female labour participation.

Social insurance in *Germany* is often characterised as the 'breadwinner-model'. Pensions are strongly linked to employment records, and there are no minimum pensions. For workers with long and stable careers, pensions are relatively generous. It is assumed that pensions should be high enough to provide for a wife without any special supplements, and consequently there are no spousal supplements to cut. Widows' and widowers' pensions are derived from the earning record of the deceased 'breadwinner'. The main qualifying conditions are that they are either caring for a child under the age of 18 or are beyond 45 years of age. Pensions are income-tested and reduced if the survivor receives income from their own work and certain other sources. This part of the German social security system has shown great resistance to reform proposals and has preserved its main characteristics during the period under study.

Unlike Germany, the pensions system of the *Netherlands* has undergone major changes during the last two decades. Dutch old age pensions are flat rate benefits. Until 1985 a full pension was 100 per cent of the minimum wage for a married couple and 70 per cent for unmarried persons. But until 1985 a married woman did not have her own independent right to a pension. Her husband was supposed to be the breadwinner, and the couple received a full pension when he reached retirement age. A major goal of the reforms of 1985 was to harmonise Dutch social security law with EC legislation concerning equal treatment of men and women. Pensions to married couples were split in two halves and married women were entitled to their own pension. To avoid reduced income in families where one partner was below retirement age, a 'partner bonus' or spousal supplement was introduced. This partner bonus has been income-tested since 1988. The same year the full bonus was also reduced and in 1998 it was decided that this element of the Dutch pension system should be removed.

Another major change was enacted in 1987, when it became no longer necessary to be married in order to be regarded as a couple. And from 1996 all categories of households were treated as if they were married. The only exception was a child–parent relationship. Today, family situation does not influence old age pensions at all; it is the household composition that counts.

Dutch survivors' pensions also experienced major reforms during the 1980s and 1990s, and a new law was enacted in 1996. Rights to benefits are now mainly limited to the generation born before 1950 or to widows/widowers with dependent children under eighteen years.

Since 1978 the *United Kingdom* has had a two-tier pension system with Nordic characteristics, although the second tier, the state earnings related pension scheme (SERPS), has always been relatively modest. But it was this element of the pension system that became the target of Margaret Thatcher's attack on state pensions. She succeeded in reducing the replacement rate from 25 to 20 per cent in 1986 and allowed members of alternative pension schemes to opt out of SERPS. Flat rate retirement pensions are now paid in different categories. The most important is category A, which requires that the person satisfies a contribution record and has reached retirement age. Category B is paid only to a married woman who up till 1978 chose not to be insured. It requires that her husband has fulfilled his contribution record and that both husband and wife are over pensionable age. It is obviously a special pension in families where the husband has been the breadwinner.

At the end of 1999 a new widows' and widowers' pension scheme was passed by the UK Parliament. It will be implemented in 2001 and gradually phased in. Today only widows can claim survivor benefits in Britain, not widowers. Full pensions require that the widow was over 55 years when her husband died. If she was between 45 (40 for older widows) and 55 years at the time of death, a reduced pension is paid.

Under the new system men and women will have equal rights. More generous benefits are to be paid at the point of bereavement, and a transitional benefit will be given for a period of six months. For widowed parents with children an allowance will be paid until the child reaches 19 years as long as still in full-time education. But there is no right to a permanent pension under the new scheme. Again we see an example of derived benefits for supported women on the retreat in Europe.

Benefits and cohabitation

The focus next shifts to the treatment of cohabiting couples. The study of how different welfare states treat cohabiting couples is an interesting question in its own right, since it affects millions of Europeans today. But it also throws light on wider issues, as discussed in the introduction. It illustrates the modern welfare state's ability to adapt to changes in the risk and need pattern in society, a problem sometimes termed 'welfare state sclerosis'. And it illustrates one of the main dilemmas in welfare policies, namely the big trade-off between distribution according to need and incentives to influence the recipient's behaviour.

Let us start with *Sweden* again. Swedish family law is built on a declared principle of neutrality between different family forms (Agell 1980), and on paper this also applies to social security. But on closer examination there are still disparities, although reforms of social security have rendered them less important. In social insurance the principle is that couples who have common children or who have been married to each other before are treated as married couples. Their pension rights are the same as legally married partners, and they have the same rights to survivor's benefits. Other cohabitants, either childless or with children they do not have together, are treated as singles in pension regulations.

Different rules apply to means-tested social assistance benefits. Social assistance is calculated on the basis of the actual household unit, whatever the legal relations of the members are. These principles did not change during the period under study.

If we are looking for inconsistencies in the treatment of cohabitants and married couples in Sweden, the interplay between social assistance and social insurance seems to provide an example. A single mother dependent on social assistance will lose her benefits if she moves in with a man who has an ordinary income and is not the father of her child. The couple are treated as if they were married. But if the man dies, she is not entitled to any survivor's benefits; she is now treated as a single.

Denmark today has a very individualised social security system, and there is little room for unequal treatment of married and unmarried couples. But their rights are not entirely the same. Thus the calculation of pensions has been more advantageous for cohabitants than married couples, although this was partly rectified in December 1998. The Social Pension Act and the Child Supplement Act were amended so that married and cohabiting couples now have the same legal status. Cohabitation is defined in the official remarks to the amendment Act as persons living in a cohabiting relationship, where the parties contribute to the common household through direct money contributions, work in the home, or otherwise. Single parents with low income are granted a special child allowance in Denmark. The concept of single parents is defined on the basis of actual cohabitation. Cohabiting couples therefore enjoy the same legal status on this point as married couples living together. The Danes usually characterise their legislation as neutral to different family forms. Today this means that they treat cohabitants as married couples in the few areas where this is relevant.

In *Norway* family-related benefits are of much greater importance than in the other Nordic countries, and the rights of cohabitants have been much discussed during recent years. To understand the Norwegian system it is necessary to distinguish between two groups of cohabitants. For couples that have children together, or have been married to each other before, the Swedish principle was introduced in 1994. This first group is treated consistently as married couples. The rights of the second group, cohabitants who do not have children together, have changed gradually over recent years. Today, basic pensions are reduced to the same level as for married couples if they have lived together one year. Transitional allowance for single parents, a minimum income guarantee from the National Social Insurance scheme, also stops if the recipient has lived with a new partner for a year. The fact that the second group are only treated as cohabitants when it is to their disadvantage has been criticised, and in 1999 a commission proposed that this group should be treated as married couples when they had lived together for a certain period, generally two years. If this proposal is implemented, all groups of cohabitants will have the right to widows'/widowers' pension and income-tested spousal supplements. Social assistance in Norway is a discretionary benefit granted by the municipalities, and the Act on social assistance has no clear rule on the treatment of cohabitants. The Ministry for

Social Affairs stresses in their guidelines that couples without any obligation to support each other should be treated as singles. Many municipalities, however, do not follow these guidelines and treat cohabitants as married couples.

In *Finland,* too, the tendency has been towards individualised social security benefits. Singles and couples largely have the same rights, and family forms are irrelevant. The levels of minimum protection are different for couples and singles, and here cohabitants are treated as singles. On the other hand survivors' pensions can only be granted to persons who have been formally married. Here Finland differs from its Nordic neighbours Sweden and Norway, where a couple with joint children qualifies for survivor's pensions. Single parents are granted higher child allowances only if they are not married or cohabiting, and cohabiting here also means living with a partner who is not the father of the child. Social assistance is granted on the basis of a family means test where cohabitants count as members of the same unit. The overall picture from Finland is that cohabitants are treated as married couples only when it is to their disadvantage. They have no right to the only important benefit that is reserved for married couples, i.e. survivors' pensions.

In the *Netherlands* all couples and other household members are treated equally in social security schemes. Whether they are married or not, of the same or different sex, brother and sister etc., is irrelevant. The basic issue is whether people are sharing costs as a household. 'Sharing a household' is important only in social security schemes that aim to offer minimum protection (social assistance, national pensions for old age, and survivors' pensions). The minimum for a cohabiting adult is lower than for a single adult, due to economies of scale of sharing with the partner. Survivors' pension is granted if the person who dies used to cohabit with the survivor; it does not matter if they were actually married or not. The Netherlands thus presents a clear picture: cohabitants and married couples are treated equally.

In *Germany* the problem of cohabitation has been vigorously discussed in a constitutional context. Article six of the German Constitution gives particular protection to marriage and the family, and an important issue is how the concept 'family' should be understood. The Green Party and a radical wing of the Social Democratic Party argue that cohabiting and homosexual couples should be included, while the Christian Democrats want to reserve the concept for married couples. The prevailing legislation favours the conservative view. This is of greatest significance for widows and single parents, since German old age pensions are calculated on the basis of previous earnings records and family situation is irrelevant. Spousal supplements do not exist. Survivors' pensions are only granted to persons who have been married. Single parents with low income receive their social security benefits in the form of social assistance; if they live in a 'marriage-like' relationship, the partner's income is taken into account as if they were a married couple.

The overall picture in Germany is that cohabitants are only treated as married couples when this is to their disadvantage. It is fair to say that this is the result of explicit policies, although these are now being debated in Germany.

In the *United Kingdom* family policies are at the top of the political agenda. Both Labour and the Conservatives want to encourage cohabiting couples to marry, but the present government has yet to propose any changes in social security law to pursue this goal. In the current British social security system, there is an important distinction between contributory benefits and means-tested benefits. Unmarried couples are not allowed to draw any benefits from their partners' contributions, entitlements to survivors' pensions being reserved for married couples. For means-tested benefits, including those for single parents, the unit of claim is the family ('family means test'), and this embraces unmarried couples living together as husband and wife. For instance, a single mother cannot claim any income support if she is living with a man on an average wage, and nor does she have a right to a widow's pension if her partner dies.

The general impression from British social security is that cohabiting couples are treated as married couples only when this is to their disadvantage. But it is hard to say whether this is a result of clear policy goals.

Summing-up policy responses

Derived social security benefits that are linked to the rights of the spouse seem to be in retreat in Northern Europe. The entitlement to widows' pensions has been reformed and limited in all the countries studied except Norway and Germany. We appear to be seeing a clear shift from derived benefits to individual benefits based on the claimant's ability to find suitable work.

Earned benefits for each individual old age pensioner also seem to be gaining ground. Spousal supplements today appear to have become an exception in social security schemes. The most widespread justification for treating singles and couples differently seems to be the 'economies of scale' argument, despite the fact that this argument applies to every household with more than one member. So far only the Netherlands has drawn this conclusion in their pension system.

The treatment of cohabitants reveals a complex picture. Sometimes they are treated as singles and sometimes as married couples. These new family forms are posing a challenge to social security, and only the Netherlands seem to have found a consistent answer.

Discussion

Returning to the introduction where a distinction was made between three types of responses, we find the formulated hypothesis only partly confirmed.

Germany clearly fits the conservative response pattern. New family forms like cohabitation are seen in a way that may be termed *negative recognition*. They get the worst of both worlds: they lose both the advantages that single persons have in some cases and that married couples have in other cases. No radical reforms have been made to widows' or old age pensions. German social security is still based on the breadwinner model where the breadwinner is legally married to his spouse.

The United Kingdom comes closest to Germany's conservative position, cohabitation being only negatively recognised. However, widows' pensions have been reformed into transitional benefits in a way that resembles Sweden. British politicians seem to accept that traditional family forms are changing and that married women should earn their own income after their husband's death.

Finland also has certain characteristics that may be classified as conservative, especially in the way it treats cohabitants, who still have no right to survivors' benefits but are treated as singles when this is to their disadvantage.

Sweden and Norway present more pragmatic responses. They have recognised cohabitants more positively, giving them some rights that are to their advantage. Cohabitants with joint children are treated as married couples.

But we find the most radical response patterns in Denmark and the Netherlands, which have advanced further towards individualised benefit systems than the other five countries. Legal family status is of little relevance for entitlement to social security benefits.

Turning to the question of feedback from social policy to family patterns, it is tempting for supporters of the conservative model to interpret Figure 6.4 in favour of their model. Germany and the United Kingdom, which only recognise cohabitation negatively, have fewer cohabitants than Sweden, Norway and Denmark, which take a more positive stand on cohabitation. But the Dutch case calls this argument into question. The Dutch do not discriminate against cohabitants, but still have relatively few couples who are living together without being legally married.

In my view we should admit that our knowledge is still too limited to explain the differences in family patterns in Northern Europe. However, there are strong signs that all Western countries are moving towards more individualism, as identified by many prominent social scientists such as Giddens (1999) and Beck (1992). People emphasise their own individual life projects and have become more independent of old classes and groups. In taxation and social security there are also strong political calls to individualise burdens and benefits, partly for economic reasons. The modern economy seems to prefer systems where benefits and tax burdens are placed on individuals. Moreover, individual systems make it easier to develop economic incentives for the labour force. Many feminists are also calling for more legislation that promotes independence and autonomy for women. The problems policy makers are facing in social security tend in the same direction. The difficulties involved in differentiating between family types disappear if the family situation is irrelevant. This means that social benefits to adults cannot be justified by their family situation. The alternative at hand is to justify all transfers on the basis of each individual's situation in the labour market. Under an individual system widows and single mothers do not receive benefits because they lack a breadwinner, but they may be granted benefits on the basis of lacking suitable work, i.e. they have no or insufficient earnings.

I conclude by focusing attention on a classic subject in social policy that is strangely little debated in connection with new family patterns. The subject is social control. When social redistribution can to a diminishing degree be based on family status, the alternative is to base it on some criteria reflecting social realities. This social reality is here termed cohabitation. It is an unclear concept both to define in law and to implement locally. It can mean sharing a household, having a common economy, having a sexual relationship. But all these dimensions touch on sensitive issues in the private sphere, which many see as protected from scrutiny by public authorities. The implementation of programmes based on such criteria imposes a difficult task for local administration. It is hard to navigate between loyalty to the legislator on one hand and respect of privacy on the other. Thus the great paradox of cohabitation is that while it is an institution justified by autonomous persons who wish to create their own lives independently of state regulations, and thereby reduce social control, it may produce the opposite result. Social control will increase if the welfare state's ambition to redistribute income between different family types is maintained.

Notes

1 My thanks to Christin Knudsen who helped me with this section.

2 I am grateful to Lotta Westerhäll (Sweden), Christian Buch Sørensen (Denmark), Wim van Oorschot (Netherlands), Jonathan Bradshaw (UK), Jochen Reinhard (Germany) and Maija Sakslin (Finland) who have helped me with data for this section, but who are not responsible for any errors.

7 Health and social care systems: How different is the Nordic model?

Tine Rostgaard and Juhani Lehto

Introduction

A central conclusion from studies of welfare models is that the Nordic countries differ widely from those traditionally associated with other welfare models. This also applies to care systems (see e.g. Anttonen and Sipilä 1996; Alber 1994). Nordic uniqueness is often highlighted for the *large public involvement,* forming what has been termed public service states. Another emphasis is on the *high degree of universalism*, along with high professional standards and the promotion of *gender equality*. Periods of economic instability, particularly in Sweden and Finland, have tended to focus critical attention on the inherent expansive nature of the welfare state, and helped create a cost-efficiency ethos. Outside the Nordic countries, social care systems have also been under scrutiny, especially in response to increased female labour force participation, with more emphasis on equal gender distribution of care work and on changing family structures. And everywhere, increased demands for more flexibility and choice are heard. An overview of the years from the early 1980s until mid-1996 therefore creates an interesting opportunity to examine whether the Nordic model is still unique.

This chapter concentrates on two basic questions:

- How homogenous and separate as a group of countries are the Nordic 'public service states' when compared to a larger group of European welfare states? Is there a Nordic 'care model' and, if so, how does this differ from other European 'care models'?
- Have trends in health and social care been converging or diverging between the Nordic nations themselves, and between the Nordic and other European countries, during the last fifteen years?

Methodological notes

Comparative analyses of care regimes have often focused on one user group (e.g. Jamieson 1991; Kamerman and Kahn 1991; Hutten and Kerkstra 1996), or included either health care (e.g. OECD 1993; Saltman *et al.* 1998) or social care (e.g. Anttonen and Sipilä 1996; Lewis 1998b; Rostgaard and Fridberg 1998). Analyses rarely focus on health and social care as well as related parts of the school system at the same time, especially in the context of more general comparative welfare state analysis. A broader approach to care systems is needed, particularly as services and other benefits in different sectors may be fulfilling more or less the same functions.

It is necessary to underline here that services and service institutions have more than one function, role or task to accomplish. Following Merton (1968), it is possible to speak about latent and manifest functions. We define some services' functions from the perspective of their manifest function – such as meeting the care needs of older people and of children. We mainly deal with the dominant manifest functions here, but we do not claim that the other manifest or latent functions of the care services are not of import in care service development.

For instance, child care systems developed on the basis of pre-school education tend to differ from those based on social care thinking. The pre-school education model tends to follow that of primary school, with less than full working days and longer holidays, whereas the social care model tends to weigh more the need of parents to obtain care for their children so they are able to work full-time throughout the year. Thus the 'pre-school education function' may be different from the 'allowing both parents to work full-time function'. Certainly maternity, paternity and parental leave schemes, too, have functions beyond that of child care, but they also have common functions as they all relate to child care.

Similarly, home help and old age homes under the social care sector, and home nursing and long-term care hospitals under the health care sector may be equivalent in terms of providing care and support in the everyday lives of older clients. However, their 'medical functions' and the professionalisation of care may make the services quite different from the perspective of other relevant functions.

We will compare the functional alternatives so that, for instance, the *école maternelle* of France is dealt with as functionally the same as the *daghem* (day home) of Sweden. Our main criterion for doing so is the number of hours children are cared for outside home, converted into full-time equivalents. We will also deal with services that provide long-term shelter and basic care for the elderly – the hospital and nursing homes of the health sector and the residential or old age homes of the social care sector – as functional equivalents. Our method of grouping them more or less together as functional alternatives is based on the literature (Lehto 1997; Lewis 1998b) indicating a trend of convergence of treatment patterns in different forms of institutional long-term care.

As provisions for older people and children may be significantly different, systematisation of a welfare state according to just one of these user groups may look different if the other user group was also included. Certain countries could have abundant care systems available for children but only few for older people, or the other way around (Anttonen and Sipilä 1996; Lewis 1998b; Rostgaard and Fridberg 1998). In order to understand the full scope of the care system, a comparison of the whole range of functional alternatives taking into account both care sectors and both user groups is advantageous.

Data

One reason for services often not being included in comparative welfare state analyses is that the available data are mostly in the form of aggregate numbers on expenditures and outputs of the service systems. There is scant comparable data on the distribution of service use within populations and on access to services. The information used here also suffers from such restrictions. We have used data gathered and made comparable by OECD, plus a collection of national data on social care[1] and other data and earlier analysis findings as mentioned in the references. We also recognise that it is problematic to use these data for international comparisons, not least because functionally equivalent services in different sectors may be dealt with differently between countries in terms of defining the borderlines of the statistical categories. It is somewhat safer to draw conclusions on the basis of comparative trends within countries, but we do so on the basis of cross-sectional inter-country figures only when there is other evidence to support the conclusion.

Differences within countries

The strong element of de-centralisation in the organisation, provision and financing of services further complicates the understanding of care benefits. Cultural, economic and political differences within a country contribute to a variety of local welfare packages. However, the countries chosen in this study benefit from having rather homogenous political and cultural structures, as well as well-developed welfare systems. The choice of countries was also made from the practical consideration that we had more data available than for other European countries. Thus the analysis includes Denmark, Finland, Norway, Sweden, France, Germany, the Netherlands and the United Kingdom (for social care, England). First, this selection enables us to make comparisons with a country usually seen as an archetype of the 'Bismarckian' welfare state (Germany). Second, we can compare with a country believed to embody the 'Beveridgean' model plus a possible impact of 'Thatcherian neoliberalism' (United Kingdom), as well as with a country that presents a mixture of the Bismarckian and Beveridgean models (the Netherlands). Finally, we are able to compare the Nordic countries with the French welfare state, which is often grouped with the 'Continental', 'Corporatist' or even 'Bismarckian' countries, but which has interesting differences, too (e.g. Bouget and Palier 1999).

'Welfare mix'

A familiar concept in international comparisons is 'welfare mix'; there may be different types of service providers and different means of financing services. Calling the Nordic countries 'public service states' does not mean that they only have public providers and public funding of services. Nevertheless, this categorisation is based on an understanding that the public sector has a much greater role in service provision and service funding than in other countries. The provider and funding types may be divided in many ways. The basic alternatives that can be used to compare the health and social care systems of the eight countries by analysing their different mixes of provider and funding types are:

Family

- Provision of care may originate from family and relatives, or the family can contribute to costs by paying user charges or private insurance premiums or by being responsible for the production costs of informal care provided within the family.

Voluntary or non-governmental non-profit sector

- This includes a great variety of providers, from mutual help groups to large national, non-governmental organisations with thousands of professional, paid employees.

Employers

- Employers may provide or fund services for employees and their family members as an extra benefit, or may indirectly fund services by supplementing the salary with family benefits, or by voluntarily insuring employees; they may also contribute to obligatory insurance, either via public or private insurance companies.

Market or for-profit sector

- The market sells health and social care services as any other commercial services. Providers who do this solely for profit may be termed the 'corporate sector'. Quite often, the market sector is formed of private practitioners or small enterprises with the primary motive of self-employment rather than maximum profit from investments.

Public

- Provision and funding from central, regional and/or local government.

A simple categorisation of service providers into these five types does not reveal much of the variation across the service pattern. The true picture is more complex, a good example being privately practising physicians. In France, these are often categorised into the non-profit sector, whereas in Finland they are placed in the market sector since they are outside the basic public primary health care provided by GPs employed by the public health centres. In Denmark, they are often assigned to the public sector, because their contracts with local authorities are not that different from public employment and because they are the main gatekeepers to the public health care system.

We also find a welfare mix in the financing of services, although the alternatives here are not much more 'pure' than the provider alternatives. For instance, forms of public support for families may include tax deductions and care allowances. The difference between government funding (tax funding) and insurance funding may be great if the insurance systems are far from universal and much more restricted, while the state gives almost completely universal insurance.

Health care and care for the elderly

While Western European health care systems are often divided into Bismarckian and Beveridgean models (OECD 1993; Saltman *et al.* 1998), care for the elderly has been much longer based in the tradition of poor relief. In comparative health care research the United Kingdom tends to be grouped with the Nordic systems, the model often being called an NHS (National Health Service) model rather than a Nordic model (Saltman *et al.* 1998; Guillén 1999, Hassenteufel 1999). Comparative research on systems of care for the elderly is rare and clear models have seldom been presented. Those that have are social care models, which often draw more from the characteristics of child care systems than from systems of care for the elderly (Anttonen and Sipilä 1996; Sipilä 1997). There seems to be some controversy between 'more general' comparative welfare state researchers and those who have contrasted discrete sectors of service or care systems. The generalists are more likely to assume a clear Nordic model than the specialists, particularly when it comes to health care (see also Alban and Christiansen 1995).

Differences and trends in expenditure

A significant political concern is expenditure on health, both public expenditure and total expenditure, including the costs of private insurance to individuals or employers, and user charges. The issue continues to fuel the argument for the need to reform the health care systems in the eight countries (Saltman *et al.* 1998). Until the 1990s, Finland and Norway had lower public health expenditure per capita than both Denmark and Sweden, particularly the latter. The latecomers have since joined the prosperous Nordic trend, but all four countries have decreased the proportional burden of health care on their national economies in recent years.[2] The concurrent development in the other four countries has been the opposite (Figure 7.1a), with the increase fastest in France and Germany and slowest in the Netherlands. In 1997, Germany and France had the highest public health expenditure of the eight countries and the United Kingdom – even after a significant increase – the lowest.

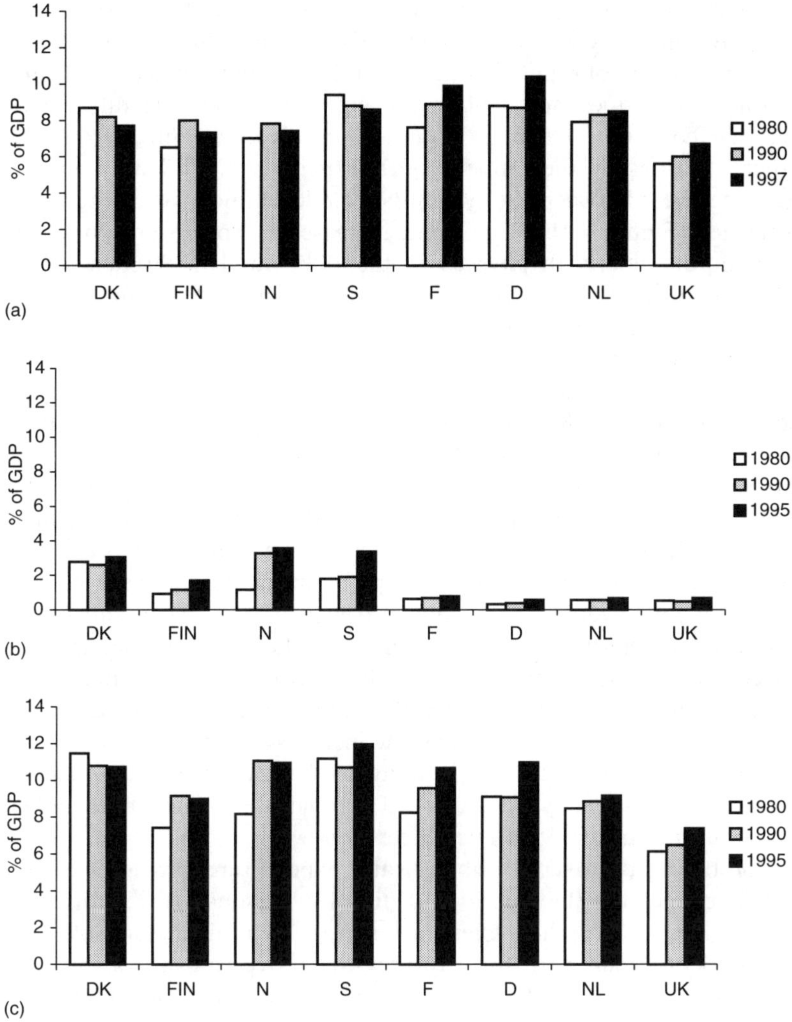

Source: OECD 1998a.

Figure 7.1 (a) Total health expenditure as percentage of GDP in 1980, 1990 and 1997. (b) Public expenditure for social services for the elderly and disabled persons as percentage of GDP in 1980, 1990 and 1997. (c) Expenditure for health and public expenditure for services for the elderly and disabled persons as percentage of GDP in 1980, 1990 and 1997

Public expenditure on care services for the elderly and the disabled[3] has grown in all the countries under study, both absolutely and in terms of its proportion of GDP. The ageing of the populations is a significant factor, but it does not explain the entire trend or the differences between countries. Denmark, Sweden and Norway differ from the other countries by their much higher expenditure. Finland seems to be somewhere between the typical Nordic level and that of the other countries (Figure 7.1b). The rapid increase in expenditure on social care for the elderly in Norway in the 1980s, and in Sweden in the 1990s, may be explained by administrative shifts of certain services and their expenditures from the health services to the social care budget (Lehto *et al.* 1999).

All the countries under study finance most of their expenditure on health care and the formal care of the elderly by public funding. Five of the countries – the Nordic nations and the United Kingdom – have mainly tax-funded systems, while Germany, France and the Netherlands use obligatory insurance as the main method (Saltman *et al.* 1998). In this context the Dutch sickness insurance system is interesting. In the Netherlands, people with income above a certain level are not covered by the obligatory insurance. They can either take private health insurance, which is the choice of the majority, or cover their health care costs themselves. More than one-quarter of the population is thereby outside the public insurance. However, the privately insured mainly use the same insurance companies, hospitals, doctors and other services as the obligatorily insured. The coverage of private insurance may be the more complete, provided that higher contributions are paid (van der Meer 1998).

Combining the overall public health expenditure with that of the social services for the elderly and disabled persons gives a different picture (Figure 7.1c) than when these sectors are looked at in isolation. Denmark, Sweden and Norway are still above the others, but the differences have significantly diminished. France and Germany belong in the second category while Finland, the Netherlands and the United Kingdom have the lowest public expenditure. If we define the Dutch private sickness insurance of the upper-middle classes as 'semi-public' and include its expenditure in the picture, the Netherlands rises to the second category with France and Germany. The Nordic countries are also different from Germany, France and the United Kingdom in their diminishing trend of sum expenditure in the 1990s.

Public vs. private expenditure

Denmark, Norway, Sweden and the United Kingdom tend to have the highest proportion of public funding of total health expenditure, with Finland, Germany and France in the intermediate group. The Netherlands has had the lowest proportion, for reasons explained above. Expenditure has tended to slightly decline in all countries other than France since the 1980s. As the trend has been somewhat stronger in the countries with the highest proportion of public funding on expenditure, the differences, particularly between the Nordic countries and Germany and France, have tended to decrease (Figure 7.2).

Comparing the proportion of private funding of total expenditure for the social care of the elderly is even more difficult. The funding systems involved tend to be more fragmented, with components from institutions such as pension funds, sickness insurance, the housing allowance system, social assistance funds and various local, regional and central government funds. Social care systems are also more dependent on the extent of unpaid care than are health care systems. On the basis of available studies (e.g. Hutten and Kerkstra 1996;

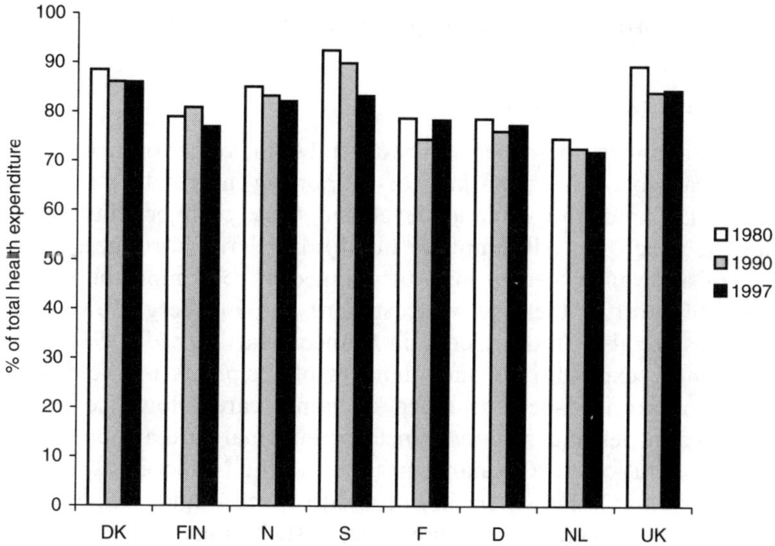

Source: OECD 1998.

Figure 7.2 Proportion of public expenditure of total health expenditure in 1980, 1990 and 1997

Wistow *et al.* 1996; Rostgaard and Fridberg 1998; Breuil-Genier 1999; Lehto *et al.* 1999; Österle 1999), the following characteristics, differences and trends may be identified:

- There is more means testing and discretion at entry to social care for the elderly, and more income-related user charges than for health care. The quality of services also tends to vary more in social care. The elderly with good income thus either have to pay significant user fees or use totally private alternatives.
- In Germany and France there is a legal obligation for children to take care of their parents or to pay, on a means-tested basis, for their public care. The other countries no longer have any such legal obligation.
- The proportion of private funding of total expenditure on social care for the elderly is probably lowest in Denmark, at an intermediate level in Sweden, Finland and Norway and higher in all the non-Nordic countries. However, the available data do not allow firm conclusions on this.[4]
- The stated policy in all eight countries is to shift the balance in the expenditure on care for the elderly from institutional care to care in the community. Success in this shift would also mean an increase in the proportion of private funding of total care expenditure.

Cash benefits for informal care

In all the countries there seems to be a trend to introduce or increase the role of cash benefits earmarked for supporting informal care for the elderly. England and Finland developed these cash benefits earlier than the other six. All countries but France have introduced some form of allowance or care insurance aimed at reforming the overall system of care for the elderly (Rostgaard and Fridberg 1998). Such proposals are also on the agenda in France (Martin *et al.* 1998).

Currently, expenditures and numbers of recipients of these 'cash instead of services'-benefits (such as home care allowance in the Nordic countries and care insurance for informal care at home or in private institutions in Germany, France and the Netherlands) remain quite low (*ibid.*). However, if not tightly needs- and means-tested they have the potential to expand very fast, because the 'reserve' of unpaid care is extensive in all the countries. Public payment for informal care work may also be seen as a new layer of state regulation of care responsibilities within families, as well as a new layer of atypical jobs with its attendant problems related to rights and social security of 'paid informal workers' (Lehto 1999). These are also important questions from the gender perspective, as most informal carers are women.

The mix of service providers

The welfare mixes in health service provision are quite different. The Nordic countries and the United Kingdom may be termed public service states. Germany, the Netherlands and France are obvious private–public mixes, where private means a hospital sector which is partly public and partly private non-profit, and which includes out-patient care given by physicians who are in private practice. There is not a very strong corporate sector in any of the health care systems under study, as occurs in the USA (OECD Health Data 1998; Saltman *et al.* 1998).

There was not a substantial change in the balance between public and different kinds of private providers of health care in the eight countries in 1980–97 (OECD Health Data 1998). The traditional differences between the 'health insurance countries' and 'tax funding countries' seem to have persisted.

With regard to care for the elderly, the welfare mixes have differed in the same way. The role of public provision has been for more significant in the Nordic countries and the UK. In Germany, France and the Netherlands the role of non-governmental and mainly non-profit organisations has been much more significant (Table 7.1). The UK has clearly undergone a radical change in its welfare provision mix for the elderly during the last fifteen years (Wistow *et al.* 1996). The role of the private for-profit sector has expanded rapidly. Most private providers in the UK are still small local units dependent on contracts with the public sector (Rostgaard and Fridberg 1998).

The gradual trend towards more private providers in many countries results from a reduction of the role of traditional institutional care in nursing homes and old age homes, and an increased emphasis on care at home and new types of residential care such as residential and sheltered housing. These new forms of residential care are more often run by private non-profit or for-profit providers in countries such as the Netherlands, the United Kingdom, Finland, Sweden and Denmark (Rostgaard and Fridberg 1998; Lehto *et al.* 1999; Österle 1999). Both home help and new types of residential care are also areas where many countries are pursuing job creation policies by providing partial public funding for small-scale private providers via public unemployment funds or tax deductions (Lehto 1999).

Table 7.1 Providers of formal social care for the elderly in 1996

Country	*Providers of home help*	*Providers of institutional care*
Denmark	Mainly municipal, some contracted for-profit agencies	Public (73%) and contracted private (27%) agencies
Finland	Municipal (90%) and non-profit and for-profit agencies (10%)	Public (81%) and contracted non-profit (19%) agencies
Norway	Mainly municipal, some non-profit and for-profit agencies	Mainly public, some non-profit and for-profit agencies
Sweden	Municipal (96%) and contracted public or private agencies	Public (84%) and private (16%) agencies
France	Non-profit agencies or persons on unemployment schemes. Some municipal agencies	Public (57%), non-profit (29%) and for-profit (14%) agencies
Germany	Non-profit and for-profit agencies	Non-profit (64%), for-profit (18%) and public (18%) agencies
Netherlands	Mainly non-profit and some for-profit agencies	Non-profit (60%) and public (40%) agencies
England	Public (77%), contracted for-profit (19%) and non-profit (4%) agencies	Private for-profit (45%), non-profit (40%) and public (15%) agencies

Sources: Rostgaard and Fridberg 1998; Lehto *et al.* 1999.

Another gradual trend seems to be a reduction of differences between the different formal care provider organisations. The popularity of New Public Management has meant conscious adoption of aspects of competition, entrepreneurship and private sector management methods by the public social and health care organisations (Ferlie *et al.* 1996; Klausen and Stahlberg 1998). So how different from public providers are the private non-profit hospitals in the Bismarckian countries? They, too, are under public control, are tied to public (insurance) funding, have politicians in the highest decision-making bodies, are large bureaucratic organisations and have health care professionals in the dominant positions within the hospitals, at the various levels of government, and in public debates (e.g. Hassenteufel 1999). There are also many indications that as contracted private non-profit organisations develop, their disparities with public and for-profit organisations tend to diminish (Wistow *et al.* 1996).

The role of unpaid informal and voluntary care as a functional alternative to formal health and social care has traditionally been very significant in all eight countries. It seems that the role of care by spouses and children is most significant in Germany. Possibly it is also more common in the UK, Finland and France, while in Denmark and Sweden formal home help seems to be a more frequent facility for older people than elsewhere. The role of voluntary help seems to be very minor in all countries, although not insignificant in Germany, the Netherlands, the UK and France (Rostgaard and Fridberg 1998).

In summary, the differences between countries in terms of welfare mix appear to have remained rather stable from the 1980s to the mid-1990s, with the exception of the radical attempts to reform social care provision in the United Kingdom during the Thatcher years. However, shifting the balance from institutional care to care in the community means a gradual decline in public provision in favour of both new and traditional alternative providers. Changes in the management of public service providers also seem to reduce the disparities between different types of providers. Even informal providers are being drawn into the systems of managed care, not least by the new schemes for paying for informal care.

Changes and differences in service use

The most visible change in service provision is the reduction in hospital care (Figure 7.3). The exception is Germany, which may be partially explained by the inclusion of the former GDR, which used to have a high rate of hospital beds per population. Germany and the Netherlands had far fewer psychiatric beds in the 1980s and all the others have significantly reduced these since then. All countries except Germany have also reduced the number of acute hospital beds (OECD Health Data 1998). The UK, France, and particularly Sweden, have compensated for some of the reduction in hospital bed numbers by an increase of beds in social care institutions.[5] The others have reduced their number of social care beds (Rostgaard and Fridberg 1998, Lehto *et al.* 1999). The overall impression is that the proportion of the elderly being cared for in social and health care institutions has decreased. Denmark and the United Kingdom seem the most de-institutionalised countries among the eight, while Finland has experienced the most rapid de-institutionalisation. One may conclude that the countries with an insurance-based health care model tend to be slower in changing their care structures than those with a tax-funded public health care system.

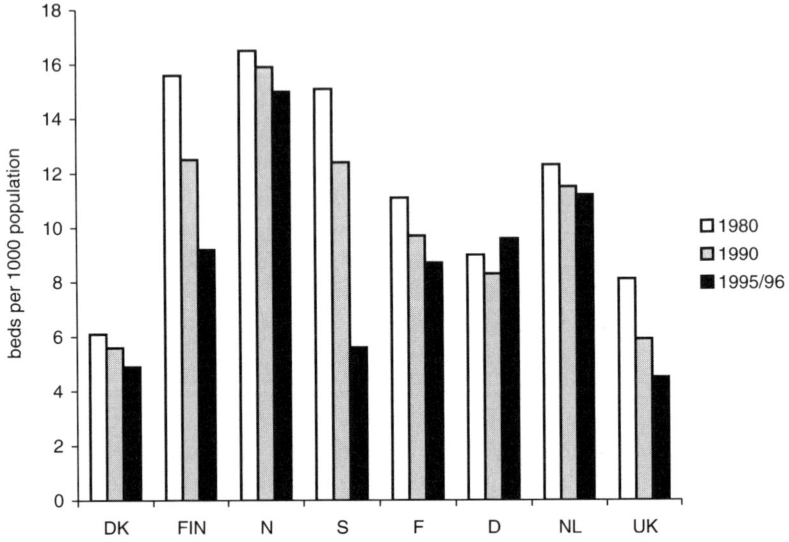

Source: OECD 1998

Figure 7.3 Inpatient care beds per 1000 population in 1980, 1990 and 1997

All the countries studied have a policy aimed at changing the balance in care for the elderly from institutional to more 'home-like' settings. However, only Denmark seems to have pursued this policy consistently by boosting the coverage of home help. Sweden, Denmark and Norway these days clearly provide more home help than the Netherlands, Finland and the UK, measured in service hours per elderly person (65 or over) (Rostgaard and Fridberg 1998; Lehto *et al.* 1999).

Over the last two decades all the countries increased consultations to physicians as well as the number of highly educated employees (physicians and nurses) in their health care (OECD Health Data 1998). Thus what may have been saved by reductions in bed numbers has often been used for more intensified, professional and high technology outpatient and inpatient treatments.

Service rights and standards

The service rights of citizens are (legally) less ambiguous in the countries more reliant on health insurance and private provision. In the Nordic countries and the UK political pressures to define the rights of citizens to health services more precisely have increased.

Reforms such as 'citizens charters' in England (Ferlie *et al.* 1996) and treatment guarantees in the Nordic countries (Lehto *et al.* 1999) address this issue, though they are not as solid as the legal rights in the insurance systems. Disparities in the legal definition of rights may be one explanation for the different trends in health care expenditure in the Nordic and Continental countries.

In the health insurance models service rights are basically restricted to the insured. Basically, health insurance is earned in the labour market in Germany, France and the Netherlands, although compensatory funding arrangements exist for people outside the labour market. Thus the insurance coverage in the countries under study is quite large, almost 100 per cent for the 'normal' population. In this sense, there appear not to be great differences with regard to the universalism of the health care systems (Saltman and Figueras 1997). The exclusion from health care funding is higher for immigrants, particularly if 'paper-less'. This problem seems to be greater in the health insurance countries (Ritsatakis *et al.* 2000).

Service rights in care for the elderly are more weakly developed in all the countries. England, in particular, has rather tight means-testing at entry to publicly funded care for the elderly (Rostgaard and Fridberg 1998; Österle 1999). Means-testing is also used in determining access to care for those people not covered by care insurance in the three continental countries under study (*ibid.*). The rights of the elderly to care are restricted in the Nordic countries by needs-testing and by income-related user fees. This weakness of social rights is most clearly indicated in the declining numbers of home help recipients in Finland and Sweden in the 1990s (Lehto *et al.* 1999). So it is difficult to claim true universalism in the care for the elderly in any of the countries, with the possible exception of the institutional care and free-of-charge home help in Denmark.

It is quite difficult to compare service standards in health care and care for the elderly between countries. In terms of the number of physicians per capita and the length of their training the disparities have decreased (OECD Health Data 1998) and there does not seem to be any particular Nordic model. During the 1990s all eight countries also emphasised the management and improvement of service quality. As medicine is quite international both as a scientific discipline and in practice, we assume no major differences in terms of medical standards.

There seems to be more variation in the quality of long-term care for the elderly, both within and between countries. While the professionalisation of care work is evident in all eight countries, the Nordic nations and the Netherlands seem to require higher average professional education for personnel caring for the elderly (Rostgaard and Fridberg 1998).

Care for children

Differences and trends in terms of expenditure

Sweden tops the expenditure league with 1.83 per cent of GDP spent on day care in 1996. France,[6] Finland and Denmark came next, spending 1.07–1.35 per cent of GDP on day care. The remaining countries spent between 0.32 and 0.47 per cent of GDP on formal day care. With the exception of Norway, the Nordic countries thus seem to confirm their label of 'service states'. Looking at the proportion of GDP spent on maternity or parental leave benefits, a similar characteristic emerges. Again, the Nordic countries allocated proportionally more of GDP, from 0.60 to 0.84 per cent, to leave benefits (Table 7.2).

When the expenditure figures are indexed per capita (Table 7.2, left columns), it becomes apparent that the Nordic countries not only expanded in terms of per capita expenditure for day care, but also per child under six years, in the period 1982–96. Expenditure for leave benefits rose more than day care in this period in Denmark and Norway. In Finland and Sweden, expenditure for leave benefits also increased until the early 1990s' recession, when benefits were cut. Some of the decline was due to decreasing birth rates. Spending in the non-Nordic countries generally increased for day care, especially in the UK and the Netherlands, while Germany also raised expenditure fairly strongly for leave benefits. Significant for the Nordic countries is thus that spending as a proportion of GDP is high both in terms of expenditure for formal day care as well as for leave benefits, and recent years have witnessed a further increase, especially for leave benefits.

Private expenditure

There are several ways to subsidise the use of day care services. The Nordic model mainly favours municipal subsidies for establishing and running day care centres, while in countries such as France, costs for day care are mainly subsidised through monetary benefits. French parents thus receive a subsidy to pay the social security for a privately-hired child care provider, and also an allowance when using family day care. It is thus hard to exactly specify subsidies for day

Table 7.2 Index of social expenditure for maternity and parental leave cash benefits and formal day care per capita at pre-school age, 1982–96 (1982 = 100), in 1990 prices

Country		*1982*	*1985*	*1990*	*1995/96*	*1995/96 % of GDP*
Denmark	Maternity and parental leave	100	177	240	333	0.73
	Formal day care	100	107	125	151	1.35
Finland	Maternity and parental leave	100	124	225	196	0.84
	Formal day care	100	136	211	208	1.15
Norway	Maternity and parental leave	100	97	201	345	0.54
	Formal day care	100	97	199	326	0.42
Sweden	Maternity and parental leave	100	109	180	105	0.83
	Formal day care	100	120	130	124	1.83
France	Maternity and parental leave	100	79	122	225	0.35
	Formal day care	–	100	127	199	1.07
Germany	Maternity and parental leave	100	70	233	240	0.25
	Formal day care	100	102	114	162	0.39
Netherlands	Maternity and parental leave	100	104	139	–	0.05
	Formal day care	100	95	102	138	0.51
England	Maternity and parental leave	100	97	134	163	0.07
	Formal day care	100	138	149	205	0.32

Sources: Rostgaard and Fridberg 1998; Barn-og Familjedepartementet 1999 pers. comm.
Notes:
1995/96: 1995 for France, Germany, England and Netherlands, 1996 for other countries.
Netherlands: 1990 = 1989 for maternity and paternity leave
England: 1983 = 100 for maternity and paternity leave
France: 1988 = 100 for formal day care
Germany: 1982, 1985 and 1990 is for West Germany
France and Germany: calculations based on 0–5 year olds
England and Netherlands: calculations based on 0–4 year olds
Denmark, Finland, Norway and Sweden: calculations based on 0–6 year olds

care use. Estimations can take account of the share of costs paid by parents when using day care; although this does not allow a comparison of actual parental fees paid per child it does provide a sketchy picture of the size of parental fees in comparison to public subsidies and other income sources (Figure 7.4).

Parents pay the highest proportion of costs in the UK, where there are few subsidised places, and in the Netherlands and Norway, where parental fees cover around 40 per cent of costs. Most of the British children involved are in private for-profit care where fees are relatively high, covering 90 per cent or more of costs. However, nursery schools and other services for 3–4 year olds provided within the education system are free of charge. In Norway, part of the reason for the relatively high parental fees is the higher sums paid for privately-owned day care, which accounts for half of the total public provision. The high parental fee in the Netherlands is mainly explained by the predominance of private day care centres, which seldom receive public subsidies. Here, subsidies are mainly from employers, who pay for a day care place for the child of an employee. As in the UK, there are no fees paid for children aged 4–5 attending nursery education in the primary schools. France and Denmark constitute a middle group in

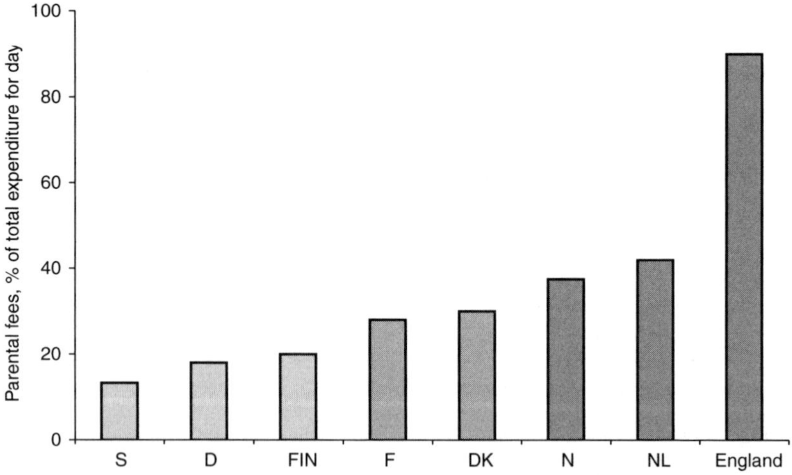

Sources: Bradshaw et al. 1996 for England; Rostgaard and Fridberg 1998 for other countries.
Note: Information concerning fees from various years between 1994–96.

Figure 7.4 Parental fees as a proportion of total expenditure for day care at day care centres in mid-1990s

this respect, with 28–30 per cent of costs paid by parents, not including the free nursery education in France's *l'école maternelle*. French day care for 3–4-year-olds, and sometimes also 2-year-olds, is thus free. Sweden, Germany and Finland have the lowest parental fees, with parents paying one-fifth of costs or less.

Public financing of child day care in terms of the share of fees paid by parents to day care centres does not, therefore, seem to be a strong feature of the Nordic model. Significant determinants of the proportion of client fees of total expenditure seem to be the balance between for-profit private and non-profit or public provision, and between education and social care. The lowest (or no) client fees are in day care provided by the education sector, and the highest in private for-profit social care.

So when formulating a model of the public service states, there are several characteristics of the day care systems in the Nordic countries that should be considered. Private provision with public funding is normal, though the share of fees covered by the state varies across the countries. It is also characteristic in the Nordic countries that the day care systems are used by all social groups alike, whereas public day care for small children in the non-Nordic countries tends to be dominated by disadvantaged families (Rostgaard and Fridberg 1998). At the same time, significant trends among the non-Nordic countries should be noted. These include the increase in public expenditure for day care provision and the expanding role of the public sector as a provider, regulator and funder of day care services – characteristics which place these countries nearer the Nordic model.

Towards more pluralism in the welfare mix

Common to all the countries under study is that a process of pluralism has occurred. This is evident in the increasing use and funding of service provision from private, for-profit and non-profit providers. It is also evident in the promotion of individual responsibility for welfare provision through cash benefits for informal care, similar to the development of care allowances for older people and their carers.

With regard to the increasing use of non-public provision, it is fair to say that use of day care from non-public providers is not a new phenomenon in the Nordic countries, whose many day care centres are in fact run by non-profit organisations or individual providers. Thus in Denmark, non-profit day care institutions cover 40 per cent of total public day care provision. For-profit provision of core social services, on the other hand, has often met opposition in the Nordic countries, although less so in the field of child care. A few municipalities contract out service provision to for-profit providers, though these are still thin on the ground. In Sweden, where for-profit provision is most widespread in the Nordic region, private for-profit provision for children accounts for only 2 per cent of all child care arrangements (Socialstyrelsen, 1996b). In contrast, countries with scarce public provision of day care such as the UK and the Netherlands typically have a relatively large, private for-profit sector within day care, due both to the unmet need for day care provision and to the ideological support for private solutions. In Britain, public day care for younger children is only provided for children considered to be at risk; most 0–3-year-old children in day care are therefore in private, for-profit centres.

Sometimes, the responsibility of employers is promoted, and here Dutch developments in day care for children provide the obvious example. Under the so-called 'Stimulative Measure', employers are now expected to co-finance provision of day care, which thus increasingly becomes a labour market issue and the employee's labour market position determines access to day care. Funding of day care provision for children of employees is now stipulated in over 220 collective agreements (van Dijk 1996). Moreover, large companies are increasingly offering child care for their employees at the workplace itself. In France, employers rarely provide day care directly but they contribute with up to one-quarter of the costs of day care in the welfare system (Rostgaard and Fridberg 1998). In the Nordic countries, the wider provision of public day care has not created the same impetus for employers to provide day care services, although the reconciliation of work and family life is gaining more emphasis here, too. So within day care, both private providers and employers are gaining ground as significant welfare providers.

Public involvement in day care has intensified in some of the countries, especially those that previously had limited state involvement in providing or funding day care services for small children.[7] We therefore see no straightforward development towards more non-public responsibility. In most countries, central government policy-making reflects concerns about variation in standards and range of provision. Regulation is being stepped up and standards made more binding. In some countries, especially those outside the Nordic region, the state thus seems to be assuming a larger role in providing stimulation through funding and setting delivery goals.

Indirect financial support for non-public provision is used to stimulate private provision. In Britain, a new Childcare Tax Credit to cover some of the costs of child care[8] came into operation in October 1999. In France, the main two schemes for supporting private day care provision subsidise the parental costs of wages and social security contributions for privately hired day carers. In the Nordic countries, too, private provision of day care is indirectly supported through public subsidies. In Denmark, for example, a new scheme allows parents to choose between a subsidy for private day care and the use of municipal day care services. Similar schemes exist in Finland and Norway.

Furthering of individual responsibility for welfare provision via cash benefits for informal care is emphasised as the last element to increase pluralism. In all countries this has occurred by improving existing leave schemes and the introduction of new ones. Parents' opportunities to care for their children at home have thus been improved as maternity leave periods have lengthened and parental leaves have been introduced.

Right to child day care

As already mentioned in the context of social care for the elderly, social services have seldom been governed by any rights criteria. Allocation has mainly been based on local, discretionary decision-making, according to available resources and without legal rights such as appeal attached. During recent later years, however, the right to child day care has been made explicit in a number of Nordic countries.

The first country to introduce such a day care guarantee was Sweden where a Parliament decision in 1985 established the right to day care. This entitled children from 1½ years till school age a place in municipal day care by 1991. The benefit applies to children of working parents or students. Finland was the next country to pass day care legislation.[9] The Danish Social Democratic government then announced in 1993 that a public day care guarantee for all children aged one to five years was to be introduced from the beginning of 1995 (Rostgaard and Fridberg 1998). Norway has so far not introduced a specific guarantee of day care provision except for handicapped children. The government did state that child care should be made universally available during the 1990s, but this was not to be considered as a legal right (Halvorsen 1996).

However, the introduction of day care guarantees is not a unique Nordic feature. Other countries have made similar moves, especially for older pre-school children. Thus since 1992, German children have in principle been guaranteed a place in nursery school from the age of 3½ years, and a further undertaking to expand the number of places for under 3-year-olds has been made. Likewise, in England since September 1998, all 4-year-olds have been guaranteed in principle a place in 'early years' education, with future expansion to 3-year-olds. France, like Norway, has no specific day care guarantee, but since 1982 as part of its early childhood policy has stressed the aim of ensuring the necessary number of places in day care and pre-school provision. Also, as all French children aged three to four and sometimes as young as two years can attend *l'école maternelle*, in principle a day care guarantee does exist for the older pre-school children. Likewise, Dutch pre-school children can attend nursery education from the age of four till the compulsory school age of five years.

The entitlement to social care is less institutionalised than that to cash benefits or education. In Sweden and Denmark, the guarantee is a central policy proposal which municipalities can choose to adhere to. The fulfilment of the guarantee depends on available local resources, which means that waiting lists form in many places. Local differences may also occur, and in Sweden, for example, unemployed parents may not have the right to a place in day care for their children (Socialstyrelsen 1996a). The Finnish approach of institutionalising the day care guarantee as a legal right is firmer than the Swedish and Danish arrangement and has also reduced waiting lists and local differences more rapidly. In the non-Nordic countries, too, access to nursery education is often arranged on a more compelling universal right basis.

Provision of day care for children has grown in all countries (Figure 7.5), most markedly in Norway, where total provision has increased from 19 per cent to 46 per cent of pre-school children, mainly as a result of expansion within day care centres. Denmark and Sweden have both expanded day care coverage, too, while the number of Finnish children attending day care centres even increased during the severe economic recession of 1990–94. Dutch provision has expanded, largely as a result of the financial stimulus introduced in the early 1990s, while German and French provision has strengthened, too, especially for older children. In France, the same trend has particularly involved better-off employed parents.

Does the development of day care provision ultimately lend support to the theory of a Nordic model of welfare? Looking at how they were placed in 1982 compared to 1996 as regards provision of day care groups, the countries can be divided into three groups of high, middle and low provision of day care. It is perhaps not surprising to find Denmark and Sweden as high providers of day care. But France is also in this group due to the relatively high number of children attending nursery education. Greater changes have occurred in the middle group of countries. From including only Finland and Germany in the early 1980s, this group now also embraces Norway and Britain, while Dutch provision of day care still lags behind the other countries. Yet all countries over the 15-year period expanded the number of full-time day care places quite significantly. Day care provision thus seems to accompany the increase in female labour force participation, which occurred throughout these years and in all countries.

Figure 7.5 does not show the age composition of the children in day care. The provision is generally high in the Nordic countries for smaller children aged 0–2 years, with between 20–40 per cent attending day care. French provision is also high for this age group, of whom around 35 per cent attend day nurseries and *l'école maternelle*. Thus at least France is here blurring the clear distinction between the Nordic and non-Nordic countries.

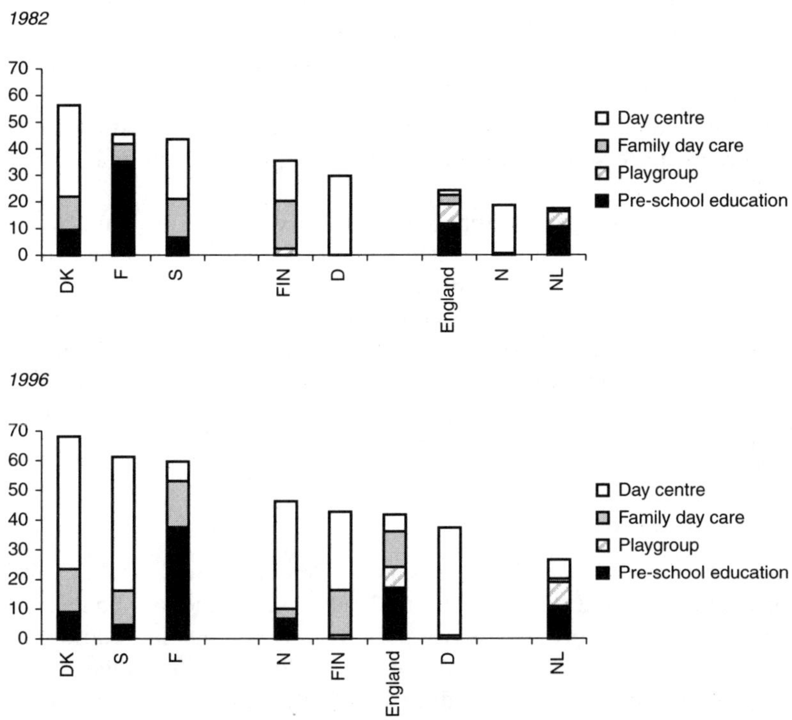

Source: Rostgaard and Fridberg 1998.

Figure 7.5 Proportion of children in day care in 1982 and 1996

Standards

The Nordic countries are, on the other hand, distinctive in terms of standards within day care services. First, day care provision is generally full-time, which covers the whole day as well as holiday periods. Parents who so wish can also opt for part-time day care. In contrast, nursery education in England, France and the Netherlands is commonly part-time; schools are often closed during lunch breaks, have shorter hours on Wednesdays, and are only open during term time. Obviously, this does not always favour parental employment.

A second distinguishing feature of the Nordic countries is high professional standards; day care provided by the social welfare systems has higher staff/child ratios and smaller group sizes than the nursery education systems elsewhere. In Britain, for example, the services provided within the education system for 3–4-year-olds have group sizes of 22–30, compared to 15–20 for the same age group in Denmark. The recommended staff ratio differs correspondingly with one adult per 10–13 children in the UK compared to one per six in Denmark. However, actual staff/child ratios may be considerably lower than those recommended (Rostgaard and Fridberg 1998). On the other hand, the professional level of staff tends to be higher in the educational services as more staff members hold formal qualifications than in the welfare system.

So some advantages are apparent in the provision of day care by the welfare system – and thus characteristic of the Nordic countries; these include full-time, year-round provision, with relatively smaller groups of children and higher staff/child ratios. Nevertheless, provision within the educational system has certain advantages as regards educational qualifications. The Nordic model therefore tends to benefit provision for smaller children particularly, whereas care models based on nursery education have certain other advantages.

Leave entitlements

The picture of child care systems is incomplete without also taking into consideration the extent of parental leave entitlements. Today, all Nordic countries provide leave periods for parents in relation to birth and during the first years of the child's life. But there is no common Nordic model regarding length of leave. The non-Nordic countries also differ significantly from each other (Figure 7.6). French and German leave benefits are similar to the Norwegian and Finnish in offering parental leave until the child is 3 years old. In France,

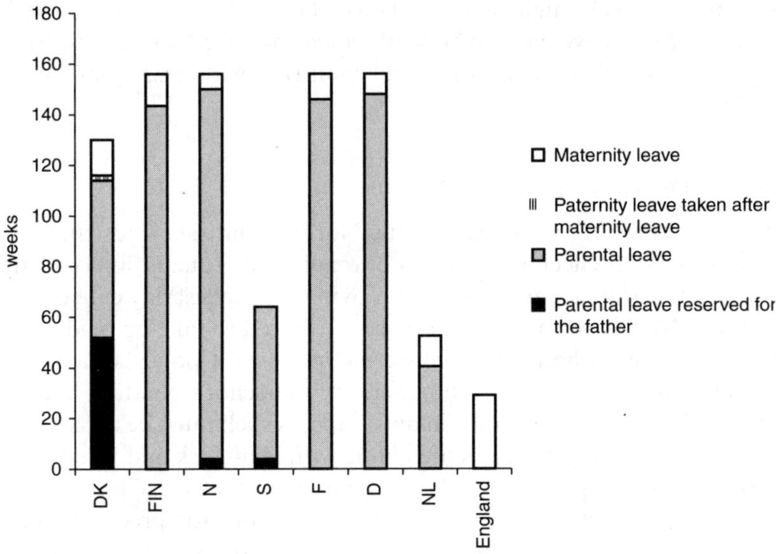

Sources: Rostgaard and Fridberg 1998; Barne-og Familiedepartementet 1998.

Figure 7.6 Length of leave after birth, weeks

however, this applies only to parents with two or more children. Britain committed itself to improve its parental leave policies in 1999 as a signatory of the European Social Charter; prior to that certain employees were only entitled to fourteen weeks of maternity leave.[10] Britain was thus the country where parents had the shortest period of leave among the countries in the period under study (Rostgaard and Fridberg 1998).

One issue is the length of leave periods, another the cash benefit parents receive during parts or the whole of the leave. If the benefit is small, the leave scheme is obviously less attractive to parents. One can consider this by including total leave entitlements in the comparison, i.e. the relation between the compensation rate and the length of leave (Rostgaard and Fridberg 1998). Traits associated with the Nordic model thereby emerge as somewhat more pronounced than before, as compensation rates multiplied by the maximum possible length of leave place Norway, Finland, Denmark and Sweden closer together than in the previous figure showing leave lengths alone. The Nordic countries are only surpassed by France, where compensation rates are relatively high (*ibid.*).[11] Thus, there are five countries with relatively good leave entitlements, of which four are Nordic countries, and a group of three non-Nordic countries with less good leave entitlements.

Gender equality

The aim of providing day care in the Nordic countries is to stimulate children both intellectually and emotionally, but equally importantly to facilitate parental employment. Enjoying the highest day care coverage rates, Nordic women should be better placed to take up paid work than women elsewhere. But France has pursued a policy which also provides day care for large numbers of pre-school children – even more so than in Norway and Finland – and as such must be considered as a woman-friendly welfare state in line with Denmark and Sweden, in particular. Although it should be borne in mind that French provision is mainly within part-time nursery education and for predominantly older children, gender equality in terms of the ability to take up work would seem to be better facilitated in these three countries.

There is also the question of whether the other facet of day care policies, the leave schemes, offer gender equality in their institutional set-up. Leave benefits are generally given as individual rights whereas entitlement depends on being a parent and not on marital status. This also applies to leave benefits in countries outside the Nordic realm. However, the low compensation rates offered in their leave schemes mean that it is mainly women who make use of them.

Unique to the Nordic countries is the introduction of a special leave for the father, sometimes termed 'daddy-days'. In the Norwegian leave scheme fathers are allowed four weeks off, and in Sweden parents may share the parental leave or choose that only one use it. Thirty days are reserved for the other parent, but if he/she does not use them they are lost. In Denmark, 12 of the 52 weeks of the child care leave are reserved for the other parent – in reality meaning the father – and fathers have recently been awarded fourteen days extra paternity leave in excess of the maternity leave (Rostgaard and Fridberg 1998). The daddy-days reflect a new emphasis on shared care responsibility and the importance of the child also spending time with the father; this phenomenon is unique to the Nordic countries.

Discussion and conclusions

Are the Nordic countries different?

With regard to health care, the eight countries do not cluster in obviously separate groups in terms of universal access, professional quality or the role of public funding. Nevertheless, there are clearly two models of financing and managing health services: the 'Bismarckian' model based on obligatory insurance funding and a greater role for non-profit providers, and the 'National Health Service' (NHS) model based on tax funding and a greater role for public providers. The United Kingdom is grouped with the Nordic countries in this perspective.

The Nordic group splits in two when it comes to care for 3 to 6-year-old children and the criteria for the degree of universalism. Denmark, Sweden and France have a high degree of universalism in practice, while Norway and Finland are left in the intermediate group. Regarding the care for children under 3 years of age, the Nordic countries are once more distinct, with more public day care, more generous parental leave schemes and novel leave for fathers of new-born children.

In terms of social care expenditure for the elderly, the Nordic countries again differ from the other four. However, when the care provided within the health sector and the variation between them are taken into account, the differences between the Nordic countries may be as great as those between the 'least universal' Nordic countries and the 'most universal' non-Nordic countries.

Much of our analysis indicates that the 'Nordic model' – if understood as the average of the four countries – is a moving target. In some respects, only Denmark and Sweden met the demands of the model in the early 1980s, e.g. in child day care and parts of the health care system. Subsequent developments in the Nordic region are often characterised as Finland and Norway accomplishing, as latecomers, the construction of their own 'Nordic' welfare state. Day care for children is a special case, because the forerunners are continuing to expand their service provision. And at the same time even the latecomers of Continental Europe have widened their child care systems to a coverage very close to the Nordic level of the early 1980s. Thus, looking at the numbers at a given moment may not be the most reliable way of generating empirical evidence for different models.

Convergence . . .

Our analysis of the health care systems reveals that differences in terms of universalism were much greater in the 1970s (OECD 1993) than in the late 1990s. There are also many indications of parallel trends in social and health care, such as:

- De-institutionalisation of long-term care for the elderly and the mentally ill, including a shift of balance from hospitals to outpatient care, from medical to non-medical care and from public to private care; also policies to create economic incentives for informal care.
- Extension of the public responsibility for care for children and the elderly, including expansion of public funding and/or provision of day care, and expansion or introduction of care insurance or care allowance schemes.
- Cost-containment and managerial reforms in the public sector – both in public provision of services and publicly funded private services, including attempts to introduce forms of competition between providers and responsiveness to user preferences.

. . . or different trajectories?

The Nordic countries and the UK have had a strong separate professional social service sector, in contrast to a much weaker independence of social care from the health and education sectors in the Continental welfare states. From the perspective of institutional structures, the insurance-based non-governmental health care structures may also be contrasted to the tax-funded governmental health care structures in terms of representation of trade union, employer and professional interests (e.g. Hassenteufel 1999; Salter 1998). These disparities in institutional structures seem to be quite persistent, even if the strong wave of New Public Management has created pressures to reduce the differences between public and the different kinds of private producers of care services.

It seems that the various institutional and political structures are tending to maintain the different developmental trajectories of their respective care systems so that the converging and parallel trends are not resulting in a more general convergence. It should also be noted that the Nordic institutional structure seems to ensure better equality between different regions and between urban and rural areas (e.g. OECD 1993; Therborn 1995; Rostgaard and Fridberg 1998; Saltman *et al.* 1998; Lehto *et al.* 1999).

With regard to health care, the Nordic systems seem more capable of containing cost expansion. We assume this is related both to the stronger development of the social care system which helps to deal with the ageing population, and to the stronger rights to the health care services. While all the countries under study are meeting the challenge of the rapid ageing of the population, the differences between the Bismarckian and Beveridgean health care systems is likely to become ever more visible.

The social service sector trajectory of the Nordic countries has led to the present significant difference between the Nordic and other welfare states. The other four countries in this regard do not show evidence of a similar trajectory, being less detached from the direct influence of the health and/or education sectors and from the residualist traditions of local social welfare. This leads us to assume that the clearly separate Nordic model of caring for the elderly will persist in the near future. The expected trajectory of care for the elderly based on care insurance modelled on sickness insurance will probably be different from the trajectory of the Nordic local public service model.

It is also quite obvious that child care systems developed from the perspective of nursery education tend to differ from those based on social care thinking. The Nordic model has led to a significant difference from other countries in terms of care for the youngest children, and this is expected to persist. There is a stronger tendency towards convergence in care systems for 3 to 6-year-old children. These systems are strongly expanding outside the Nordic countries, too, and at least Sweden, Finland and Norway also started to link this care more closely to their education systems in the 1990s.

Do politics matter?

Thus it is possible to find convergence, parallel development with different timing, and different trajectories all at the same time. And depending on one's perspective, the overall conclusion may be different. Our own conclusion tends to underline much parallel development on different trajectories and less convergence, which emphasises the differences in institutional and political structures.

Different historical service system trajectories also have their roots in the different political objectives of governments. The stronger role of the trade unions and employer organisations in shaping social policy in Germany and France has probably contributed to their difficulties in containing health care expenditure (Hassenteufel 1999). Moreover, the strong separate social care system of the Nordic countries may, at least partly, be related to the stronger role of women in the political decision-making in these countries and to perceiving the development of social care services as an important factor in advancing gender equality (Sipilä 1997). The Thatcher governments in the UK succeeded in making a difference, at least in the social care system.

It also seems that politics do matter in terms of the pressures for Western European convergence. The ideological impact of EU institutions and policies may be perceived in at least two aspects of the social and health care sector. The first is the growing support in numerous EU documents for policies – including social care policies – to facilitate female participation in the labour market. The second is the role of the EU, together with the OECD and other intergovernmental organisations, in promoting public sector reforms in line with the New Public Management ideas.

Notes

1 Collected by the Danish Social Research Institute for a comparative project on the European welfare states; main results published in Rostgaard and Fridberg (1998).
2 In Sweden, and particularly Finland, this has meant almost a complete halt in the expansion of public health expenditure during the economic recession of the early 1990s. In Denmark and Norway public health expenditure expanded more slowly than the GDP.
3 It is even more difficult to develop reliable data that would allow international comparison of expenditures on care for the elderly. Quite often it is not possible to separate expenditure on care services for the elderly from those on care services for disabled persons. We use here data from OECD Social Expenditure Data (1998). The overall numbers given in these data do not differ very much from the more detailed data collected directly from the countries and presented by Rostgaard and Fridberg (1998).
4 We assume that the proportion of private funding is highest in France, Germany and United Kingdom due to targeting public funding more tightly by socioeconomic criteria (Lewis 1998b; Rostgaard and Fridberg 1998).
5 The explanation of the radical drop in the number of hospital beds in Sweden (Figure 7.3) is due to a large number of nursing homes from the health sector being shifted to the municipal social care administration in the early 1990s (Lehto *et al.* 1999).
6 French expenditure on day care provision is, however, even higher than noted here, as expenditure for fiscal benefits is not included.
7 As mentioned earlier, countries such as England, France and Germany have had extensive public day care for pre-school children in their nursery education system.

8 Tax credits for families with children are found in most countries, but it is rarely specified that the credit is to be used for day care costs, as it is in the English scheme.
9 Parents of children 0–2 years have the right either to a place in day care or to a Home Care Allowance, whereas parents of children 3–6 years have the right to a day care place.
10 Maternity leave was 29 weeks for employees who had worked for the same employer for at least two years, for all others fourteen weeks. A proposal to extend this period to eighteen weeks with a one-year qualifying period has recently been made.
11 French average production wage (APW) base is relatively low in comparison with the other countries because of a high proportion of unskilled workers in the manufacturing industries. French compensation rates are therefore relatively high.

8 Towards activation? The changing relationship between social protection and employment in Western Europe

Bjørn Hvinden, Matti Heikkilä and Ilkka Kankare

Introduction[1]

In this chapter we examine how the relationship between employment and social protection policies was restructured in Western Europe in the course of the 1990s. We address the changes that took place on two different levels. First, we analyse the new ideas about the relationship between employment and social security arrangements, as these ideas were expressed through two supranational bodies: the Organisation for Economic Co-operation and Development (OECD) and the European Union (EU). Second, we are interested in the extent to which the new policy discourse on these issues was matched by changes in policy practice in a number of European countries, i.e. the measures and provisions aimed at people out of work.

During the 1990s the EU strengthened its involvement in the interrelated fields of employment and social protection. It formulated fairly ambitious programmes of reform and set up complex new procedures to co-ordinate, monitor and assess actual changes in the policies of member states. However, there is controversy over how much membership of the Union has so far affected the policies of member states in these areas. Until recently the dominating view was that formal decisions made by the EU have only a limited impact on the social policies of member states. For instance, there have been uncertainties over the EU's competence and the principle of subsidiarity. Member states may have been reluctant to allow the EU to take over national social policy, as this has been assumed to be an important source of legitimacy for governments. On the other hand, one may argue that processes of convergence have been under way, in spite of these formal hindrances, as member states have had to make similar adjustments to the demands of the internal market and, more generally, to fiercer international competition. More recently, it has been suggested that the procedures set up in relation to the employment strategy represent a significant step towards a *de facto* co-ordination of member states' policies.

Arguably it is still too early to assess the possible effects of such processes of convergence and co-ordination empirically. Nevertheless, we are interested to see whether various empirical indicators suggest that the policy practice of Western European countries converged in the course of the 1990s, or whether divergence and separate trajectories dominated the picture. More specifically, we ask whether there were still signs of a distinct 'Nordic model' at the end of the decade.

The new policy discourse in Western Europe

It is possible to discern three major developments in the emerging European discourse concerning the activation of social protection arrangements.

The *first* trend may be called the Europeanisation of social policy. This refers to the higher profile adopted by the EU on matters of social and employment policy previously seen as the sole responsibility of member states. In these respects an important source of inspiration has obviously been the research and recommendations made by OECD since 1990. The European Community, later the European Union, focused from the start on economic issues: promoting the free movement of commodities, labour, services and capital. But as persistent problems of unemployment and exclusion seem to hamper the progress of economies across the Union, employment issues have moved to the top of the European agenda.

A *second* central line of development is the stronger emphasis given to the inter-linkages between labour market and social security policies. Drawing on the results and recommendations already formulated by the OECD, the EU has within its employment strategy called for a shift from passive to active measures. Here 'passive measures' basically refers to cash transfers to people out of work, i.e. unemployment compensation and early retirement for labour market reasons. 'Active measures' comprise practical efforts to assist people to find or remain in paid employment and thus improve their prospects in the labour market. Such efforts range from providing opportunities for acquiring new qualifications through vocational training, offering guidance and information about vacancies, improving job-seeking skills, to various forms of job-creation through wage subsidies and placement in specially constructed job openings. Similar initiatives have been taken within the EU's programme to reform the social protection systems of member states, in order to make them more sustainable and 'employment-friendly'.

A *third* trend is the stronger emphasis on the effective use of limited resources within the social protection system of member states. This trend is partly expressed in proposals to tighten eligibility criteria, reduce the maximum benefit period and/or level of benefits, and in attempts to strengthen or reinforce conditions or requirements attached to receipt of benefits. The latter change has for instance been justified in terms of notions of reciprocity or by slogans like 'no rights without responsibilities/obligations'. In practice this means that if claimants turn down a work or training course they will be exposed to negative sanctions, such as having their benefit reduced or stopped. But the same trend has also emerged in calls for targeting resources towards those in greatest need, e.g. through greater use of income-tested benefits. We trace these three trends in somewhat greater detail.

The employment strategy

In response to growing political concern about persistent high levels of unemployment, the ministers of the OECD countries gave the organisation a mandate in 1992 to analyse the causes and consequences of high and persistent unemployment and propose effective remedies to deal with the problem (Martin 1998). Here, the need for an urgent shift from passive to active labour market measures was first put forward. Within the EU similar concerns were subsequently expressed in the common European Employment Strategy. Like the OECD, the 1994 Essen European Council emphasised the importance of examining the combined effects of the tax and income transfer systems on the job creating process (Bosco and Chassard 1999).

In 1995 the Madrid European Council recommended that the social protection system must never function as a disincentive to seeking work. This marked an important shift in the discourse, as a direct link was drawn between social protection and employment, with the social protection system now given a role in promoting labour market participation. This was elaborated in the 1997 Luxembourg and Amsterdam Councils, where the task of promoting employability was given first priority. It was argued that efficiency and equity gains were to be achieved by turning benefit systems into proactive systems seeking to improve the employability of workers. Similar aims were also expressed in the decisions made at the 1997 Luxembourg Jobs Summit. This meeting adopted the 1998 Employment Guidelines and decided that member states were to submit National Employment Action Plans (NAPs). These were to be reviewed and assessed by the Commission and other member states, as steps towards the co-ordination of member states' employment policies (EC 1997b). Later amended guidelines have been adopted for 1999 and 2000 (EC 1998a, 1999c).

In this strategy the EU has sought to encourage national governments to integrate their systems of education, taxation and income support, and to effectively involve all the relevant players (including employers and non-governmental organisations), especially at a local level. All social transfers are to be examined to see whether they could be used more effectively in promoting rehabilitation, reintegration, training and work experience. According to the 1999 Employment Guidelines each member state is expected to increase significantly the proportion of persons benefiting from active measures to the average of the three most successful member states or at least 20 per cent of the unemployed (EC 1998a). The guidelines do not call for an increase of overall expenditure but rather a restructuring of expenditure, a reform of benefit and taxation systems and a move from passive income support measures to proactive policies so as to maximise the return on existing budget outlays, and a preventative approach (EC 1997a).

Legitimising the ideological shift

The primary impetus behind the EU agenda on employment is economic: higher levels of employment are necessary to make the economies of member states more viable, as well as to finance welfare state provisions. Policy documents also emphasise the social goals of the employment strategy. Surveys across Europe have indicated that people wish to live in a healthy and affluent society, based on solidarity and equality. The new 'Social Europe' should provide citizens with opportunities for a good life, with work being considered a major factor in achieving this. The purpose of economic growth should be to improve citizens' standard of living. At the same time, people are seen to be happiest when actively involved in their social environment, in the community, and this is achieved most effectively if they are in work (EC 1997b). In combination, these assumptions provide the rationale for pursuing all possible means of reducing unemployment and increasing labour market participation. Here, the policy documents seem to imply that the individual cannot always be expected to know what is best for him or her. Thus it is the obligation of the state to assist and guide the individual, sometimes even through sanctions. Arguably, the EU's need to legitimise its employment strategy stems partly from its entry into a field previously left to national governments, and partly because it proposes that public authorities should infringe more directly on individual rights and autonomy. Legitimisation via pure economic arguments would be insufficient or problematic. By adopting the highly acceptable goal of promoting a good life for all the people of Europe, the most obvious criticism against limiting the individual's rights and freedom could be countered in advance.

An important assumption behind the recommended tightening of income maintenance schemes aimed at the unemployed has been that the benefit systems of the member states have become too accessible through eligibility rules and too generous in terms of benefit level and duration. It is assumed that these systems have negative effects both on employment and productivity. The combined result of high levels of compensation, high marginal tax rates and additional entitlements for those out of work is high net replacement rates and these are assumed to create poverty traps. For a small but significant minority of the workforce the financial incentives to find work are claimed to become negative. However, even the international organisations dealing with these issues have expressed different opinions about how important disincentives are. While the OECD (e.g. in its Jobs Study, OECD 1998d and 1998e) has more or less explicitly asserted that high replacement rates represent a real work disincentive, the International Labour Organisation (ILO 1995) has maintained that their effects are of limited impact (Bosco and Chassard 1999).

It has also been maintained that many low-skilled workers have been 'priced out' of the labour market as a result of wage floors created by relatively high minimum wages and/or relatively high welfare benefits (OECD 1998b). From this perspective an expansion of low-paid employment is part of the cure for high and persistent unemployment, and not part of the problem. At the same time long-term structural changes are believed to have diminished the opportunities for the low qualified part of the labour force. So far adult education and active labour market policies have to a small extent been able to modify this. Adult training only extends to a few, and rarely to those in the growing area of non-standard jobs; on average, only 10 per cent of the unemployed are offered training. The limited role of active efforts in many countries has been related to an understanding of unemployment as basically cyclical. Job losers were laid off temporarily until the economy picked up again and they would be rehired. This process was expected to take some months and that was how long the unemployment benefit lasted. But recent years have shown that much unemployment does not fit this model but is structural and long-term. Such unemployment is associated with diminishing employability and may lead to permanent exit from the labour market. Similarly, young people, especially those with low formal qualifications, may find it difficult to move from education to employment. For a number of reasons the educational system may be unsuccessful in providing many young people with the knowledge and skills in demand in the expanding parts of the labour market.

As there appears partly to be a qualification gap, and partly a mismatch, between the qualifications available in the labour force and those in demand, the natural solution would seem to be more vocational education, labour market training, etc. Doubts have been raised, however, about how suitable some of the existing training provisions have been for improving employability, for instance because they have been too brief, superficial and general. Both the OECD and the EU have therefore recommended a more individualised approach. Based on a thorough assessment of the unemployed person's needs and prospects, a tailor-made training plan is to be developed. The emphasis on individualisation of labour market policies is one of the major new developments in the European level discourse. Individualised services, however, are resource-intensive. Since increased spending on social benefits is out of the question, member states are advised to target their resources on those in greatest need. Many of those who have previously participated in active measures would probably have obtained a job anyhow. By contrast, many of those most in need have often been left without active measures, partly because frontline operators have recruited those they believed had the greatest chance of success in finding work, and partly because some benefit recipients have themselves been reluctant to take part (OECD 1998c).

In most Western European countries the emphasis in social protection arrangements for those out of work has traditionally been to shield people from a complete loss of income. The granting of cash benefits has rarely been linked to obligations to actively seek employment, or such obligations have not been enforced and therefore easy to evade. In the new strategy the emphasis is on active support to help people maintain or improve their skills during periods of unemployment. It seeks to promote any activity, work or training, whether full or part-time, to keep the unemployed in touch with the labour market and preserve or increase their employability, even if a job cannot be offered in the short-term perspective. This is called 're-employment insurance' in contrast to the traditional income support insurance.

While the term 'Social Europe' accentuates the social goals behind the strategy, these goals are almost exclusively approached from the direction of employment. The underlying message is that the social value of an individual is primarily determined by his/her potential contribution as a worker. The overarching operational aim is to get those able to work working and those unable to work enabled.

Modernising social protection

Many of the concerns of the employment strategy are reiterated within the EU's programme for modernising the social protection systems of member states, while others are also added. We will here concentrate on those aspects relating to the *public income maintenance* of member states. The EU's impetus has partly been the growing costs of these systems and the threat they are perceived to represent to public budget balances both in the short and long run. Some of the costs are directly related to higher levels of cyclical and/or structural labour market problems, such as spending on unemployment compensation. But there has also been considerable concern about increased costs of other parts of the income maintenance system. These prospects have in themselves led to a general search for ways of controlling the growth and perhaps even of reducing the costs of income maintenance schemes. Key objectives have been to make income maintenance systems more sustainable (particularly pension schemes) and make work pay, i.e. to prevent social protection schemes from creating disincentives to work.

Furthermore, the EU has emphasised that member states need to make better use of the resources available for income maintenance and other forms of social protection. These systems are also to promote social inclusion, for instance by 'fostering active rather than passive measures and by providing incentives and pathways to (re) integration into the labour market and society' (EC 1999a: 14; see also EC 1997c). By integrating social protection and taxation these systems are to be developed into an integral part of an active employment policy (EC 1997c: 3 and 10–11). Finally, it is worth noting that the European Commission in other contexts has referred also to the overall structure of income maintenance systems of member countries. For instance, it has observed that 'although attempts have been made in most member States to target social protection on those most in need, benefits subject to means-testing . . . still account for *only a small* proportion of spending across the Union' (EC 1998c: 68, our emphasis).

Was the emerging discourse equally 'new' to all?

Thirty years of comparative analysis of the welfare states in Western Europe have demonstrated far more variation and divergence than trends towards convergence (see overviews by Finer 1999; Mabbett and Bolderson 1999). A differentiated picture has emerged from research using quantitative cross-sectional data, as well as from more detailed case studies based on historical and qualitative material. This variability suggests that the Western European welfare states had extremely different points of departure in relation to the new policy discourse, as we have outlined it here.

Generally speaking, the new discourse represented less of a break with previous understandings and existing practices in some countries than in others. More specifically, the Nordic countries, and Sweden and Norway in particular, had a long tradition of activist and employment-oriented social policies (Rehn 1988; Wilensky 1992; Hvinden 1994, 1999; Lindqvist and Marklund 1995; Drøpping *et al.* 1999). In both Sweden and Norway the whole income maintenance system from its start fifty to sixty years ago was based on many of the ideas currently presented as 'new'. In both countries one spoke about the 'work option' in contrast to the 'benefit option'. According to the 'work option' there should be direct links between the income maintenance system (both the nationalised social insurance and the local social assistance parts) and the labour market services. For instance, it was an important part of the mandate of the income maintenance schemes to maximise labour market participation. No person was supposed to be granted long-term public income support until all possibilities for making the person self-sufficient through entry or return to employment had been exhausted. This principle was closely related to the governments' commitment to full employment and active labour market policies (ALMP). Such policies were originally adopted as an integrated part of attempts to facilitate and speed up structural change in the labour market. By means of guidance, job brokerage, job subsidisation, training measures and support to move to another part of the country, ALMP were designed to stimulate both labour demand and supply, and improve the match between them. Admittedly, these work-oriented policies were exposed to various forms of policy erosion after they were originally formulated, partly by design and partly through adjustments by the agencies responsible for their implementation. Still, what happened from the late 1980s was not really the invention of a new policy, but largely a return to or a revival of policies with a long tradition in Norway and Sweden. In the two other Nordic countries it may seem more appropriate to talk about a shift in the policy discourse, especially in Denmark (cf. Drøpping *et al.* 1999).

If we turn to the other Western European countries a discontinuity from earlier policies was even more evident. In some of these countries, e.g. the United Kingdom, the balance between income maintenance and labour market policies was notably different, and the boundaries between them more sharply drawn, than in the Nordic countries. Here the long-term separation between these and other public provisions and services had partly been based on notions about the integrity of the individual and the inviolability of his or her entitlement to cash benefits. Consequently, ideas about 'linking welfare and work' and making the social protection system 'more employment-friendly' represented a more dramatic challenge to established ideas, principles and perceptions in these countries.

How did policy practice change in Western Europe in the 1990s?

The national governments of Western Europe have had different options for responding to the concerns and recommendations that have emerged in the recent discourse. The options have been constrained by various factors: the history of national protection systems, existing configurations of provisions, institutionalised expectations from different corporate actors, political constellations, as well as dissimilar financial pressures and degrees of freedom. It is important to emphasise, however, that hardly any government has been dictated to solely by circumstances but has had some element of choice. Although they might have moved more or less in the same direction governments were also likely to have given dissimilar weight to various considerations and aims, and consequently constructed somewhat different 'packages' of measures. On the basis of the recent discourse on social protection for people of working age, we can assume that national governments have considered taking the following steps:

- giving more emphasis to active efforts;
- reducing the level of cash benefits;
- reducing the maximum length of benefit periods;

- tightening eligibility criteria or enforcing such criteria more stringently;
- strengthening conditions for the continued receipt of benefits;
- shifting the emphasis from non-means-tested to means-tested benefits.

We will examine the extent to which the governments in sixteen Western European countries introduced such policy measures in the 1990s. In this examination we are constrained by the quality, completeness and comparability of existing macro-data. In principle we would have preferred to be able to collect original data from national sources. But available resources have not permitted data collection in all the sixteen countries. Being faced with the choice between using data collected by others, mainly the OECD and the EU/Eurostat, and concentrating on a smaller number of countries where we could have collected data ourselves, we have in this article opted for the first alternative. The main reason is that we are interested in drawing a general picture and in identifying some important overall trends. This means that various forms of simplification are called for, and that we will have to disregard much of the inter-country nuances in the processes we are dealing with.

One critical question is of course how to operationalise a shift to more active efforts in social protection. In the absence of better indicators we will use a change in spending on active measures, as percentage of the gross domestic product (GDP). The idea here is that the size of the GDP determines the amount of resources a national economy has available for different purposes, and that the proportion of GDP spent on active measures is a crude expression of the priority given to activation policies.[2] Obviously this proportion does not say anything about how sensibly or wisely the resources are spent. It would have been good to have other and supplementary indicators, e.g. the proportion of people out of work who are taking part in active measures. Although the European Union has started to request member states to provide this kind of information as part of their NAPs, no time series for the 1990s exist. Moreover, even this indicator has its limitations, as it says nothing about the duration of participation or the quality of the training, etc., provided.

Doubts may also be raised about the comparability of the figures for unemployment rates and labour market participation ratios. The OECD has sought to standardise the figures they collect from national sources. Still one may wonder whether the OECD has succeeded in correcting for all the variations in how national employment statistics treat various groups at the margin of the labour market (e.g. students, homemakers or disabled people who would prefer to work or work more than they do). But for the purposes of this article we assume that the OECD's figures give a fairly reliable picture of the overall trends in the labour market of Western Europe in the 1990s. Thus we presuppose here that the level of unemployment was higher in 1997 than in 1990 in most Western European countries. The exceptions were Denmark, Norway, the Netherlands, Ireland and the United Kingdom (Table 8.1). In the same period, the overall labour market participation is taken to have increased – to a smaller or greater extent – in half of the countries (Norway, France, Germany, Luxembourg, the Netherlands, Greece, Spain and Ireland). This implies that the labour market trends of the 1990s did not fall into any simple and straightforward pattern conforming with the usual groupings of welfare states (e.g. the four-fold division between Nordic, Continental, Mediterranean and Anglo-Saxon countries adopted in this chapter).

Spending on active measures

Governments appeared to have spent more on active measures in 1997 than in 1990 in a majority of eleven countries (Table 8.2). But these figures for spending on active measures are misleading if we do not take into account that the unemployment rates were higher in eight of the eleven countries in 1997 than in 1990. Moreover, we see that in six of the eleven countries expenditure on passive measures had also grown in the same period. Thus it is not clear that the overall balance between spending on active and passive measures changed in the direction recommended by the OECD and the EU.

Arguably, if two countries have the same level of spending on active efforts it is reasonable to see the country with the lowest unemployment rate as the more 'activist' of the two, *ceteris paribus*. One way to take into account that levels of unemployment are dissimilar from the start and change differently in the countries and period under study, is to standardise the expenditure figures.[3] We may calculate what the expenditure figures would have been *hypothetically*, if all countries had an unemployment rate of 10 per cent *and* spent the same amount of resources for each per cent unemployed as they did with their actual level of unemployment. We do not have strong reasons for believing that the countries would have had this level of spending if their unemployment rate had been 10 per cent, as this would depend

Table 8.1 Labour market performance: Standardised unemployment rates, overall labour market participation rates for sixteen Western European countries in 1990 and 1997 (both sexes) and per cent change from 1990 to 1997

	Unemployment			*Overall labour market participation*		
	1990	*1997*	*% change*	*1990*	*1997*	*% change*
Denmark	7.7	5.6	−27	83.1	80.8	−3
Finland	3.2	12.7	297	77.1	72.6	−6
Norway	5.3	4.1	−23	78.0	80.6	3
Sweden (c)	2.4	9.9	313	82.7	75.0	−9
Mean	*4.7*	*8.1*	*74*	*80.2*	*77.3*	*−4*
Austria	3.0	4.5	50	67.4	66.8	−1
Belgium	6.7	9.2	38	61.9	66.6	3
France	9.0	12.3	37	66.6	67.2	2
Germany (a)	4.8	9.9	106	69.1	68.5	−1
Luxembourg	1.7	2.8	65	62.1	62.5	1
Netherlands	6.2	5.2	−16	58.2	63.8	10
Mean	*5.2*	*7.3*	*40*	*64.2*	*65.9*	*3*
Greece	6.4	9.6	50	59.0	60.8	1
Italy (b)	9.1	12.0	32	58.9	57.7	−2
Portugal	4.6	7.3	59	72.2	68.2	−6
Spain	16.2	20.8	28	61.3	62.3	2
Mean	*9.2*	*12.4*	*37*	*62.9*	*62.3*	*−1*
Ireland (b)	13.4	11.6	−13	61.9	64.2	4
UK (c)	8.0	7.6	−5	76.4	75.3	−1
Mean	*10.7*	*9.6*	*−10*	*69.2*	*69.8*	*1*

Sources: OECD 1999a: Table A and OECD 1999b: Table 1.1 for unemployment; OECD 1998g: Annex Table 19 for labour market participation.

Notes:

a 1990 figures refer to West Germany before unification.

b 1996 figures instead of 1997 figures.

c 1990 figures are averages of 1990 and 1991 figures, for the United Kingdom the 1997 figure is an average of 1996 and 1997.

on other factors (e.g. political priorities or concerns about the deficit in government finances). Rather, the point of calculating these contrafactual figures is to be able to compare the overall profile of different countries' expenditure. Moreover, the standardised figures highlight how spending on active and passive measures has changed in the sixteen countries *relative* to their levels of unemployment. The results of this standardisation exercise are presented in Table 8.3.

Table 8.2 Unstandardised expenditure on active and passive labour market measures in sixteen Western European countries in 1990 and 1997 as a proportion of GDP and per cent change from 1990 to 1997

	Active labour market measures			*Passive labour market measures*		
	1990	*1997*	*% change*	*1990*	*1997*	*% change*
Denmark	1.26	1.80	43	4.40	4.02	–9
Finland	1.01	1.57	55	1.16	3.21	177
Norway	1.01	0.98	–3	1.18	0.70	–41
Sweden (c)	1.69	2.09	24	0.88	2.16	145
Mean	*1.24*	*1.61*	*30*	*1.9*	*2.5*	*32*
Austria	0.31	0.45	45	0.97	1.28	32
Belgium	1.17	1.29	10	2.65	2.67	1
France	0.80	1.37	71	1.87	1.80	–4
Germany (a)	1.03	1.25	21	1.10	2.55	132
Luxembourg	0.36	0.30	–17	0.73	0.67	–8
Netherlands	1.04	1.65	59	2.17	3.63	67
Mean	*0.39*	*1.05*	*34*	*1.58*	*2.1*	*33*
Greece	0.50	0.35	–30	0.43	0.50	16
Italy (b)	0.65	1.08	66	0.84	0.88	5
Portugal	0.72	0.87	21	0.42	0.91	117
Spain	0.76	0.56	–26	2.42	1.88	–22
Mean	*0.66*	*0.72*	*9*	*1.03*	*1.04*	*1*
Ireland	1.51	1.66	10	2.88	2.42	–16
UK (c)	0.61	0.42	–31	0.95	1.05	11
Mean	*1.06*	*1.04*	*–2*	*1.92*	*1.74*	*–9*

Source: OECD 1994: Table 1.B.2; 1998c: Table 1 and 1999a: Table B.

Notes:

a 1990 figures refer to West Germany before unification.

b 1996 figures instead of 1997 figures.

c 1990 figures refer to the financial year 1990–91, for the UK 1997 figure refers to the financial year 1996–97.

Only six countries – Denmark, Norway, France, the Netherlands, Italy and Ireland – increased their standardised spending on active measures between 1990 and 1997 (Table 8.3). Why was this so? One interpretation is that decision-makers in the majority of the sixteen countries primarily saw increased active efforts as representing increased total social protection costs in the short-term perspective and an investment where the possible return was uncertain and/or not likely to appear until much later. Not only did most of the countries

Table 8.3 Standardised expenditure on active and passive labour market measures in sixteen Western European countries in 1990 and 1997 as a proportion of GDP and per cent change from 1990 to 1997

	Active labour market measures			*Passive labour market measures*		
	1990	*1997*	*% change*	*1990*	*1997*	*% change*
Denmark	1.64	3.21	96	5.71	7.18	25
Finland	3.16	1.24	−61	3.63	2.53	−30
Norway	1.91	2.39	25	2.23	1.70	−24
Sweden (c)	7.04	2.11	−70	3.67	2.18	−40
Mean	*3.44*	*2.23*	*−35*	*3.81*	*3.40*	*−11*
Austria	1.03	1.0	−3	3.23	2.84	−12
Belgium	1.75	1.40	−61	3.95	2.90	−27
France	0.89	1.10	24	2.08	1.46	−30
Germany (a)	2.15	1.26	−41	2.29	2.58	13
Luxembourg	2.12	1.07	−50	4.29	2.39	−44
Netherlands	1.68	3.17	89	3.50	6.98	99
Mean	*1.60*	*1.50*	*−6*	*3.2*	*3.2*	*−1*
Greece	0.78	0.36	−54	0.67	0.52	−22
Italy (b)	0.71	0.90	27	0.92	0.73	−21
Portugal	1.57	1.19	−24	0.91	1.25	40
Spain	0.47	0.27	−43	1.49	0.90	−40
Mean	*0.88*	*0.68*	*−23*	*1.00*	*0.88*	*−15*
Ireland (b)	1.13	1.43	27	2.15	2.09	−3
UK (c)	0.76	0.55	−27	1.19	1.38	16
Mean	*0.95*	*0.99*	*5*	*1.67*	*1.70*	*4*

Sources: For original (unstandardised) expenditure figures see OECD 1994: Table 1.B.2, OECD 1998f: Table 1 and OECD 1999a: Table B. For standardised figures for unemployment see OECD 1999a: Table A and OECD 1999b: Table 1.1.

Notes:

a 1990 figures refer to West Germany before unification.

b 1996 figures instead of 1997 figures.

c Expenditure figures for 1990 refer to the financial year 1990–91, for the UK 1997 figure refers to the financial year 1996–97.

become less activist, we can also observe a trend towards less dispersion in the degree of activism between the sixteen countries over the period studied here.[4] Thus there appeared to be a trend towards convergence, but not in the direction recommended by the OECD and the EU.

It is also worth noting that the inter-country pattern of changes in degree of activism cuts across the four-fold grouping of welfare states mentioned previously: two Nordic countries, two Continental countries, one Mediterranean and one Anglo-Saxon country became more activist. However, if we compare the situations in 1990 and 1997, the average level of standardised spending on active measures remained highest in the Nordic group throughout the period. The level of active spending continued to be somewhat lower in the Continental group, with the Anglo-Saxon and Mediterranean groups in third and fourth place, respectively (Table 8.3).

If we turn to the expenditure on passive measures, we see that ten of the sixteen countries reduced their spending, relative to their level of unemployment, in the same period. The exceptions were Denmark, Germany, the Netherlands, Portugal and the United Kingdom. Again, the countries in question were scattered across the four groups of welfare states. But the average level of spending on passive measures remained highest in the Nordic group during the period from 1990 to 1997. The Continental group followed closely behind, while the average levels of expenditure were considerably lower in the Anglo-Saxon and Mediterranean groups throughout the period.

All in all, the sixteen countries appeared to be more successful in limiting their expenditure on passive measures than on broadening their active efforts, when we take into account their official levels of unemployment. Two countries stand out: Denmark and the Netherlands; in relation to the recommendations from the OECD their achievements appear ambiguous, as in the period under study they increased their spending on *both* active and passive measures. To the extent that the figures presented here reflect reality we would expect that many of the sixteen countries had reduced benefit levels or length of benefit periods, tightened eligibility criteria or conditions, or achieved some combination of such measures.

Benefit levels[5]

The findings of OECD (1999b: 49 and 111, 1999c: 93–4) surveys indicate that the level of cash benefits for the unemployed was cut back in ten of the sixteen countries during the 1990s. The exceptions were spread across the four groups of welfare states (Norway, Luxembourg, Greece, Italy, Portugal and the United Kingdom, cf. Table 8.6). In one country, France, the reduction in benefit level was later to some extent reversed. Similarly, Sweden reversed changes introduced in the early 1990s. Payment benefits and other unemployment-related benefits were increased in Greece and Italy, albeit from very low levels.

OECD estimates reveal substantial variations in the net replacement rates at the end of the period. The net replacement rate refers to the calculated proportion of expected income from work that is replaced by unemployment and related benefits after tax (Martin 1998: 23). The estimated net replacement rate for a single person for the first month of unemployment ranged from 33 per cent (Ireland) to 86 per cent (Luxembourg), with an average of 65 per cent (OECD 1999b: 112). If we take into account different family types and compare the average level of net replacement within the four groups of welfare states, the Nordic and Continental groups appeared to be about equally generous, while the Mediterranean and Anglo-Saxon groups were somewhat less so (*ibid.*).

Benefit duration

The OECD surveys (1999b, 1999c) indicate that the maximum duration of unemployment benefit was reduced, during the 1990s, especially for young unemployed people, in seven of the sixteen countries. Again, those in question were scattered across the four groups of welfare states (Denmark, Norway, Belgium, Germany, the Netherlands, Greece and the United Kingdom, cf. Table 8.6). In contrast, France increased the duration of unemployment benefit for older unemployed persons (fifty years and over).

Eligibility criteria

The OECD (1999c: 93–4) suggests that nine of the sixteen countries made eligibility criteria for unemployment benefit stricter in the course of the 1990s. This happened in all four Nordic countries and in some of those in the other three groups (cf. Table 8.6). Four of the nine countries also introduced stricter conditions for sick pay and invalidity benefit, as did two additional countries (OECD 1999b: 49).

Conditions for continued receipt of benefits

Ten of the sixteen countries introduced stricter conditions of 'work availability' or 'willingness to work' during the decade (OECD 1999c: 93–4). Such changes took place in the majority of both Nordic and Continental countries, and in half of those in the two other groups (cf. Table 8.6).

Role of means-tested assistance

There were striking differences in the proportion of all social benefits expenditure paid out as means-tested support between the sixteen countries, and these differences remained surprisingly stable in the 1990s (Table 8.4). Ireland, the United Kingdom and Finland had the highest mean-tested benefits share; in the former two this was related to the low level of old age pensions (Ditch 1999). In the case of Finland the flat-rate old age pension was reformed in 1996 to become income-tested. In many countries the number of lone parents claiming social assistance increased, with their proportion of all recipients being particularly high in the United Kingdom and Finland.

Moreover, some countries also had a high proportion of unemployed people claiming means-tested assistance in the 1990s, either as their main source of income or as supplement to other benefits. This is related to the design of the overall income maintenance systems for people out of work. Means-tested unemployment assistance had no or only a marginal role in the Nordic countries (except Finland[6]), in Continental countries like Belgium, France and Luxembourg, and in Mediterranean countries such as Greece and Italy. In Finland, a means-tested scheme, 'labour market support', was introduced in 1994. In the Netherlands, Ireland and the United Kingdom means-tested unemployment assistance played a key role in the 1990s and became more important in Austria and Germany (EC 1998c: 69). The proportion of total expenditure on benefits related to unemployment provided as unemployment assistance more or less increased in nine countries in the period from 1990 to 1997 (Table 8.4). As already indicated, these nine countries were spread across the four groups of welfare states.

Was there a distinct Nordic model at the end of the 1990s?

One way of approaching this question is to examine the extent to which countries belonging to the four groups of welfare states exhibited traits usually associated with the 'Nordic model'. Broadly speaking, the Nordic model could be said to be associated with the following characteristics (e.g. Esping-Andersen 1990, 1999):[7]

- strong emphasis on active efforts;
- generous income maintenance for people out of work;
- low reliance on the use of means-tested benefits;
- low level of unemployment;
- high level of labour market participation.

Table 8.4 Expenditure on means-tested benefits as proportion of (a) total social benefit expenditure and (b) total expenditure on benefits related to unemployment in sixteen Western European countries in 1990 and 1997, and per cent change from 1990 to 1997

	All expenditure on means-tested benefits as percentage of total benefit expenditure			*All expenditure on particular means-tested benefits to unemployed people as percentage of total expenditure on benefits related to unemployment*		
	1990	*1997*	*% change*	*1990*	*1997*	*% change*
Denmark	3	3	10	–	–	–
Finland	12	15	28	16	23	40
Norway	3	2	−16	–	–	–
Sweden (b)	7	6	−6	–	–	–
Mean	*6*	*7*	*4*			
Austria	4	4	0	19	22	19
Belgium	5	4	−19	–	–	–
France	9	12	27	8	9	7
Germany (a)	8	10	15	14	17	22
Luxembourg	–	–	–	–	–	–
Netherlands	10	7	−23	56	49	−13
Mean	*7*	*7*	*3*			
Greece	6	9	49	1	3	177
Italy	8	6	−16	–	–	–
Portugal	7	7	−4	22	23	5
Spain	14	13	−6	24	25	3
Mean	*9*	*9*	*0*			
Ireland	32	33	3	69	71	4
UK	17	19	12	43	45	3
Mean	*25*	*26*	*6*			

Source: Eurostat 2000.

Notes:

a 1990 figures refer to West Germany before unification.

b 1990 figure refers to 1993.

Again we use standardised spending on active measures as an indicator of degree of activism or emphasis on active efforts. We use standardised spending on passive measures as a proxy for overall generosity of the income maintenance system for people out of work. Clearly it is not a goal in itself for any government to have a high expenditure on such benefits. Broadly speaking, the standardised spending on passive measures will be a product of the average level of benefits and the average length of the period in which people receive benefits. In this sense a high proportion of long-term unemployment will inflate the spending figure.

Table 8.5 summarises and simplifies the information previously provided in Tables 8.1, 8.3 and 8.4. First, we see that the four Nordic countries all in all came close to the Nordic ideal-type in 1997, given the way in which we have operationalised the five characteristics here. Finland emerged, however, as the least 'Nordic', on account of its reliance on means-tested support and level of unemployment in the late 1990s.

Second, we note that the Continental group of countries had several of the assumed 'Nordic' characteristics, especially in terms of their level of expenditure on passive measures, in 1997. Given the limitations of the indicator adopted here, it is significant that the OECD estimates referred to previously did not show any clear differences in net replacement rates between the Nordic and Continental groups of welfare states (OECD 1999b: 112).

Third, we can observe that the countries belonging to the Mediterranean and Anglo-Saxon groups had very few, if any, of the assumed 'Nordic' characteristics in 1997.

In conclusion, Table 8.5 suggests that there was a rough correspondence between the ideal-type Nordic model and the empirical characteristics of the Nordic welfare states of the late 1990s in the field of social protection for people out of work. At the same time, the Continental countries also exhibited several of the characteristics of this model. On this basis, doubts may be raised about how *distinct* the situation in the Nordic countries was at this particular point of time and in this area of social protection.

Strategies of reform: alternative or complementary options?

We are interested in the extent to which the sixteen Western European countries adopted the same overall strategies in response to the challenges they faced in the 1990s, or whether there were distinct differences between the policy choices of their governments. More specifically, we ask whether these choices emerge as *alternatives* or as *complementary*. When choices are regarded as alternatives, this roughly means that governments choose between option A *or* option B (*or* option C, etc.). When choices are perceived as complementary, it implies that governments may consider different *combinations* of options as most appropriate and desirable (e.g. option A *and* option B, option A *and*

Table 8.5 Summary Table: Levels of expenditure on active and passive measures, reliance on means-tested support for the unemployed, and unemployment and labour market participation in 1997 in sixteen Western European countries

	A. Expenditure active measures	*B. Expenditure passive measures*	*C. Reliance on means-tested support*	*D. Unemployment rate*	*E. Labour market participation rate*
Denmark	High	High	Low	Low	High
Finland	High	High			High
Norway	High		Low	Low	High
Sweden	High	High	Low		High
Austria		High		Low	
Belgium	High	High	Low	Low	
France			Low		High
Germany	High	High			High
Luxembourg		High	Low	Low	
Netherlands	High	High		Low	
Greece			Low		
Italy			Low		
Portugal				Low	High
Spain					
Ireland	High				
UK				Low	High

Explanation:

'A. Expenditure active measures' – level of standardised spending on active measures (cf. Table 8.3)

'B. Expenditure passive measures' – level of standardised spending on passive measures (cf. Table 8.3)

'C. Reliance on means-tested support' – level of expenditure on particular means-tested support for the unemployed, as proportion of total benefit expenditure related to unemployment (cf. Table 8.4)

'D. Unemployment rate' – level of standardised unemployment rate (cf. Table 8.1)

'E. Labour market participation rate' – level of overall labour market participation rate for people of both sexes (cf. Table 8.1)

'High' if level above median (in the cases of columns A, B and E) and 'Low' if level below median (in the cases of columns C and D). Only the coding of these values are presented as they are associated with the ideal-type 'Nordic model', and since we want to render a visually clear impression of the degree of 'Nordicness' of the four groups of welfare states.

option C, etc.). More specifically, we ask to what extent governments appeared to have seen a shift towards more active efforts and various forms of tightening the income support system for unemployed people as alternative or complementary options in the 1990s. The following discussion refers to the summary presented in Table 8.6.

First, we note that in the cases of Luxembourg and Portugal no adoption of specific policy instruments is reported in the sources available to us. Thus there seems to be no change in the overall policy configurations in these countries, as measured here. Obviously this also amounts to a form of choice, but we still exclude Luxembourg and Portugal from further discussion.

Second, we start with the four different forms of changes in the income maintenance benefits for the unemployed (columns 2–5 in Table 8.6). All fourteen countries adopted at least one of these measures, and eleven introduced two or more of them in the 1990–97 period. We interpret this as meaning that a majority of the governments perceived these measures as complementing each other, not as mutually excluding alternatives. We find these governments spread over all four groups of welfare states.

Third, we note that in four countries the introduction of changes in the income support system for the unemployed was accompanied by a greater take-up of special means-tested assistance for the unemployed (column 6). Admittedly, in the case of Greece such assistance continued to have a small and marginal role. In the cases of Finland, Austria and Germany we are talking about more significant increases, which may or may not be the result of planned changes in the overall income maintenance system for people out of work. However, in these three countries a *de facto* move towards greater reliance on means-tested support appeared to complement the attempts to tighten up the unemployment benefit system.

Fourth, we draw attention to the relationship between increases in spending on active measures (column 1) on the one hand and attempts to tighten up the unemployment benefit system (columns 2–5) and/or *de facto* greater reliance on social assistance (column 6) on the other hand. We can here make the observation that all six countries that expanded their active efforts (relative to their unemployment levels) *also* undertook changes on the income maintenance side (Denmark, Norway, France, the Netherlands, Italy and Ireland). For these countries the two kinds of measures were clearly *complementary*. In the eight other countries changes in the income maintenance system appeared to have played the main role (Finland, Sweden, Austria, Belgium, Germany, Greece, Spain and the United Kingdom). Thus for a majority of the countries, attempts to tighten up the unemployment benefit systems served largely as an *alternative* to an expansion of active measures. We also note that the two groups of countries cut across the four-fold classification of welfare states.

Finally, we can also observe that four of the six countries adopting the complementary strategy (Denmark, Norway, the Netherlands and Ireland) *decreased* their level of unemployment from 1990 to 1997. This was the case with only one of the eight countries (the United Kingdom) pursuing the alternative strategy (column 7). Moreover, four of the six countries adopting the complementary strategy (Norway, France, the Netherlands and Ireland) *increased* their overall labour market participation rate in the same period. However, this was also the case for three of the eight countries in the other group (Belgium, Greece and Spain). Thus adoption of the complementary strategy was weakly correlated with an increase in participation. Finally, these findings suggest that many countries found it difficult to decrease unemployment *and* increase labour market participation *at the same time* (compare Denmark and France in the group adopting the complementary strategy, and Belgium, Greece, Spain and the United Kingdom in the group pursuing the alternative strategy).

How were policy changes related to the structure of the benefit system?

We have seen that there were substantial variations in the role that means-tested financial support played within the overall income maintenance system of the sixteen countries under study. There could be reasons for expecting that countries with a large proportion of social benefits provided as means-tested support would be more concerned to tighten up the income maintenance system for people out of work. Beneficiaries of social insurance or contributory schemes have usually been seen as enjoying greater legitimacy and 'deservingness', and thus clearer entitlement, than recipients of means-tested assistance. More specifically, the use of work requirements and negative sanctions against those who do not comply with such requirements – 'work for benefit' or 'workfare' schemes – have tended to be associated with means-tested assistance (e.g. Hanesch 1999; Lødemel and Trickey 2000).

On the other hand, beneficiaries of social insurance, such as unemployment insurance, have in many countries enjoyed somewhat more generous levels of payment than those who must rely solely on social assistance. One could therefore argue that governments might

Table 8.6 Summary Table: Policy measures adopted during the 1990s and overall labour market trends between 1990 and 1997 in sixteen Western European countries

	Measures adopted ('policy inputs')						*Labour market trends ('outcomes')*	
	1. Increased active efforts	*2. Reduced benefit levels*	*3. Reduced benefit duration*	*4. Tighter eligibility criteria*	*5. Tighter availability criteria*	*6. Increased role of means-tested benefits*	*7. Reduced unemployment*	*8. Increased labour market participation*
Denmark	X	X	X	X	X		X	
Finland		X		X	X	X		
Norway	X		X	X			X	X
Sweden		(x)		X	X			
Austria		X		X		X		
Belgium		X	X		X			X
France	X	(x)			X			X
Germany		X	X	X	X	X		
Luxembourg								X
Netherlands	X	X	X	X	X		X	X
Greece			X			X		X
Italy	X				X			
Portugal								
Spain		X		X	X			X
Ireland	X	X					X	X
UK			X	X	X		X	

Explanation:
'1. Increased active effort' – increased standardised spending on active measures (cf. Table 8.3)
'2. Reduced benefit level' – reduction in unemployment benefit levels (OECD 1999b and 1999c)
'3. Reduced benefit duration' – reduction in maximum unemployment benefit duration (OECD 1999b and 1999c)
'4. Tighter eligibility criteria' – tightening of eligibility criteria for unemployment benefit (OECD 1999b and 1999c)
'5. Tighter availability criteria' – tightening of work availability criteria for continued receipt of unemployment benefit (OECD 1999b and 1999c)
'6. Increased role of means-tested benefits'– expenditure on particular means-tested assistance for the unemployed, as proportion of total benefit expenditure related to unemployment, increased by more than 10 per cent (cf. Table 8.4)
'7. Reduced unemployment' – standardised unemployment rate reduced more than 10 per cent (cf. Table 8.1)
'8. Increased labour market participation' – increased overall labour market participation rate for people of both sexes (cf. Table 8.1)
X if yes, (x) if change later reversed to some extent

Note:
Even if no reform (columns 1–6) is reported in the cases of Luxembourg and Portugal, in the sources adopted here these two countries are still included as a matter of completeness. Even a lack of (reported) reforms is significant, as illustrated by Luxembourg, which nevertheless increased its labour market participation in the period.

have perceived a greater 'need' to tighten up social insurance schemes and/or introduce mechanisms to prevent people remaining beneficiaries for a long time, for example, by strengthening requirements about availability or actively seeking work. As we have seen, however, the trend towards tightening up benefit schemes was so general (Table 8.6) that it is impossible to identify a greater tendency to do so among countries with a high or low proportion of spending on means-tested assistance. But without exception the countries that increased their active efforts were different from those where spending on means-tested assistance grew in the 1990s (Table 8.6). This lends additional support to the idea that governments had *alternative* courses of action available to them in the 1990s.

Building on Ditch (1999), we can identify some general characteristics and trends in the conditions set for eligibility and continued receipt of means-tested assistance. All the Western European countries operated some form of 'work test' for people of working age claiming means-tested benefits. In the great majority of countries, this usually required that recipients register as unemployed and establish that they were actively looking for work. Work tests could also be applied informally through the basic conditions of eligibility. In virtually all countries, work tests were not applied, or were more relaxed, for people who were ill or experienced disabilities, or who were over or approaching retirement age. The major variations related to single parents, in particular to those with young children who exempted them from the requirement to actively seek work. Remarkably liberal provisions applied in the United Kingdom, where single parents were not required to seek work until their youngest child was sixteen years (or older) (Eardley *et al.* 1996). Germany was also relatively liberal in this respect, single parents normally being required to seek part-time work when their youngest child was at school and full-time work when the child was fourteen or over.

Most means-tested assistance schemes employed sanctions against those who failed the work tests. Sanctions ranged from full loss of benefits either through ineligibility or suspension, or loss of part of benefits for defined periods. There were, however, also schemes offering positive incentives to return to work or to set up as self-employed. Specific incentives could be identified, e.g. in the Netherlands, Norway, Sweden and the United Kingdom. In most cases, these appeared to be small extra supplements, or lump-sum grants, although a number of countries also made available loans and grants under their various special assistance arrangements for people wanting to start up in self-employment.

In summary, there appeared to be a general trend towards stricter enforcement of 'availability for work' and 'actively searching for work'. This was, however, not only the case for those living on means-tested benefits but also for the beneficiaries of unemployment insurance schemes. Similarly, stricter sanctions were adopted against those who refused offers of jobs or training, or who left jobs 'without good cause'. More attention is now given to all forms of 'benefit abuse' – broadly understood – and abuse is also reacted against more actively through prosecution, disentitlement to benefits for extended periods, etc.

At the same time we may ask to what extent the recent trend towards negative sanctions and coercion was experienced more strongly by people claiming means-tested assistance than by social insurance beneficiaries. Ultimately, this question can probably only be answered through studies of local-level practice in each country. We would want to study how and to what extent the various types of requirements or conditionalities were actually implemented in practice. What degree of choice or form of co-determination was the individual provided with? How frequently were benefit payments actually reduced, suspended or stopped as a sanction against non-compliance with agency requirements? The likelihood of this happening would probably be affected by the fact that means-tested assistance is meant to be a 'last resort' scheme, when all other sources of income, including social insurance benefits, have been exhausted.

In his survey of the recent developments toward activation in Danish social policy, Abrahamson (1998: 14–15) argues that there are significant differences in emphasis between activation measures related to the social insurance system and those organised by local municipalities for recipients of social assistance. Within the former, relatively more weight is given to improving the individual's prospects of getting a job in the mainstream labour market and promoting ordinary education. In the local measures for social assistance recipients operational objectives are more limited, being directed towards participation in employment-*projects* and more short-term job training courses. Abrahamson also claims that the coercive or disciplining element is more pronounced within the latter system. Beneficiaries of social assistance will be at greater risk of losing their right to cash benefits than recipients of social insurance if they refuse to participate in an activation offer. Thus the relationship between rights and duties tends to be different in the two cases: the social insurance beneficiary may choose between *different* offers, while the social assistance beneficiary may be expected to accept *any* offer.

Finally, it may be noted that a recent OECD summary of *The new social policy agenda* linked the concept of 'workfare' to on-going reforms of social assistance schemes in member countries (OECD 1999c: 101–2):

> Social assistance has been made *conditional* on individual behaviour taking a certain form. Policy in many countries is moving towards *reciprocity*, with assistance (in the form of both cash and services) being made conditional on efforts of the assistance recipients. [emphasis in original]

Two target groups are mentioned in this context: young people and single parents (*ibid*.: 89, 91, 102). On the basis of these and similar trends the OECD's secretary-general argued that, 'we can see emerging across OECD countries a new balance of the rights, obligations and opportunities of individuals . . . including developments such as workfare' (*ibid*.: 4).

Conclusions

This chapter has addressed the changing relationship between employment and social protection policies in Western Europe through the 1990s.

First, we examined the key assumptions underlying the new discourse on such policies, as they emerged on the basis of an analytical reading of EU and OECD documents. By and large the survey of the European-level discourse showed three trends: the Europeanisation of national employment and social protection policies, a desire to shift from passive to active measures, and a move towards targeting of resources through a tightening of eligibility criteria and greater reliance on means-tested support. The analytical reading of key texts revealed that when the stated objective of the new Social Europe is to provide citizens with better opportunities to live a good life, the primary instrument to promote this objective is integration through participation in paid work. Hence it is only a 'Europe at work' that can provide the good life. This assumption forms the basis for the now frequent claim that governments have both a right and obligation to take practical steps to promote employment, even if this may reduce the autonomy and self-determination of the individual.

Second, we presented a number of aggregate indicators of the changes in policy practice in sixteen Western European countries. We found that only a minority of these countries had made any significant increase in their active measures, gauged by the expenditure on active measures relative to the unemployment rate of each country. On the other hand, the great majority of the countries had introduced changes to tighten up their income maintenance schemes aimed at unemployed people. Thus the sixteen countries appeared to have been more successful in reducing their expenditure on passive measures – relative to their level of unemployment – than in strengthening active efforts which might provide the unemployed with new resources and opportunities. The exact combination of measures to tighten up income maintenance schemes varied significantly between the sixteen countries. More detailed research at local level in each country is called for to assess to what extent these variations are real or just artefacts created by the monitoring and reporting systems of the OECD and the EU. Our analysis indicates that countries adopting a complementary strategy (combining active efforts *and* a tightening of the income maintenance system) were by and large more successful in improving their labour market situation than those relying mainly on a tightening of their income maintenance system for people out of work.

Third, we focused on the relative role of means-tested assistance within the overall income maintenance scheme for unemployed people and the implications for the policy changes undertaken. During the 1990s means-tested assistance played an increasing role in the overall income transfers to people out of work in several countries. On an aggregate level there was some indication that countries chose *either* to spend more on active efforts (relative to their level of unemployment), *or* to give means-tested assistance a more important role. At a less aggregate level one may argue that beneficiaries of *both* social insurance and means-tested assistance became exposed to more stringent rules and administrative regimes, for instance expressed in stricter requirements about availability for work, demonstration of active job searching and participation in work or training measures. In this sense, to participate in active measures became for both categories of beneficiaries 'an offer you cannot refuse' (Lødemel and Trickey 2001). At the same time it might still be the case that people claiming means-tested assistance experienced more coercive and punitive sanctions than recipients of social insurance benefits. There are some indications that social assistance recipients were left with less choice between various options than social insurance beneficiaries when required to take part in active measures, and that such measures less frequently provided them with any substantial improvement in vocational qualifications. Arguably, the consequences of refusing to participate in measures might be more negative for social assistance recipients than for social insurance beneficiaries, as social assistance is usually supposed to function as a last-resort safety net. To the extent this was so, it obviously adds to the coercive element in the particular activation efforts aimed at social assistance recipients. Again, more detailed and local-level studies of implementation are called for.

Finally, we examined in various ways whether the development in the Nordic countries during the 1990s was systematically similar or different from the trends in the Continental, Mediterranean and Anglo-Saxon groups of welfare states. Our conclusion was that in most instances we could not trace a particular and common 'Nordic' path in this period. The recession in the first part of the 1990s had a stronger and more lasting impact in Finland and Sweden than in Denmark and Norway. As a consequence the two pairs of countries were faced with different constraints in their choice between various policy options, and they followed slightly different trajectories in the 1990s. By and large, the choices and changes made in the Nordic countries were not systematically different from those undertaken in a number of other Western European countries. But at the end of the decade the four Nordic countries still exhibited traits usually associated with the 'Nordic model' and more so than those in the three other groups of welfare states (although the countries in the Continental groups came fairly close). In this sense the Nordic model in terms of social protection for people out of work appeared to have survived the 1990s.

Notes

1 We wish to thank John Ditch for helpful and encouraging comments on an earlier version of this article. Johan Fritzell, Mikko Kautto, Jon Kvist and Hannu Uusitalo have contributed with important clarifications and stimulated the authors to sharpen their arguments.

2 Some authors have expressed reservations about using proportion of GDP to study changes or trends, as the GDP is likely to increase or decrease over time (e.g. Clayton and Pontussen 2000: 326). But even so, the GDP can be interpreted as a crude indicator of the total resources available in a country in any year. Among the sixteen countries studied here only Finland and Sweden experienced a reduction in real GDP for more than one year in the 1990–97 period (OECD 1999d, annex table 1).

3 The European Commission has undertaken a similar standardisation in recent documents, cf. EC 1998c: 110 and EC 1999c: 21–3.

4 The standard deviation for the standardised expenditure on active measures decreased from 1.5 to 0.9 between 1990 and 1997.

5 Differences between and trends in the unemployment benefit schemes of Denmark, Finland, Norway, Sweden, Germany, the Netherlands and the United Kingdom are discussed in greater detail by Clasen, Kvist and van Oorschot in their chapter in this book.

6 In this context it should be noted that a substantial proportion of people claiming general means-tested social assistance in the other three Nordic countries in the 1990s were out of work. For instance, in Norway in 1998 31 per cent of the recipients of social assistance were registered as 'unemployed' by the local authority social services departments administering this assistance. Another 6 per cent were registered as 'participating in labour market measures operated by state or local authority agencies' (Statistics Norway 2000).

7 This list of 'Nordic' characteristics is not meant to be exhaustive. For instance, a high degree of universalism in income maintenance benefits (see Chapter 8) or redistributive effect of such benefits (see Chapter 2) are other important 'Nordic' characteristics. If these characteristics had been included in the analysis, it would probably have produced greater contrasts between the Nordic and Continental groups of countries.

9 On condition of work: Increasing work requirements in unemployment compensation schemes

Jochen Clasen, Jon Kvist and Wim van Oorschot

Introduction[1]

A number of recent comparative studies suggest the existence of some common tendencies in national welfare state reforms (see e.g. George and Taylor-Gooby 1996; Ploug and Kvist 1996; Clasen 1997; Daly 1997; Ferge 1997). To differing degrees, access to universal protection schemes has become limited and solidarity ties in social insurance systems (between good and bad risks and higher and lower income groups) have been shortened. Apart from a few exceptions (such as the introduction of long-term care insurance in Germany), the role of means-testing has become more important, more stringent definitions of what constitutes unemployment and disability have been implemented, and measures have been introduced that reduce the level and duration of benefits. In short, it appears that collectively organised income protection systems are becoming less universal and more selective, with the effect that those confronted with a social risk and/or dependent on cash support are having to fulfil stricter qualifying conditions.

A common trend in reforms of national social security systems for jobless people is increased emphasis on work and training, either as replacing or at least accompanying social security provision. Some countries have been moving slowly but steadily in this direction for some time (e.g. the United Kingdom, the Netherlands), others have rapidly caught up since the early 1990s (e.g. Denmark) while others have moved in the same direction but have yet to make more than hesitant steps (e.g. Germany). The new emphasis is reflected in populist policy slogans such as 'welfare to work' (United Kingdom), 'work before income' (The Netherlands), 'active line' (Denmark), and 'work line' (Norway). These slogans are translated into central elements of welfare reform programmes that are aimed at stimulating labour market participation of unemployed and other groups, such as (partially) disabled social security claimants or single parents (e.g. Thornton *et al.* 1997).

Beyond national boundaries, catch phrases such as 'making benefit systems more employment friendly' (EC 1999b) or transforming passive into active types of social protection (e.g. OECD 1994) suggest a broad consensus about the direction in which income maintenance systems should move (see Chapter 8). Employment and training – whether ordinary or subsidised – are increasingly seen as a superior way of providing social protection compared to a so-called 'passive doling out of money'. At the same time, work-conditionality, reflected in claimants' past employment histories as well as certain conditions attached to continuous benefit receipt, is becoming an increasingly important determinant of eligibility and entitlement to social protection.

Within the emphasis on work and training in unemployment policy two major components can be distinguished. The first is active labour market policy, i.e. public programmes which seek to qualify and (re)train in order to make beneficiaries more active and increase their 'employability' in the labour market. Active labour market programmes are not new policy instruments but have existed alongside unemployment benefit schemes in many countries for some time. However, in some countries they seem to be acquiring a new function as either a substitute or principal condition for receiving cash benefits and in this sense are 'linking welfare and work' (European Foundation for the Improvement of Living and Working Conditions 1999).

As active labour market policies were discussed and compared in the previous chapter, this chapter focuses on the second, much less documented component, i.e. the work-conditionality within social security transfers *per se*, as exemplified by unemployment compensation. Broadly, work-conditionality refers to the range and degree to which benefit eligibility and entitlement are dependent on (mostly paid) employment. Traditionally, paid work has been a central reference point for determining access, level and duration of unemployment benefits. Criteria such as past employment and (insurance) contribution record, previous earnings, availability for work, suitability criteria regarding job and training offers and requirements regarding the intensity (and type) of job-seeking behaviour regularly function as gateways to unemployment compensation. For example, benefit claimants with a paid employment record of less than a specified number of months might not be entitled to (full) benefits or only to a shorter duration.

Equally, the refusal to accept a job offer which is administratively defined as 'suitable', or the failure to engage in appropriate job-seeking behaviour, might lead to benefit loss, reduction or suspension.

While the work-conditionality of benefit criteria is self-evident in unemployment compensation, the concrete specification of criteria, and the degree to which they determine access, level, duration and obligations attached to benefit receipt, may differ across national schemes and welfare regimes, with variation over time. Against the backdrop of the 'welfare to work' trend discussed above, it might be assumed that work-conditionality within unemployment benefit schemes has become more rather than less explicit, since this would signal the growing relevance of work at the expense of 'welfare' as a means for income security. This is what the chapter seeks to explore. More specifically, it aims to assess the profile and degree of work-conditionality within unemployment insurance and assistance schemes in the Nordic countries and to compare them with the situation in three other Northern European countries: Germany, the Netherlands and the United Kingdom.

The following section examines the reasons for suggesting that a distinctive regime of work-conditionality in the four Nordic countries might be expected. This is followed by a comparative assessment of separate criteria of work-conditionality within national unemployment compensation systems. The findings suggest that a Nordic profile does not seem to be apparent across any of these criteria if considered in isolation from each other. However, if considered as a whole, a distinctive Nordic manifestation of work-conditionality can indeed be identified. With the aim of exploring the notion of a distinct world of Nordic work-conditionality further, the final part of the chapter reviews major reform trends in Denmark, Norway, Sweden and Finland and contrasts them with policy changes in the other three countries.

Unemployment regimes and work-conditionality

As 'social-democratic' welfare states, Norway, Sweden and Denmark occupy a distinct position in Esping-Andersen's typology of welfare regimes (Esping-Andersen 1990, 1999). Characteristically these countries combine a high degree of decommodification of labour with low income inequality as a result of extensive state intervention in the production of welfare. A previous 'laggard', Finland joined the Nordic family in the 1980s (Kangas 1993). Since a welfare state's potential for decommodification and reducing inequality can be assumed to depend on the accessibility of social security transfers, as well as on benefit level and duration, one would expect a distinctive Nordic pattern within the specific domain of unemployment compensation.

Most recently, this has also been inferred by Gallie and Paugam (2000), who argue that the Nordic countries form a 'universalistic' regime type of unemployment protection. Compared to their three other regimes, the 'universalistic' regime is characterised by a more comprehensive benefit coverage, high levels and duration of benefits and extensive active employment policies. Work-conditionality is not a separate criterion for their typology, although they imply that it is most explicit in countries such as France, Germany, Belgium and the Netherlands (forming the 'employment-centred' type). In these countries, it is argued:

> the coverage of the unemployed remains far from complete as a result of the principles of eligibility for compensation. These are primarily defined in terms of previous employment experience. The system is concentrated on those who have accumulated the most rights. . . . It is a type of regime that will disadvantage people who have only been able to obtain temporary jobs or those with little work experience.

The 'liberal/minimal' regime, which applies in the United Kingdom, for example, is portrayed as distinctive in terms of its incomplete coverage, low compensation levels and the extensive role of means-testing.

Based on this typology one could take as an initial hypothesis that work-conditionality in Germany and the Netherlands is likely to be both more explicit and more selective than in the universalistic Nordic countries. Qualifying for benefit, for example, might require a longer attachment to the labour market than in the Nordic countries. Also, it can be assumed that benefit eligibility and entitlement are more strictly determined by individual records of participation in paid employment. On the other hand, given their extensive use of active employment policies, obligations to participate in paid employment on the part of benefit recipients can be expected to be more pronounced in the Nordic countries. Indeed, work-conditionality in terms of obligations on the part of beneficiaries is one of the most direct tools for linking welfare to work, and has traditionally been the core of the Nordic, or at least the Swedish, model of social protection.

The respective position of the United Kingdom as a 'liberal/minimal' regime (Gallie and Paugam 2000) is not immediately obvious. Whilst 'citizenship' is the guiding principle for Nordic social protection, and 'merit' or 'contribution record' plays a central role in the insurance-based unemployment schemes of Germany and the Netherlands, the principle of 'need' has had a major influence on policies shaping British protection schemes (Kvist 1998; see also Janoski 1998). Thus, one would not necessarily expect work-conditionality to be a dominant feature regarding benefit accessibility. Instead, the extent of need resulting from unemployment should be central, particularly since contributory benefits are relatively low and flat-rate. On the other hand, work-conditionality might be elaborate because this would reflect the notion of public provision as the last and inferior resort compared with market or individual and family support. Equally, the receipt of unemployment benefit might be strongly coupled with work-conditionality, since job search obligations should be crucial instruments for stimulating beneficiaries to take up individual responsibility for their subsistence.

In short, there are reasons why a distinct Nordic profile could be expected. In comparison with Germany and the Netherlands we would assume work-conditionality to be weaker regarding access, level and duration, but stronger regarding obligations and sanctions on the part of beneficiaries. Compared with the United Kingdom, the Nordic profile might manifest itself as having somewhat less pronounced accessibility criteria, with a comparable strictness of work obligations and related sanctions. Overall, Nordic policies of unemployment compensation may be characterised by a high degree of universality as reflected by relatively easy access to benefits and relatively generous benefits in terms of levels and duration (although egalitarian principles render high income groups less well covered than low income groups), and a strong emphasis on active labour market policies as visible in strict obligations (Kvist 1999).

Some organisational and institutional features

Putting the subsequent assessment of the degree of work-conditionality across countries into context, some appropriate background information suggests a distinctive Nordic approach in terms of organisational and institutional criteria. Unlike in other European countries, Nordic unemployment insurance schemes are organised and financed according to the Ghent model, i.e. they are tax subsidised, voluntary and affiliated to trade unions. Norway is an exception since it has a mandatory national insurance scheme and a public employment service (for the historical development of unemployment insurance schemes see Alber 1981; Carroll 1999). However, the state covers the marginal risk of unemployment through taxes in all the Nordic countries.

Indeed, membership fees cover only a relatively small share of expenditure in Denmark (20 per cent), Finland (6 per cent), and Sweden (5 per cent). In contrast, contributions cover the main bulk of expenditure on unemployment insurance in Norway, Germany, the Netherlands and also the United Kingdom (for the minority of unemployed who are in receipt of insurance-based benefits, i.e. contributory Job Seekers Allowance).

Because of the historical link to trade unions in Sweden, Finland and Denmark, a minimum period of trade union membership is required before eligibility for unemployment insurance is established, i.e. ten months in Finland and twelve months in Denmark and Sweden. Partly due to the voluntary nature of these schemes, not all unemployed persons are dependent on unemployment insurance in these countries, but may also receive unemployment assistance and/or social assistance. Indeed, social assistance provides an important means of subsistence for the unemployed in many countries. Moreover, there are many other social security schemes which may provide an income for non-employed people (see also Blöndal and Pearson 1995; Group of National Experts 1995; Kvist 1998). In the 1990s, the share of those in receipt of unemployment insurance benefits out of all registered unemployed was 50–60 per cent in Finland, 53–73 per cent in Norway, 68–78 per cent in Denmark, and 71–80 per cent in Sweden (Torp 1999). Recent changes to the Finnish system mean that today virtually all the unemployed receive one of the three possible unemployment benefits (Lilja and Savaja 1999). By comparison, the share of unemployed with insurance-based unemployment benefit is below 20 per cent in the United Kingdom, about 35 per cent in the Netherlands and about 30–35 per cent in Germany, with a similar percentage receiving earnings-related unemployment assistance.

Unemployment assistance schemes can be found in Germany, the Netherlands and the United Kingdom. However, it should be pointed out that Germany's scheme is somewhat special. It caters almost exclusively for those who have exhausted their claim to unemployment insurance and provides benefits that are proportional to previous earnings (insurance principle), while benefit eligibility is dependent on a family income test (assistance principle). This means that there are some unemployed who are not in receipt of unemployment benefit but are on local social assistance. This is very different to the situation in the United Kingdom, where the vast majority of the unemployed (over 80 per cent) rely on the means-tested Job Seekers Allowance which is identical to the general social assistance (Income Support) system in all but name. The Dutch unemployment assistance scheme resembles that of Germany in that it functions as a safety-net for those unemployed whose entitlement to insurance benefit has expired (or who do not qualify for it at all), but eligibility as well as entitlements are subject to a household means test.

Within the Nordic countries, neither Norway nor Denmark have unemployment assistance schemes. By contrast, since 1994, Finland has had an unemployment assistance scheme (*työmarkkinatuki, arbetsmarknadsstödet*) parallel with the unemployment insurance scheme, providing flat-rate, means-tested benefits with no limit to the benefit period. Finland used to have another unemployment assistance scheme (*peruspäiväraha, grunddagpenning*), but in 1994 this became integrated with the unemployment insurance scheme as a mandatory part, and its means-tested element was replaced by the new scheme. In 1998, Sweden also made its previous unemployment assistance scheme (*Kontant Arbetsmarknadsstöt, KAS*) a mandatory part of the otherwise voluntary unemployment insurance.

Work-conditionality within unemployment compensation in seven European countries

This section compares the extent of work-conditionality inherent in unemployment insurance and unemployment assistance schemes in the seven countries. As outlined at the beginning of this chapter, work-conditionality can be assessed in relation to four criteria, i.e. to benefit access, benefit level, benefit duration and obligations on the part of benefit recipients. Basic information on the current legal situation regarding these four criteria in the seven countries is provided in Appendix Table 9.2 at the end of the chapter.

Access

Both employees and self-employed are covered by unemployment insurance in the Nordic countries, except for Norway where a large group of self-employed in seasonal work, such as fishermen and -women, can take out insurance. Only employees are covered in Germany, the Netherlands and the United Kingdom. In all seven countries, unemployed must be able, willing, and looking for work, as set out by the ILO criteria. Of course, it has to be recognised that administrative practices which seek to establish how far these criteria are met might differ between and perhaps even within countries. For example, following the Ghent model, the question of whether trade unions in Sweden, Finland and Denmark actually do monitor and report insured members who are not available for work has repeatedly become an issue in public debates. Unfortunately, administrative procedures cannot be captured in this chapter. Instead, this section concentrates on legal differences specifying the relevance of a record of paid employment for benefit eligibility. Such a requirement is generally established to limit unemployment benefits to people in the official labour market as opposed to, for example, those working in the household or participating in education and other activities. The relevance of previous work requirements is expressed in four factors:

- *A minimum work record*, as an expression of affiliation to the labour market. It can be measured by length of time spent in work, contributions made, or income earned. Persons with no or only a short previous work record are less likely to qualify for insurance benefits than people with long work records.
- *A relevant work period*, which stipulates the period within which the minimum work record has to be established. Obviously, longer relevant work periods make it easier to qualify for unemployment benefit.
- *The work intensity*, which measures the extent of previous labour market attachment. This is typically expressed as the number of weekly working hours or level of income. People with shorter weekly working hours or low income might find it difficult to qualify for insurance benefit.
- *The work concept*, which denotes what is considered as 'previous work' in a given social security scheme. For example, in some countries only non-subsidised paid work might be acceptable for benefit qualification, whereas in other countries caring for relatives or other non-paid activities might have the same status as paid employment.

In the following we use the ratio between the minimum work record and the relevant period as a shorthand way of presenting the degree of previous work requirements and changes therein. For example, access to unemployment insurance in Germany requires a period of at least one year insured employment within the past three years, giving a ratio of 0.33. The respective ratio is also 0.33 in Denmark and 0.41 in both Finland and Sweden. In Norway previous income rather than length of time spent in previous employment is relevant. The demand of 125 per cent of the basic amount corresponds to 20–40 per cent of income from full-time work, depending on wage level (Torp 1999), and is hence not radically different from the other Nordic countries, perhaps somewhat more lax. In Norway, it is also possible to qualify by having an average of 100 per cent of the basic amount in the three preceding years. In the United Kingdom a certain number and amount of paid and credited contributions is required before benefit eligibility is established. This means that better income earners and full-time employees qualify sooner than those with low income, or part-time workers. Essentially, two years of employed work are required before eligibility is established, which is relatively strict. With a ratio of 0.66 for the short-term benefit and 0.80 for the long-term benefit the Netherlands has by far the toughest work-conditionality of access to unemployment insurance and this places it in a group of its own. This 'Dutch toughness' also manifests itself in the fact that individual work records not only influence benefit access, but level and duration as well.

Work intensity requirements may modify the above country ranking. Indeed, the apparently lenient Danish work demand of 52 weeks within 3 years (a ratio of 0.33) applies to work of normal duration, i.e. 37 hours a week. This is more than double the work intensity of Sweden, where the work has only to be of 70 hours per month, just under half the number of hours in an official working week. In Germany, work averaging 18 hours per week is sufficient for benefit qualification. In the Netherlands, the country with the toughest work-conditionality, a person has to work only 52 days in each of the required 4 years as compared to typically 260 days per year. As far as work intensity conditions are concerned, it is Norway where access to unemployment benefit depends less on past employment than in any of the other countries. In short, taking work intensity into account, countries such as Denmark and the Netherlands may in fact lie closer together than their marked differences in minimum work records imply. Again, it is very difficult to identify a Nordic profile.

Finally, a strict work-conditionality in terms of benefit access might be weakened by treating certain activities as fully or partly equivalent to paid employment, i.e. by broadening the *work concept*. This is the case in the Netherlands, for example, where caring for children is taken into account, full or partial credits being given depending on the age of children. In the United Kingdom, insurance credits are granted for certain activities but become irrelevant if not accompanied by actual paid employment for at least some time. In the Nordic countries, caring for children does not count towards entitlement. However, participation in 'activation offers' is equal to paid employment in Sweden, which results in a virtual never-ending benefit period.

Indeed, the possibility of renewing benefit periods varies across countries. Overall, then, it seems difficult to identify a distinct Nordic degree or profile of work-conditionality regarding benefit access. If anything, countries with long minimum work records and short relevant periods tend to have less strict requirements on work intensity and broader concepts of what counts as work.

Level

The level of flat-rate benefits is by definition less conditional on paid employment than earnings-related transfers which, to some extent, reflect previous work records. What is more, the degree of work-conditionality within the latter is stronger the fewer criteria are involved, other than previous earnings and length of work record, in determining the level of benefit. In other words, minimum benefit floors or maximum benefit ceilings, for example, might significantly weaken work-conditionality, as can benefit differentiation according to age or supplements granted for dependants. However, there are other, less overt, aspects. Earnings-related benefits usually represent a proportion of earnings, averaged over a certain period. Here, the length of the relevant earnings period is important, as is its definition. For example, until recently only standard earnings were recognised in Germany, thus excluding regular bonuses such as holiday and Christmas pay, or regular overtime pay. The less such components of regular paid employment are taken into account, it could be argued, the less benefit systems are work-conditional.

Except for the United Kingdom all countries run earnings-related unemployment insurance schemes. There is some variation in the earnings-replacement rate, benefit ceilings, and minimum benefits. Combined with different tax systems, this results in varying net replacement rates and income compensation profiles. In 1997, claimants with previous earnings equal to an average production worker would receive unemployment insurance benefit equal to 20.2 per cent of those earnings (after taxes) in the United Kingdom, 58.4 per cent in Germany, 60.7 per cent in Finland, 67 per cent in Denmark, 70.8 per cent in Sweden, and 72.6 per cent in the Netherlands (Hansen 1999; unfortunately no comparable data exists for Norway).

Schemes with flat-rate benefits and earnings-related benefits with a low benefit ceiling do not reflect work to the same extent as earnings-related benefits with no or a high ceiling. The latter type of scheme can be seen as tightly related to work since benefits reflect the former earnings record also for people with high incomes. This contrasts with flat-rate and earnings-related benefits with a low ceiling. For example, in Sweden and Denmark income compensation decreases for claimants with previous income above the level of the average production worker, whereas the compensation rate remains constant in Germany and the Netherlands up to levels of, respectively, 1.7 and 1.5 times the level of the average production worker (Hansen 1999). In this regard, the Dutch and even more so German unemployment insurance schemes (with no benefit floor) reflect previous work performance to a much greater extent than the Nordic and British schemes. The use of minimum benefits or benefit floors has a similar effect on work-conditionality since they can undermine the relation to previous work for those on lower earnings. For example, the Danish benefit floor, pegged at 82 per cent of the maximum unemployment benefit, implies that transfers are only related to previous work for people with incomes between 0.53 and 0.64 times the level of the average production worker – a *de facto* flat-rate benefit for the majority of unemployment insurance beneficiaries.

The above suggests a distinction between two groups of countries. The first group consists of the United Kingdom and the Nordic countries, where benefits relate to previous work only for low and middle income groups, and only to the extent that this is not ruled out by minimum benefits. In the second group, consisting of Germany and the Netherlands, a higher degree of work-conditionality is expressed as benefit levels are much more dependent on previous earnings for a much larger group of claimants, including groups with higher incomes. Finland can be seen as a hybrid between the two in having guaranteed minimum benefit coupled with decreasing earnings-replacement rates without a ceiling.

Duration

Work-conditionality regarding benefit duration refers to how much the period during which benefit is payable is determined by individual employment records, i.e. by the length of time spent in previous employment, work period and/or work intensity. We distinguish these, often objective and measurable, *ex-ante* criteria, from those which might arise as a result of claimants violating their obligations for job search, etc., with administrative discretion usually playing a much larger role in the latter. Some countries might not attach work-conditionality to benefit duration. In other words, once access has been established, the maximum benefit duration does not vary according to individual employment records. In contrast, other countries may apply work-related criteria that can lengthen or shorten benefit entitlement.

The maximum period for receiving insurance-based benefits is six months in the United Kingdom and twelve months in Germany, while in the Netherlands it is sixty months for those who qualify for standard benefit, but only five months for those on short-term benefit. However, the latter two countries allow people above a certain age significantly longer benefit periods. In Germany this applies to claimants aged 45 and older, reaching an overall maximum of 32 months, depending on age and length of contribution record. In the Netherlands benefit duration is extended for those 57.5 years of age and over. Differences in re-qualification criteria and 'transitionary' schemes in Germany make it possible to receive unemployment assistance for longer periods: in principle indefinitely but at decreasing benefit levels.

Within the Nordic countries, the length of maximum benefit periods ranges from 14 months in Sweden to 23 months in Finland, 36 months in Norway and 60 months in Denmark, with considerably longer periods for people above a certain age. However, the seemingly significant variation in maximum periods masks differences with respect to both the possibility of benefit re-qualification, where Sweden has the most lenient conditions as described above, and the transition into other unemployment compensation schemes, while Finland today has the only Nordic 'transitionary' unemployment assistance scheme.

In summary, the United Kingdom stands out as the country with the shortest period by far. Together with Denmark, Finland and Sweden, the duration of benefit receipt has a low degree of work-conditionality. Thus, we cannot distinguish a Nordic group, given that in Germany, the Netherlands, and even in Norway, the extent of previous work has an impact on the length of the maximum period. For example, in Germany and the Netherlands it is a combination of age and individual contribution records which determines the respective maximal length of benefit duration. In Norway the amount of previous earnings is the determining factor. Work-conditionality of duration is thus visible for this subset of three countries. Indeed, one can speak of a degree of individual work-conditionality or 'work-relatedness' of income maintenance, i.e. a correspondence between individual labour market participation and benefit entitlement. No such stratification is observable in the remaining Nordic countries or in the United Kingdom.

Obligations

Unemployed persons have certain obligations to fulfil in order to gain and maintain benefit eligibility. The primary obligation is to be available for and to seek employment, but also to accept 'suitable' work offers. There are marked differences as to how countries implement these conditions. 'Suitable work', for example, refers to different dimensions of mobility which are deemed acceptable for claimants. The latter might include stipulations as to the level of earnings in relation to previous earnings or benefit (wage mobility), the length of time or distance between home and work (geographical mobility), and obligations to accept work outside previous work experience or qualification (occupational mobility).

The different types of mobility requirements may co-exist and be combined in various ways. An additional obligation might be willingness to participate in 'suitable' training, work experience, or other types of active labour market programmes. Whether, in which ways and how frequently these obligations are actually applied might depend on individual circumstances and administrative practice. This posed a problem for this study since it proved impossible to gather representative and comparative data on policy implementation, not least since administrative routines can differ significantly across regions within a single country. We therefore limit ourselves to comparing current legislative frameworks and to analysing recent developments.

As we argued in the preceding section, if anything we would expect the Nordic countries to be at least as prescriptive as other countries regarding obligations for work and training imposed on beneficiaries. An important assumption is that there are considerable differences with regard to work incentives in a scheme with easy access and generous benefits, depending on whether this is combined with lenient or strict obligations and sanctions for participation in the labour market. The easier the access to benefits, coupled with lax obligations and sanctions, the more a scheme will resemble a basic income or citizen wage, which has never been the aim of the Nordic welfare state.

All the Nordic countries expect unemployment beneficiaries to accept offers of 'suitable' work, and participation in active labour market programmes. Unfortunately, we do not know much about how authorities interpret and implement the notion of 'suitable' work, although general practice is believed to vary widely between regions, and, for the three countries following the Ghent model, between different trade unions. In both cases one may assume that the intra-country differences are as wide as the cross-country differences.

Nevertheless, judging only from formal rules, there seem to be some distinctive cross-national differences with regard to the requirements of geographical, occupational, and wage mobility. For example, both Norway and Sweden demand full geographical mobility within the country. This is not the case in Denmark, where geographical mobility requirements may not be enforced in case of 'good reasons', in particular when the claimant has sole responsibility for dependants. In principle, full occupational mobility is required in Norway and Sweden at the onset of the unemployment period. Again, this is not the case in Denmark. Full wage mobility is not required in any of the Nordic countries. In Denmark and Norway jobs offered should not pay less than the relevant wage agreement, and in Sweden the wage offered should be no more than 10 per cent less than the benefit received. In sum, Norway and Sweden have stricter official obligations to accept work with regard to geographical and occupational mobility than Denmark, and none of the Nordic countries requests full wage mobility.

Obligations on the part of job seekers are also fairly strict in the United Kingdom. There is no full geographical mobility, but after 13 weeks of unemployment there is full wage mobility and no restrictions on the type of occupation. Fortnightly interviews and a range of work tests put a strong onus on benefit claimants to demonstrate that they are actively seeking work, and training or work experience schemes are mandatory for some groups (particularly the young and long-term unemployed) and can be used to test willingness to work for others. By comparison, obligations are less prescriptive in Germany, but vary between different groups of unemployed, influenced by the type of benefit received and individual circumstances. For example, recipients of unemployment insurance have to participate in appropriate training schemes when offered, and accept job offers with specified but declining earnings in accordance with lengthening unemployment (but not below benefit), as well as a maximum travelling time to and from work per day. For claimants of unemployment assistance the same obligations apply, but wage mobility is greater because of declining benefit rates in accordance with the length of unemployment. Recently, restrictions on occupational mobility have been abolished for both groups. In the Netherlands 'suitability of work' is defined in detail and (except for school-leavers) depends on level of education, former job and wage, as well as on unemployment duration. After 1.5 years of unemployment all work is regarded as suitable for all unemployed.

In sum, with regard to formal obligations all countries impose requirements on being willing, and able for work and looking for it. However, we can distinguish between three regime–specific ways of implementing such obligations. In the Nordic countries, there is generally more emphasis on geographical and occupational mobility than in the Netherlands and Germany. However, the Nordic countries do not, at least initially, place the same emphasis on wage mobility as in these countries and, in particular, the United Kingdom. Indeed, the latter stands out as having the toughest obligations imposed soon after the onset of benefit receipt. Germany and the Netherlands have a 'moving' interpretation of obligations where the different types of mobility requirements become stricter as the duration of benefit receipt lengthens. This reflects the status-preserving element of the employment-centred model in these countries, whereas the Nordic countries can be seen as having more of an egalitarian approach whereby all claimants within the country are met with equally tough obligations.

A Nordic profile?

As far as the degree and type of work-conditionality within unemployment compensation schemes are concerned, we conclude from the discussion that it seems possible to distinguish three types or groups, broadly reflecting Esping-Andersen's (1990) categorisation of welfare regimes and Gallie and Paugam's (2000) typology of unemployment protection schemes. Based on the previous section, Table 9.1 depicts profiles of work-conditionality within three broad types, the Nordic countries, Germany and the Netherlands, and the United Kingdom with a distinctive profile. Of course, Table 9.1 provides a stylised

Table 9.1 Profiles of work-conditionality

	Access	*Level*	*Duration*	*Obligation*	*Guiding principle*
Nordic countries	±	–	–	+	Egalitarian
Germany/ Netherlands	±	+	+	+	Merit/status
UK	+	–	–	+	Need

Explanations:
+ equals strong degree of work-conditionality;
– equals weak degree of work-conditionality.

picture. Yet the grouping seems justified on the grounds that cross-national differences appear smaller between countries within the same group than between groups.

Table 9.1 indicates the difficulty of identifying a Nordic profile when each of the four criteria is considered in isolation. Briefly, access to benefit seems comparatively easy in some Nordic countries, but also in Germany. However, the relatively strict work-conditionality in countries such as Sweden and the Netherlands is softened because of the recognition of non-paid employment as constituting benefit qualification. As to the level of benefits, the dependence on previous work and earnings is weakened in countries such as Denmark and Sweden due to benefit floors and ceilings which leave relatively fairly narrow corridors in which benefits reflect former earnings. The equivalent corridor is much wider in the Netherlands and even more so in Germany because of the absence of a benefit floor or ceiling. In other words, the Nordic countries are not unique in the *level* of benefits when contrasted with Germany and the Netherlands, but rather in the *setting* of benefits, where the link between former work and benefit is much stronger in the latter group of countries than in the Nordic nations. The United Kingdom operates flat-rate benefits, and thus a weak expression of work-conditionality, but stands out with the lowest level of benefits in all groups. However, it should be noted that the above focuses on unemployment compensation only, i.e. it does not take into account the salient role played by housing and other benefits, which, if included, would bring the United Kingdom closer to the other countries as far as total benefit level is concerned.

Benefit duration is perhaps the area where national schemes differ most, at least when considering the maximum period for unemployment insurance. Germany and the Netherlands in particular stratify the length according to previous work record. By contrast, the maximum period is the same for all eligible in Sweden, Finland and Denmark. Moreover, all countries but the United Kingdom provide older unemployed with longer periods of compensation. Again, it is not so much the potential length of maximum benefit periods which distinguishes the three Nordic countries from Germany and the Netherlands, but rather that periods are not determined by the length of previous participation in the labour market. Illustrating the difficulty of distinguishing a Nordic profile according to a single indicator, Norway is the exception here, even though the correspondence between individual labour market participation (expressed as level of earnings) and length of entitlement is less pronounced than in the two Continental European countries. The United Kingdom shares the egalitarian approach to benefit periods, but has a far shorter maximum contributory benefit period.

Finally, Table 9.1 indicates an equally strong degree of work-conditionality as far as obligations on the part of unemployed people are concerned. This is justified only if obligations are interpreted as a composite criterion of work-conditionality. As the discussion has shown, the Nordic profile combines relatively strong requirements regarding geographical and occupational mobility with weaker expectations in terms of wage mobility. The United Kingdom has the strongest obligations regarding the latter indicator while obligations imposed on German and Dutch job seekers vary according to type of benefit or length of time spent in unemployment.

To sum up, while there seems to be no clear Nordic profile with respect to individual indicators of work-conditionality, the notion of a distinctive Nordic orientation within unemployment compensation can be justified if all four criteria are considered as a whole. The overall egalitarian approach in the Nordic countries shows up not so much in terms of eligibility but of entitlement, i.e. by not (or not to the same extent) linking levels of benefits and benefit periods to previous work performance. This is distinctively different to Germany and the Netherlands, where benefits are based on merit or status (reflecting previous earnings or labour market attachment) to a much larger extent. The comparatively generous benefit levels distinguish the Nordic countries not from the latter two countries, but from the United Kingdom where benefits are flat-rate but also very modest and of short duration.

Trends

Having established a cross-sectional picture of the relative degree of work-conditionality within the seven countries, the remainder of this chapter will investigate trends and patterns over time. Have conditions of benefit eligibility and entitlement systems become more or less influenced by aspects of labour market participation? Within social security reforms over the past twenty years or so, has work become an increasingly prominent factor in benefit qualification and entitlement? Are there cross-national distinctions between the Nordic and other countries?

Of the Nordic countries Denmark has had the longest experience with high and long-term unemployment. During the first half of the 1980s the policy response was primarily to reduce benefit generosity by way of not fully indexing unemployment benefits. As a consequence the purchasing power of the maximum benefit in 1987 was only 82 per cent of the level in 1976 (Knudsen 1987). The maximum benefit ceiling has since been raised, but remains low compared to the other Nordic countries.

Following on from experiments with activation schemes in the late 1980s, the Labour Market Reform in 1994, and subsequent revisions, gave a new impetus to the so-called move from passive to active labour market policies, with the (re)design of the unemployment insurance scheme playing a major role. Since then, policies have aimed not so much at changing benefit levels but restricting access to benefits, shortening duration, and especially increasing the emphasis on the obligation to work, or, more generally, to participate in activities. Policies included an extension of the minimum work record for benefit eligibility and a maximum entitlement period (84 months). This maximum period has subsequently been further reduced (to 48 months in 1999). As an example of the tighter relation between rights and obligations, the division of the overall entitlement period, between the first 'contact' period and the second 'activation' period, has been significantly changed. In 1999, the first period was fixed at one year compared to four years in 1994, while the second period, when the unemployed has both the right and obligation to participate in activation schemes, was three years. The increased emphasis on obligations goes hand in hand with more activation, and today around one-third of all unemployed are in some sort of activation scheme at any one time (see also Langager 1997; Madsen and Loftager 1997; Larsen and Langager 1998; Madsen 1999). In short, the politics of retrenchment during the first half of the 1980s has gradually been replaced by a more proactive employment policy involving a firmer link between benefits and employment.

The Finnish welfare state matured in the 1980s (Kangas 1993). In the area of unemployment compensation this was particularly true with the introduction of a new unemployment insurance and assistance scheme in 1985. The new Finnish unemployment insurance scheme could in many ways be interpreted as more generous and displaying a higher degree of work-conditionality than other Nordic schemes at the time. This was due to its minimum floor and an earnings-replacement rate which gradually decreased as income rose, but without upper limits. In contrast, the Swedish and, in particular, Danish schemes both had relatively low benefit ceilings.

However, the dramatic economic crisis in Finland in the first half of the 1990s did not leave the unemployment compensation system untouched. To reduce the cost of the surge in unemployment the earnings replacement rate was reduced in 1992, and the base for calculating benefits was gradually diminished in the following years, while the supplements for children were not indexed (fully) or, in the case of child supplement while receiving unemployment assistance, even nominally reduced. Access was made stricter in 1997 by increasing the work demand from 26 to 43 weeks of work within two years, and it also became more difficult to re-qualify for new benefit periods by participating in active labour market schemes. However, the self-employed were included in the unemployment insurance scheme in 1995 (KELA 1999). Recently, there has been renewed emphasis on active labour market policies in Finland, and these are becoming closely connected with the design of the unemployment compensation scheme, in particular with the administration of job seekers' obligation to participate in such schemes. For example, the benefit waiting period for not accepting activation offers was generally raised from six weeks to two months in 1998. In sum, the development in Finland was characterised by more generous benefit schemes in the 1980s, whereas the reforms in the 1990s aimed at reducing costs, and in linking benefits more firmly with work. Hence, the 1990s saw reduced benefit levels and access made more difficult through stricter work requirements, while greater obligations to work and participate in active labour market schemes went hand in hand with increased sanctions for not accepting job and activation offers.

In Norway, a clear line can be drawn between policy debates surrounding the introduction of the 'work for all' in 1974 (Halvorsen 1990) and present debates which indicate a stronger emphasis on incentives, obligations, activation, and the 'good life' as involving participation in work (see, for example, Halvorsen *et al.* 1986; Hatland 1994a). Yet it is more difficult to identify a consistent development with regard to work-conditionality in unemployment compensation. In 1984, the maximum duration was extended from 40 weeks, repeatable after 12 weeks of no benefit, to 80 weeks repeatable after 26 weeks of no benefit (in 1991 reduced to 13 weeks and possibility of dispensation). The periods without benefits were intended to provide the unemployed with a strong financial incentive to find work. In 1997 the no-benefit period was abolished and the maximum period fixed at 156 weeks for people with previous income above twice the basic amount, and at 78 weeks below it. Hence, the current maximum benefit period is almost four times longer than it was in the early 1980s and without the work incentive mechanism of the no-benefit periods (see also Hatland 1994b). This can be interpreted as a move towards less work-conditionality. So can the development towards making benefit levels markedly less dependent on previous work. In 1989 maximum income taken into consideration when calculating benefits was halved from twelve to six times the basic amount (in 1999 equal to 46,950 NOK). At the same time, however, the linkage between previous work and length of maximum benefit period (introduced in the 1997 reform) can also be seen as increasing the level of work-conditionality. Moreover, the same reform also meant that access became slightly more dependent upon previous work as the income requirement for eligibility was increased from 0.75 to 1.25 times the basic amount. As a consequence, very low income earners, in particular students and some groups of primarily elderly women in seasonal work, have found it increasingly difficult to qualify for unemployment insurance. With regard to the obligation to accept training and job offers, recipients of unemployment insurance in Norway have during the whole period been required to demonstrate, in principle, full geographic as well as occupational mobility. As this is from the first day of unemployment, Norway has very tough obligations compared to the other Nordic countries, but the actual implementation varies across regions, branches, and over the economic cycle. Today, unemployment is very low in Norway as a whole, and jobs are particularly being created in the Oslo area. As a consequence, the labour market can be seen as a motor generating demands for geographical mobility outside Oslo. In short, cost-cutting exercises in the 1980s resulted in benefits becoming less generous for high income earners, accompanied by extensions of benefit periods to accommodate longer spells of unemployment. The 1990s witnessed a further expansion of benefit periods accompanied by a variety of demands concerning the obligation to work and to participate in labour market measures.

The Swedish development in the 1980s may be characterised as one of 'calibration', with some programmes and areas being expanded and others reduced. By contrast, Marklund (1997) interprets the 1990s as a period of 'contraction' or even 'deconstruction'. This description also fits the area of unemployment compensation, where some improvements were made in the 1980s, but where the 1990s witnessed a number of restrictive measures. For example, with the aim of motivating participation in education or work, persons under twenty years of age were barred from eligibility to unemployment assistance (KAS) in 1986 and from unemployment insurance in 1999. Like the other Nordic countries, Sweden made work requirements stricter during the 1990s, although the concept of what is considered as work has been broadened on several occasions since 1980. In 1982, two months of participation in occupational rehabilitation became countable towards fulfilling the work demand and in 1986 any time spent in training and rehabilitation programmes became recognised as qualifying towards unemployment insurance. As a result, compared to the situation in the other six countries, the Swedish unemployment insurance scheme is, if not the most easy to access, the most difficult to exit in terms of a claimant's possibilities to requalify for unemployment insurance by participation in such programmes.

Sweden has made more frequent and visible changes to its benefit formulae than any other country, with increases in the replacement rate in the early and late 1980s followed by reductions in the mid-1990s which were reversed in the late 1990s (but not to the previous level). In the early 1990s the maximum benefit levels were lowered and fixed for five years. The level of the unemployment assistance scheme (KAS) was not indexed fully with prices and wages during the 1990s. In fact the level of KAS was frozen at 245 SEK/day in 1994, and nominally reduced to 230 SEK/day for 1996 and 1997.

Perhaps the most crucial organisational change concerns the merging of the Swedish unemployment insurance and assistance schemes. The unemployment assistance scheme (KAS), in place from 1974 to 1998, covered people who fulfilled the work demand for unemployment insurance but were not members of an unemployment insurance fund or failed to meet the one-year membership requirement. This scheme merged with the unemployment insurance scheme in 1998, but rules regarding access, benefit level, duration and obligations remained much the same. In sum, the Swedish development during the 1980s witnessed a still broader notion of work and higher benefits, whereas the 1990s saw tighter work requirements, decreasing benefit levels and a stricter administration of claimants' obligations.

The German system of unemployment compensation is highly work-conditional in all respects and has become more so due to changes introduced since the beginning of the 1980s. However, it is noticeable that there have been relatively few changes regarding benefit access or (direct) reductions in benefit level. Instead, changes have been incremental and differentiated, hitting those hardest with weak labour market attachment. For others with long work histories, and if above a certain age, the unemployment insurance system actually became more rather than less generous in the 1980s (apart from a modest reduction in benefit level). However, recent changes have reversed this tendency. Indeed, changes implemented since the mid-1990s have signalled a new trend since they call into question the traditional notion that claimants in receipt of insurance benefits are to be rewarded and reintegrated in accordance with their previous status in the labour market. For example, there is now full occupational mobility and claimants have to demonstrate a higher degree of wage mobility.

Overall, it can be argued that until the mid-1990s changes in the system were largely driven by short-term responses to the fiscal state of the unemployment insurance budget which, when in deficit, has to be tax subsidised. Improvements in the second half of the 1980s were equally contingent on the budget situation. None of these changes altered the system in any structural way but clearly concentrated social protection on core workers. In contrast, changes regarding higher occupational mobility on the part of job seekers since the mid-1990s have been officially justified as in accordance with a necessary adaptation to a more flexible labour market. However, this stops short of any move towards (compulsory) activation within unemployment insurance, which would be much harder to implement in Germany than in the Nordic countries or the United Kingdom (Clasen 2000).

Unlike the contributory-funded unemployment insurance, the German unemployment assistance scheme is tax funded, which is why governments (of whatever composition) have repeatedly singled it out for policy change. However, due to the complex policy-making structure in Germany, several attempts to downscale, abolish or integrate it with local social assistance, which would have adverse consequences for local authority funding, have been successfully vetoed. Smaller changes nevertheless indicate a clear-cut trend towards making unemployment assistance more work-conditional in terms of all four criteria applied. Unemployment assistance caters for those who have exhausted unemployment insurance and for those who have some work record but fail to qualify for unemployment insurance. Over the past two decades policy changes have been successful in terms of making the system less generous and increasingly irrelevant for the latter group. What is more, compared with unemployment insurance, the increased work-conditionality regarding obligations particularly since the mid-1990s has to be noted, although it manifests itself mainly on a discretionary basis on the part of employment offices. In practice, workfare and other work-testing options seem to create administrative problems and have therefore not been applied extensively, although there are regional exceptions. Finally, there have been attempts to make combining benefits with earnings more attractive.

In the Netherlands, there was a clear shift towards stronger work-conditionality in the 1980s and 1990s, with both eligibility and entitlement criteria becoming more closely determined by personal work histories. The 1987 reform of the unemployment insurance scheme made the duration of prolonged benefit (which comes into operation once the standard benefit has expired) dependent on work history. At the same time access to the prolonged benefit period became dependent on a further requirement (on top of a work record of 26 weeks in the previous year) of having worked at least three years in the previous five. After expiry of the prolonged benefit a follow-up benefit was paid for a period depending on age. In 1995 eligibility criteria for the standard benefit were tightened. Now claimants have to have a work record of 26 weeks in the previous 39 (rather than 52) weeks, and four instead of three years within the previous 5-year period. Most significant, however, is that both conditions are now combined, which implies that nowadays it is rather difficult to be entitled to the standard benefit. It is estimated that only about 45 to 50 per cent of present workers would meet the new combination of criteria. Those who meet the first criterion only (26 out of 39 weeks) are entitled to short-term benefit of just 70 per cent of the minimum wage. The unemployed who fail to meet any of the criteria have to rely on means-tested social assistance.

The 1987 reform also converted the traditionally earnings-related insurance benefit for long-term unemployed who had exhausted their rights to the standard and prolonged benefit into a flat-rate payment equivalent to 70 per cent of the minimum wage. In 1995 the flat-rate benefit was also introduced for those whose standard benefit had expired. In other words, benefit levels became increasingly linked to individual work histories. The maximum duration of unemployment insurance has been extended from 2.5 years (for those under 60 years of age) to a maximum of 7.5 years. However, the work history requirements for entitlement to prolonged benefit have been tightened strongly. In other words, the position of unemployed with extended work records has improved, while for those with shorter work records it has become more difficult to receive (wage-related) benefits for more than six months. Overall, compared with the early 1980s, becoming unemployed nowadays implies lower benefits for shorter periods of time. As a result, remaining in work or finding jobs has become more important and compelling to workers. In addition, stricter definitions and implementation of obligations, such as ‘suitability of work’, have been introduced which accord with the much increased degree of work-conditionality within the Dutch unemployment compensation system.

Finally, access to contributory benefits in the United Kingdom became more dependent on longer work histories in the 1980s, contributing to a gradual but steady erosion of insurance coverage throughout the past two decades (to below 20 per cent by the end of the 1990s). As a result, means-testing and thus 'need' rather than 'work history' have become even more important criteria for benefit receipt than they already were in the 1970s. At the same time, and irrespective of the type of benefit received, there has been a growing emphasis on work-conditionality as far as obligations on the part of benefit claimants are concerned. Benefits for unemployed people in the United Kingdom have never been generous. However, unfavourable benefit indexing since the 1970s, the abolition of the earnings-related supplement in the early 1980s and a number of small changes thereafter have led to a decline in value in relation to net average wages, particularly for people under the age of twenty-five.

Since the end of the 1980s, a dominant thrust of social security reforms in the United Kingdom has been to make work-conditionality of benefit receipts more explicit, as manifested in tighter controls, more prescriptive job-seeking requirements and stiffer sanctions for non-compliance (Finn 1997). Intensifying this emphasis on work-conditionality and placing it in a broader context of a redefinition of rights and responsibilities within the British welfare state, the Labour government continued this trend after 1997. In essence this project involves the propagation of a new 'contract' between citizens and the state, with the latter offering different types of assistance for labour market integration and the former being obliged to accept this assistance (Department of Social Security 1998). The most prominent of the mandatory labour market participation programmes has been the 'New Deal' for young unemployed people, which requires the transition from benefit receipt to a subsidised job in the private or public sector, or full-time education. The focus on labour market integration is also evident in other New Deal programmes (e.g. for single parents) and in a range of social security and tax policies (Deacon 1997, 1998).

In sum, this section has demonstrated an overall shift towards a stronger element of work-conditionality for unemployed people across all seven countries over a period of twenty years or so. Despite some countervailing policies, particularly in the 1980s and early 1990s, and especially in Norway, the general tendency since the early 1980s has been one of unemployment systems becoming more rather than less work-conditional. However, two important qualifications have to be made when assessing the four criteria of work-conditionality separately. First, it is particularly benefit access and obligations imposed on job seekers which have become more explicitly linked to work-related criteria across all countries. In fact, despite remaining cross-national differences, some degree of convergence can be observed with respect to obligations imposed on benefit claimants, with countries such as Germany, the United Kingdom and the Netherlands, but also Denmark, catching up with the traditionally more prescriptive Swedish and, arguably, Norwegian 'work-line' approach towards unemployed benefit recipients. However, the mandatory approach to 'activation' still remains more pronounced in the Nordic countries and the United Kingdom than in the two continental welfare states, which can be explained on institutional, economic and ideological grounds (Clasen 2000). Second, as far as the other two criteria are concerned, it is noticeable that in the Netherlands and in Germany the level of benefit and, to some extent, the maximum duration of benefit receipt have become more work-conditional over time, thus stressing the traditional merit and status orientation even more. By contrast, irrespective of benefit increases or decreases, benefit levels in the United Kingdom and the Nordic countries (with the exception of Norway) now reflect previous earnings less than they did in the early 1980s, thus decreasing the work-conditionality in this respect.

Conclusion

From regime theory we expected that the Nordic countries would form a distinct group characterised by relatively easy access to unemployment compensation, i.e. approaching a universalistic regime where benefit receipts are not strongly dependent on having participated in working life (Gallie and Paugam 2000). We also assumed that the egalitarian approach in the universalistic regime would imply little differentiation within the level and duration of benefits received by claimants. Finally, we assumed claimants' obligations to work and training would be relatively strict, with the exception of wage mobility. In contrast, the employment-centred regime was expected to be prevalent in Germany and the Netherlands, with eligibility and entitlement stratified according to merit. This would be achieved by making access to benefits dependent on time spent in employment, by linking benefit levels to previous income and benefit periods to individual work records. In return, short spells in unemployment were expected to be accompanied by lenient obligations on claimants. Such principles would result in differentiated coverage depending on individual work histories and level of previous incomes, and thus demarcating labour market insiders from outsiders. Finally, the liberal model, as represented by the United Kingdom, was expected to manifest itself in easy access, but modest benefits for all claimants.

The main thrust of our empirical findings supports such hypotheses, although at times specific components of unemployment compensation schemes render such generalisations somewhat crude. For example, countries with strict access criteria to unemployment benefits and short benefit periods tend to operate parallel systems of unemployment assistance. Similarly, the eligibility requirement of long work history often goes hand in hand with broad conceptions of what is recognised as work. Nevertheless, when all four criteria of work-conditionality discussed in this chapter are taken into account simultaneously, the seven European countries do largely fall into regime clusters. Thus, across all four criteria as a whole, the distinctive egalitarian profile of unemployment compensation in the Nordic countries becomes distinct, but not when it comes to assessing individual criteria such as benefit generosity or benefit eligibility, for example. It could be argued that the egalitarian feature is also prevalent in the United Kingdom. However, the British system does not share either the universality or the generosity of the Nordic group.

As a consequence, those with better earnings and long-standing work careers (insiders on the labour market) are better protected in Germany and the Netherlands than in the Nordic countries, with higher benefits and (less pronounced or linked to age) longer benefit periods. In addition, despite recent changes they are exposed to fewer and less strict obligations to take up training and work than their counterparts in the Nordic countries. On the other hand, persons with less stable jobs and lower earnings are likely to be considerably better off in the Nordic countries than in Germany or the Netherlands. Consisting largely of women, ethnic minorities, low-skilled and seasonal workers, and persons in atypical and short-term jobs, these groups are likely to receive better benefit for longer periods in the Nordic countries than elsewhere, but will be required to participate in training programmes and actively look for work.

The generosity of unemployment insurance has decreased almost everywhere during the 1990s, whereas the picture for the 1980s is more blurred, with both increases and decreases in almost all countries. More relevant in the context of this chapter, there has been a tendency towards stricter work requirements as a condition for access to, and maintenance of, unemployment insurance benefits. Despite this general trend, the second part of the chapter has shown that benefit levels and duration have become more work-conditional in countries approaching the 'employment-centred' model, i.e. Germany and the Netherlands, where status and merit are stronger principles within social security arrangements than in the other countries. By contrast, benefit levels have become less differentiated and determined by previous earnings in the Nordic countries. In other words, we observe simultaneous diverging trends between different regime types along specific criteria, coupled with an overall converging trend towards making benefit entitlement and eligibility more dependent on work-related criteria.

Thus, claiming that national schemes of unemployment compensation are converging seems to oversimplify matters. It is obligations imposed on job seekers where boundaries between regime types seem to become most blurred, with new prescriptive policies introduced in Germany and the Netherlands going some way towards eroding differences between claimants according to status and merit. By contrast, other regime-specific characteristics have become even more pronounced over time. Since the 1980s, the United Kingdom has made its schemes increasingly liberal in nature. The Netherlands and Germany have strengthened many of their employment-centred aspects. The Nordic countries have, on the whole, made eligibility to benefits stricter, which could be interpreted as moving away from the universalistic notion of social security. On the other hand, changes within benefit levels and duration reinforce egalitarian principles, and there is no increased differentiation of benefits according to previous work. Overall, the growing emphasis on work in recent reforms of unemployment compensation regimes thus reflect both regime-specific features – or path-dependency – and a common concern to link rights to social security with an obligation to work.

Note

1 The authors would like to thank Sharon Wright and Andreas Mauer for research assistance in the United Kingdom and Germany.

Appendix Table 9.2

Features of unemployment compensation schemes in seven European countries in 1998

Appendix Table 9.2 Features of unemployment compensation schemes in seven European countries in 1998

Unemployment insurance

	Denmark	*Finland*	*Norway*	*Sweden*	*Germany*	*The Netherlands*	*United Kingdom*
Membership	Voluntary	Voluntary[b]	Compulsory	Voluntary[e]	Compulsory	Compulsory	Compulsory
Coverage	Employees, self-employed	Employees, self-employed	Employees[c]	Employees, self-employed	Employees	Employees	Employees
Waiting period	None[a]	7 days	3 days	5 days	None	None	3 days
Work demand for employees	52 weeks of work within 3 years	43 weeks of work within 2 years	Previous earned income at least 125% of basic amount in last calendar year,[d] or an average income equal to the basic amount in the last 3 years	5 months of work within 1 year	12 months of work within 3 years	26 weeks of work within last 39 weeks for short-term benefit; 26 weeks within last 39 weeks and 52 working days in 4 years of last 5 years for standard benefit and follow-up benefit (after expiry of standard benefit)	Minimum 25 contributions paid and 100 credited within last 2 years

Level	Earnings-related with 90% of previous earnings. Low benefit ceiling. Minimum equal to 82% of maximum benefit	Flat-rate benefit of 118 FIM per day plus earnings-related supplement between 20% and 42% of previous earnings, decreasing with income. No benefit ceiling, minimum given by flat-rate benefit.	Earnings-related with 0.24% of annual income per day for six days a week, equal to earnings-replacement rate of 62.4%	Earnings-related with 80% of previous income. Low benefit ceiling	Earnings-related with 67% of net earnings for people with at least one child (60% for others). No benefit ceiling and no minimum benefit	Standard benefit: 70% of previous wage (wage related) Short-term benefit: 70% of minimum wage (flat rate) Follow-up benefit: 70% of minimum wage	Flat-rate at £51.40 per week (for over 24 year olds); £40.70 per week (younger claimants)
Maximum duration	5 years. Longer for persons above 50	100 weeks within 4 consecutive years. Longer for persons above 57 years of age	156 weeks if former income above 2 times basic amount. 78 weeks if former income below. People above 64 years can receive benefit until official retirement age at 67	14 months, 21 months for people above 55/57. Renewal possible via job and training offers	6 months to 12 months depending on work record, but 32 months for claimants above 45 years of age. 12 months of work gives right to 6 months of benefit,	Short-term benefit: 6 months Standard benefit: 60 months (6 months plus 6 extra months for every half year of work-record) Follow-up	6 months

					24 months to 12 months, i.e. 2:1	benefit: age dependent: 24 months if < 57.5 years of age, till 65 years of age if > 57.5 years of age	
Obligations	Willing to accept 'suitable work'. After 3 months obligation to search for and accept jobs outside occupation. Geographical mobility stipulates up to 4 hours of daily commuting	Willing to accept 'suitable' work	Willing to accept 'suitable' work which is paid according to wage agreement and local custom. In principle full geographical and occupational mobility	Willing to accept 'suitable' work or training offers. Full geographical and occupational mobility required, but wage not to be less than 10% less than benefit	Willing to accept 'suitable' work or training offer. Geographical mobility of up to 3 hours of daily transport. Wage mobility: at least 80% of previous income during first 3 months, then 70% during next 3 months, and thereafter no limit. People above 57 years	Willing to accept 'suitable' work offer: job at level of highest education, previous skill and wage, max. 2 hours of daily transport. For every half year of unemployment one level down (out of three) in education, skills and wage. After 1.5 years all	In principle any type of employment is suitable. After 13 weeks on JSA any type of work becomes suitable. After 6 months of JSA the rate of pay no longer constitutes a restriction

					of age do not have to look for work	work suitable and max. 3 hours of transport.	
Unemployment assistance							
Existence	None	Yes	None	None[e]	Yes	Yes	Yes
Coverage	–	Unemployed not eligible for insurance	–	–	Unemployed not eligible for insurance	Unemployed not eligible for insurance, households with insufficient income	Unemployed not eligible for insurance
Waiting period	–	5 days	–	–	None	None	As in unemployment insurance
Work demand for employees	–	As for unemployment insurance	–	–	Either out-insured or fulfilling work requirement for insurance		–
Level	–	Flat-rate at 120 FIM/day. Means-tested. Supplements for children: 24 FIM/day for one child,	–	–	Earnings-related at 56% of net earnings for claimants with at least 1 child (53% for others), after	Means-tested: up to 100% of minimum wage for couples, 90% for single parents and	Flat-rate at same rates as above, but means-tested

		35 FIM/day for two, 45 FIM/day for three or more			passing a means-test; levels reduced by 3% for each year of receipt	70% for singles	
Maximum duration	–	Infinite	–	–	Infinite for out-insured	None	Infinite
Obligations	–	As in unemployment insurance	–	–	As in unemployment insurance and claimants may be required to participate in work and training schemes	Willing to accept 'suitable' work offer: job at level of highest education, previous skill and wage, max. 2 hours of daily transport. For every half year of unemployment one level down (out of three) in education, skills and wage. After 1.5 years all	As in unemployment insurance

						work suitable and max. 3 hours of transport	
Sanctions	–	As in unemployment insurance	–	–	As in unemployment insurance		As in unemployment insurance

Notes:

a The employers pay compensation for first two days.

b The unemployment insurance scheme consists of two parts, a mandatory basic amount, and a voluntary earnings-related part.

c Fishermen and self-employed above 64 years of age can also take up coverage.

d Equal to 20 to 40 per cent of income from full-time job depending on wage level.

e In 1998, the Swedish unemployment assistance scheme (KAS) was merged with the unemployment insurance scheme. As a result, the Swedish unemployment insurance scheme now (like the Finnish) – consists of two parts; a mandatory basic amount, and a voluntary earnings-related part.

10 Moving closer? Diversity and convergence in financing of welfare states

Mikko Kautto

Introduction[1]

While social spending and social rights lie at the core of welfare state research, financing of social protection and the 'social duties' to contribute to funding have received only modest attention. It is therefore not surprising that issues related to financing are seldom explicitly addressed in welfare state typologies, either. The Nordic model, for instance, is much more characterised by the origins, causes and nature of different welfare measures and their outcomes than by the pattern of financing. This chapter considers financing from a comparative and longitudinal perspective. It first explores recent discussions that question the permanence of present financing solutions and then empirically examines similarities, differences and changes in the financing of welfare states in Western Europe.

Although not at the core of comparative welfare state research, financing has been an eternal policy issue for welfare states. Doubts about sustainability accompanied the introduction of Bismarckian social insurance schemes (Alber 1988). Disparity between expenses and revenues became an issue of growing importance in the 1950s and re-emerged during times of economic uncertainty in the 1970s. Fiscal crisis, government overload and tax revolts were frequently used concepts to frame the issue at that time. Since the 1970s the fiscal consequences of unemployment and the ageing of Western societies have been permanently on the agenda. During the last decade concern over the sustainability of financing has increasingly been seen in the context of external pressures. Mobile capital, globalisation of investments and industries together with political deregulation at the supranational levels have been named as key factors forcing governments to reconsider their financing structures. It is now claimed that in the new environment tax systems and financing of social protection are especially subject to significant stress (e.g. Tanzi 1999), and calls to consider the extent to which changes in welfare states are related to external pressures have been voiced (e.g. Martin 1996). Concern over financing has also become topical at the supranational level, as exemplified by the first EU-level conference in autumn 1999 on financing social protection (*Financing Social Protection in Europe 1999*).

Research-wise, the enduring phenomenon of 'fiscal crisis' has attracted plenty of both theoretical and empirical interest over the years. If in the 1980s and early 1990s empirical research concluded that efforts to reduce the government's role in the economy failed everywhere (Alber 1988; Marklund 1988; Mishra 1993; Pierson 1994), there is now evidence that at least the increase in government outlays and indebtedness has halted in most countries (OECD National Accounts). Moreover, towards the end of the 1990s there was even some evidence of successful cost-cutting, especially in the Nordic countries (Heikkilä and Uusitalo 1997; Palme and Wennemo 1998). Nevertheless, there is a certain imbalance in the focus of empirical research efforts, as most investigations have examined cost-containment of expenditures rather than revenues – despite the obvious fact that balancing public budgets has led governments to reconsider both sides of the coin. While it is important to continue to monitor and examine changes in policies, there is a need to complement these research findings with evidence about developments in financing in order to better understand the present restructuring of welfare states. Here, a comparative perspective may also prove helpful.

Starting from these concerns this chapter examines *patterns* and *trends* in financing of social protection from a comparative perspective. It begins with an overview of the recent debates about the effects of external pressures on financing of welfare states. It will be argued that various external factors – together with other prevailing reasons for fiscal considerations – may restrict present financing solutions and force countries to consider their financing structures. Judging from the existing literature this is expected to result in merging of financing solutions. The research questions for the empirical part of the chapter are formulated as follows: Can countries be grouped according to financing patterns? Do the Nordic countries form a distinct group? How do financing solutions develop over time? Can we detect convergence? The chapter provides answers to these questions by examining variations in the financing of welfare states in general and in the financing of social protection in particular. After a presentation of results the chapter concludes with a discussion.

'External pressures' for convergence in financing solutions

Since the early 1990s the future of welfare states has increasingly been addressed from a perspective stressing *external pressures*. Free circulation of production factors, developments in capital and financing markets, increasing competition in the European internal (and global) market, political development at the supranational level, technological progress and global changes in the culture and identities of the people are among the main factors under the conceptual umbrella of 'external pressures'. External pressures are thus characterised in various forms, but globalisation, European integration and the European Union are the factors most often referred to. While there seems to be no uniform understanding of their specific contribution, nor about the mechanisms of how they are or should be affecting national social policy-making, one cannot escape the impression when reading the literature that external pressures pose some 'necessary' demands for welfare state adjustment. Furthermore, in many contributions these demands are supposed to encourage convergence of policy solutions. (See e.g. Kosonen 1994, 1998; Järensjö Montanari 1995; Rhodes 1995, 1996; Martin 1996; Strange 1996; Scholte 1997; Gough 1999; Tanzi 1999.)

On the other hand, there also exists another strand of literature on the relation between globalisation and the welfare state which holds that welfare states can enhance the competitiveness of national capital (e.g. Garrett 1998; Gough 1999). Globalisation does not necessarily lead to dismantling of the welfare state because the state plays an important adjustment role (Hirst and Thompson 1996). A volume edited by Dunning (1997) shows how the way national governments respond to globalisation greatly affects the competitiveness of the firms operating in that territory. Garrett (1998) argues that social-democratic corporatism and investments for redistributive policies and employment can be united with economic growth. In addition, Kosonen (1998) has shown how small countries with large welfare states also manage well in terms of internationalisation of their economies (see also Cameron 1978; Katzenstein 1985; Huber *et al.* 1993; Garrett and Mitchell 1995). This strand of literature suggests that choices in economic and social policies still matter: 'Enabling' welfare states survive the challenge of market integration, and while there are both enabling and non-enabling states, this view also suggests that variations between countries are not necessarily decreasing.

Although views on the consequences of external pressures differ, one can probably agree with Susan Strange (1996) that simultaneously with the advent of globalisation there have occurred important shifts in the quality and quantity of state power and authority. Increasing trans-border activities together with developments in the currency and capital markets have meant that states have lost 'the complete and exclusive control of the national currency and associated financial markets' (Scholte 1997) and their possibilities to exercise 'sovereign' macroeconomic policies (Scharpf 1991; Strange 1996). Moreover, changes in the structure of the international economy have created an environment where the power of private business and financial interests over the state has grown (e.g. Pierson 1996; Gough 1999). In addition, with the launching of EMU, the economic policy choices for countries belonging to the 'Euro-zone' are further restricted. As a result, nation–states have lost some macroeconomic instruments at their disposal,[2] which for some analysts is a reason why the weight of fiscal policy in the tool box of the government – and fiscal severity – has grown (see e.g. Pochet and Vanhercke 1998, 1999). These developments have undermined the authority and capacity of the interventionist state; in turn this loss is seen to constrain the room for manoeuvre regarding the formulation of welfare policies (Gough 1999).

Thus although external pressures certainly do not dictate the future of welfare states, in a general manner they could restrict the possibilities and choices welfare states have at their disposal. Rhodes (1995: 402) argues that 'state autonomy is progressively being eroded', both for internal and external reasons. The grimmest views see not only resources and political choices about how to use them as restricted, but also identify an additional effect of external pressures whereby exogenous factors are said to undermine the efficiency of different welfare programmes, or their capacity to reach designed goals (e.g. Gough 1999; Hagen 1999). In theory at least, the effects of external pressures may then impact upon different spheres of the 'welfare production' chain.

But these views are also open to criticism. The future of financing is more affected by 'internal' factors such as employment trends, the ageing of society, political choices or willingness to impose and pay taxes. Besides, there is no international authority or supranational legislation urging welfare states to design their financing or social protection schemes in a uniform way. As long as decisions concerning social protection continue to be in the hands of national authorities, relevant factors affecting the balance of revenues and expenditures can be adjusted and fiscal choices remain at the discretion of national decision makers. From a research perspective one can also ask whether it is at all possible to prove that changes, if any, in the financing of welfare states are related to external rather than internal factors. One can agree with Hagen (1999) that there is probably no way to single out specific effects that could be attributed to different external forces.

While one can thus be critical of determinist tones and question the overall significance of external factors among others, it is still feasible that external pressures may contribute to financing difficulties. It may be argued that while control of expenditure remains in the hands of the government, the revenue side is increasingly affected by factors beyond the control of nation–states (see Sinn 1990; Keen 1996). The most important factor in the vulnerability of financing solutions is considered to be the increased mobility of production factors. In a standard account of globalisation, external pressures ultimately stem from the fact that borders have lost some of their earlier significance. Most importantly, this has resulted in increased capital mobility, relocation of production and fiercer competition between firms which have consequences for employment. More than ever before, firms are exposed to international competition, and as a country's wealth and capacity for redistribution ultimately depend on the success of resident firms and their choices concerning employment, nation–states need to nurture national competitiveness and competitiveness of firms. General worries about competitiveness are supposed to lead policy makers to consider a lower cost strategy. Moreover, even if it could be shown that external pressures are not 'real' constraints, the key policy makers, as members of 'epistemic communities' (Deacon, B. 1998), are constantly subjected to this sort of argument.

Convergence of financing solutions is expected to result from equal rules for competition. UNICE, the organisation of European industry and employers, holds the view that the continued expansion of public expenditures has resulted in an intolerable tax burden with damaging consequences for production, employment, growth and competitiveness (UNICE 1998). According to UNICE, governments have so far reacted to public deficits by increasing taxation rather than reducing expenses. This has resulted in European employers having the world's heaviest burden in the form of total labour costs. UNICE strongly rejects tax-switching measures as a cure for this situation and suggests reducing public expenditure and correspondingly the tax burden instead. Non-wage costs[3] in particular should be the target if higher employment is to be facilitated.

Pressures to reconsider financing solutions in the new global environment amount to more than just speculation, the imagination of globalisation theorists and the lobbying of employers' interest organisations.

There are also more practical reasons why adjustments that would result in convergence of financing are anticipated. Big differences in taxation levels and criteria (what to tax) create room for tax competition and tax evasion. Capital owners and individuals can leverage tax differences in their favour and it is argued that it has become less viable for governments to tax mobile production factors (see e.g. Swank 1998). Most policy makers and economists agree that taxation levels in countries increasingly trading and competing with each other cannot be very different if one wants to avoid these negative effects. This is especially the case for countries belonging to the same trading bloc and political community.

In addition, the European Commission actively urges member states of the European Union to consider similar policy solutions. The completion of the internal market necessitated removal of tax barriers between member states. In the search for equal rules of competition and trade, differences between the tax systems of the member states of the European Union have occasionally been seen as hindrances to the full functioning of the Single Market.[4] It is generally perceived that European integration, driven by its key engines the European Commission, EMU and the Single Market, is thrusting member states' financing solutions towards a similar mould. As tax harmonisation has so far been considered impossible to achieve,[5] the European Commission's objective since the outset of the Single Market has been to achieve convergence of tax systems (or 'tax approximation') within fairly narrow limits (Keen 1996). While the issue of tax harmonisation has been dormant on the EU agenda for a long time, the planned incorporation into the EU of Eastern European countries with considerably lower levels of taxation has raised concerns again. Hout (1998) is not alone in arguing that tax policy co-ordination by the EU institutions will result in a convergence of tax rates and instruments of taxation.

Even without any active push from EU institutions, many EU social policy analysts (e.g. Streeck 1996; Hagen 1999; Leibfried and Pierson 2000; see also various authors in Beck *et al.* 1997) consider that the existing discrepancy between economic and social priorities and economic and social policy decision-making at the EU level[6] is affecting the future of social policy negatively. In this view social policy solutions may converge accidentally, as a spill-over reaction. Some even believe the social dimension of the EU is being 'consciously' underdeveloped to give way to market forces, which would, in the end, lead to the restructuring of the 'expensive' welfare state (see e.g. Vanhercke 1998). Economic policy, formulated more and more at the supranational EU level and beyond the democratic control of citizens (Scharpf 1997), is supposed to have implications for the scope and content of social policy. From such a wide perspective, convergence in other than social policy spheres may encourage convergence in public budgets and ways of financing welfare (e.g Kosonen 1994).

From a nation–state's perspective the processes of globalisation and European integration can hardly be analysed separately, nor is it fruitful to think of them solely as 'pressure' factors. While globalisation and European integration have opened up new possibilities for European countries and firms, the European Union in turn can be seen as a means to limit and govern the destructive forces of globalisation. Accordingly, external pressures can come in various forms and diverse routes and countries may exploit them differently. There hardly exists unanimous views regarding their nature and origins, nor an easy way to weigh the risks and opportunities. How exactly these types of external pressure affect taxation solutions of countries is an area of growing interest among tax researchers and far from fully understood. The literature on the subject is in honest disagreement about how severe this pressure is and will come to be, and how radical the reforms already executed or still needed. Neither does there seem to exist any agreement about the mechanisms. What is evident, however, is that international considerations of this type are prominent on national and supranational agendas and are already affecting the formulation of tax policy and the search for optimal taxation (see Sinn 1990; Keen 1996; Piekkola 1996; Birch Sørensen 1998).

Some conclusions from this short exploration may now be drawn for the purposes of the remaining chapter. First, while one does not need to accept any deterministic views concerning the detrimental effects of external pressures, it is acknowledged that the increased intercourse across borders and at the supranational level has resulted in limitations concerning the financing of state activities and consequently in a new precondition for welfare states to take these seriously into account. Second, governments are therefore reconsidering how to finance state activities under the new conditions. Since these conditions are more or less similar for different countries, convergence in policy responses is expected. Third, if such a restructuring of financing arrangements is currently taking place, it is generally anticipated that overall tax levels will be reduced, at least in countries with high taxation. Fourth, in addition to tax reductions, or instead of them, shifts in the way tax revenues are collected are a possible answer to the pressures.

Fifth, these concerns apply to the financing of social protection, and therefore governments may look for cuts in social protection expenditure or aim to change the relative balance in financing shares. In particular, it is anticipated that the shares paid by employers will be reduced.

Research questions, data and methodology

Talk about external pressures is often holistic in the sense that all countries should experience similar pressures and react similarly. However, the existing differences between countries mean that it makes little sense to imagine that such adjustment pressures are equally severe for all countries. Thus country responses should rather be different.

When financing has been addressed from a comparative perspective it has been emphasised how the Nordic welfare states differ from other welfare states in two important respects. First, the Nordic countries spend much on welfare. Korpi and Palme (1998) have pointed out how the 'encompassing model' (consisting of the Nordic countries) necessarily has, due to its strategy of redistribution, a bigger redistributive budget than the other ideal-types. Second, the Nordic countries are characterised by the predominance of tax financing as opposed to contribution financing (see e.g. Esping-Andersen and Korpi 1987). The size of the redistributive budget and the way this budget is financed are considered important because different solutions are supposed to have different consequences for the well-being of the population.[7] Korpi and Palme (1998) argue that encompassing schemes (which demand a bigger redistributive budget) reduce inequality and poverty more efficiently than other schemes. The redistributive outcomes of social policy programmes thus depend on how the risks, contributions and benefits are linked (Sjöberg 1999). Furthermore, the design of schemes and financing solutions behind them are also believed to have some feedback effects. It is often argued that tax financing, the universal character of social security schemes and public support for social policy are mutually reinforcing (e.g. Sihvo and Uusitalo 1995; Svallfors 1996; Forma 1999; Goul Andersen *et al.* 1999).

As financial resources at the state's disposal are a *sine qua non* for any choices over policies and in as much as there are external pressures for limiting the size of the redistributive budget and/or for changes in the balance of financing responsibilities, this is fundamentally important for the design of social policy schemes and worthy of research. Because high rather than low taxation is seen as a problem, this issue is paramount to the Nordic welfare states. It is often pointed out that the Nordic countries as the 'big spenders' with 'too big public sectors' and 'too heavy taxation' are vulnerable to external pressures and should anticipate losses in their tax revenues or renegotiate how 'social duties' are being shared (e.g. Kosonen 1994). Convergence of financing structures is thus presumed to happen by countries of high taxation and high social protection costs moving closer to the European average.

To argue that the Nordic countries are losing their distinctiveness in financing arrangements may be jumping to conclusions, as proponents of this view seem to take it for granted that in addition to similarities in policy measures and well-being of their populations they also share similar financing solutions. This is not self-evident, and for this reason there are two research topics for this chapter: the existence of different financing clusters and the presumed convergence in financing solutions. Accordingly, the chapter aims to clarify whether distinct groups of countries exist that exhibit similar financing *patterns*. Has there ever been a Nordic model of financing? Does such a model still exist? Do differences in financing patterns correspond to welfare state models? In addition, by providing and analysing data from 1980 to the latest available, the chapter illuminates *trends* in financing. Are countries becoming more similar in their financing patterns, or is it rather that solutions concerning financing are diverging?

Data and methodology

The empirical part presents data for fourteen or fifteen European countries (fourteen EU countries and Norway depending on the availability of data; Luxembourg is omitted from the examination due to its small size) allowing us to determine whether or not the Nordic countries form a group and if the trends hypothesised are unique for them. The statistics used are chosen to allow comparable data. The chapter uses new Eurostat data on social protection expenditure and receipts for 1980–97 (*Social Protection Expenditure and Receipts* 1993, 1996, 1999, 2000), data on general government accounts and statistics 1985–96 (*The Government Sector in the European Union* 1997) and data on taxation systems (*Structures of the Taxation Systems in the European Union* 1998). The examination is thus based on aggregate financing data and the unit of analysis is countries. This approach cannot reveal any differential development in different programmes.

Eurostat data on national accounts are standardised according to the European System of Integrated Economic Accounts (ESA) but collected and classified by the statistical offices of the member states. In a similar manner, data on social protection are standardised according to the European System of Integrated Social Protection Statistics (ESSPROS). These two systems are designed to enable comparisons but nevertheless contain various footnotes, warnings about problems caused by publishing of provisional data, or revisions that may follow later (for more details see the publications cited, ESA and ESSPROS manuals, and the 'New Cronos' database). There are two more serious data limitations that affect the empirical part of this chapter. First, while Norway is not included in ESA statistics it is included in ESSPROS statistics. Second, the revision of ESSPROS methodology has led to a break in comparable time-series in social protection statistics. The new manual has been in use since 1996 and the latest social protection statistics published by Eurostat include figures since 1990. However, figures for Sweden according to the new ESSPROS system are available only from 1993.

Scatter diagrams are drawn to illustrate differences and similarities between the countries. In addition, statistics are complemented by our own calculations so as to have some statistical parameters (means, medians and coefficients of variation) to rely on in the interpretations concerning group membership, direction of trends and convergence. Instead of coefficient of variation, convergence could also be measured by standard deviation as most figures used are percentage shares. Indeed, both standard deviation and coefficient of variation were calculated, and according to both these measures the trends presented later in this chapter were similar, irrespective of the choice of convergence measure. This partly reflects the fact that the means in many cases are fairly stable over time. However, as the coefficient of variation is a convergence measure of relative dispersion that allows standardisation, i.e. comparing development between the indicators, it is used throughout the chapter.

Financing of welfare states[8]

First we examine the overall financing of European welfare states between 1980 and 1996. Table 10.1 presents total taxation as percentage of GDP between 1980 and 1996.[9] The countries are listed in Table 10.1 in a conventional order that groups countries according to the welfare state model they are regarded as belonging to. Looking first at the situation in 1980, the table clearly shows that there was no major difference in total taxation between the three Nordic and five Continental countries. Sweden, the Netherlands and Denmark are at

Table 10.1 Total taxation as percentage of GDP, 1980–96

	1980	*1985*	*1990*	*1996*	*Change 1980–96*
Denmark	45.6	49.1	49.7	53.1	7.5
Finland	36.9	40.9	45.4	48.2	11.3
Sweden	49.1	50.0	55.6	54.1	5.0
Mean	*43.9*	*46.7*	*50.2*	*51.8*	*7.9*
Austria	41.0	43.0	41.3	44.2	3.2
Belgium	44.0	47.2	44.3	46.3	2.3
France	41.7	44.5	43.7	45.9	4.2
Germany	41.6	41.6	39.5	42.0	0.4
Netherlands	46.0	45.5	45.1	44.8	−1.2
Mean	*42.9*	*44.4*	*42.8*	*44.6*	*1.8*
Greece	n.a.	20.6	29.0	31.6	11.0
Italy	30.6	34.8	38.8	42.9	12.3
Portugal	25.5	29.3	32.3	37.1	11.6
Spain	25.6	29.9	35.3	35.5	9.9
Mean	*27.2*	*28.7*	*33.9*	*36.8*	*11.2*
Ireland	34.7	38.9	35.5	33.3	−1.4
UK	36.1	38.2	35.7	35.6	−0.5
Mean	*35.4*	*38.6*	*35.6*	*34.5*	*−1.0*
Median, all	41.0	41.3	40.4	43.6	4.6
Unweighted mean, all	38.3	39.5	40.8	42.5	5.4

Source: Structures of the Taxation Systems in the European Union (1998).
Notes:
Eurostat data is collected and classified by the statistical offices of the countries, comparability is ensured by their common use of ESA (European System of Integrated Economic Accounts). According to ESA 'total taxation' includes current taxes on income and wealth. capital taxes (on capital or wealth), taxes linked to production and imports (that consist of VAT and general turnover taxes, import duties and agricultural levies, excise duties, taxes on services, taxes on ownership of land and buildings, stamp, registration and similar duties, and other taxes linked to import and production) and actual social contributions (i.e. payments to acquire and/or preserve the right to social benefits).
Data for Greece is available from 1985 only, change refers to period 1985–96. Mean for Southern countries in 1980 is calculated without Greece.

the top, followed by Belgium, France, Austria and Germany. Finland comes only after these, below the European average and a little ahead of the UK and Ireland, which are at a distance from the Southern countries Italy, Spain and Portugal. Judging group memberships by the means, there are few grounds for claiming a definite Nordic group of taxation.

Throughout the period from the early 1980s until now Denmark and Sweden have been the two top countries. As taxation levels in Finland grew quickly during the 1980s, there is more justification for claiming a Nordic cluster of high taxation countries since the late 1980s. Also, the mid-1980s seem to form a watershed in the development between the Nordic and Continental countries, as between 1985 and 1990 total taxation as percentage of GDP increased in the former countries, while it decreased in the latter. Since 1990 the difference between these two groups has stayed about the same. Another interesting development pattern is revealed by comparing the Southern European countries to Ireland and the UK. In 1980 taxation was at a lower level in the Southern countries. While total taxation remained almost constant in Ireland and the UK, taxation rates grew fast in the Southern countries, especially during the 1980s. A shift in the relative position of these two groups occurred in 1992, since when Southern European countries have had a higher level of total taxation.

According to the latest available data in 1996 the Nordic countries form a clear group of their own. Continental countries seem to have remarkably similar tax rates. Italy is arguably a border case between the Continental and Southern groups of countries. Finally, Ireland and the UK may be seen as a separate group. Financing 'clusters' thus resemble typologies, but only towards the end of the period.

Figure 10.1 shows the convergence in total taxation and the development of mean taxation between 1985 and 1996 (data for Greece are missing for 1980–84). The lower the coefficient of variation (the y-axis on the left), the more similar the countries are. Accordingly, a downward trend shows convergence, whereas an upward trend reports countries are becoming less similar. Looking at Figure 10.1, one can see that the coefficient of variation in 1996 is lower than in 1985: over the period countries definitely became more alike. However, the trend is not linear and there are two turning points. In the period between 1985 and 1988 the situation was rather stable; between 1988 and 1992 the countries were converging, whereas since 1992 convergence in total taxation has stopped. Contrary to what could be expected, actual developments in the 1990s do not show any 'convergence impact' from external pressures, in fact since 1992 the opposite is more the case. Figure 10.1 also shows that convergence occurred at the same time as total taxation as percentage of GDP on average has gradually increased (right-hand y-axis). Convergence is mainly caused by increases in total taxation in the Southern countries.[10]

In conclusion, between 1980 and 1996 tax levels continued to grow in most countries. The growth was most marked in the Nordic and

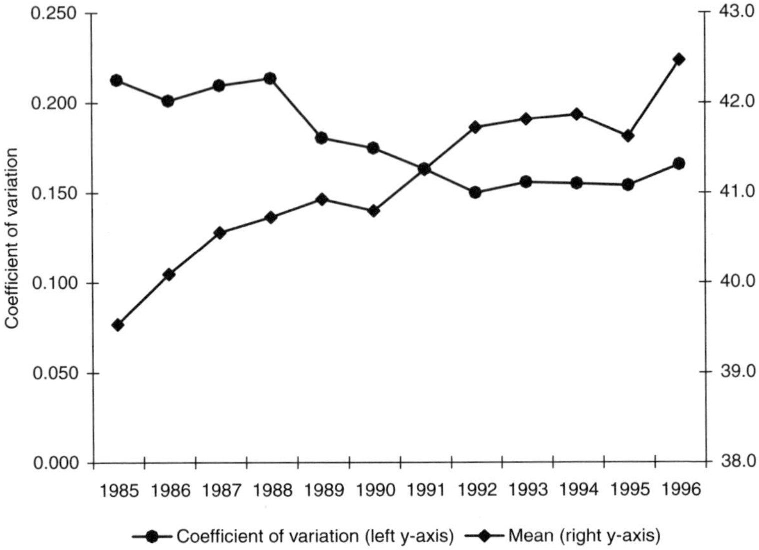

Source: Own calculations based on data from *Structures of the Taxation Systems in the European Union* 1998.

Figure 10.1 Convergence and European averages in total taxation, 1985–96

Southern countries, whereas it was slower in the Continental group of countries. In Ireland and the UK taxation first increased and then decreased to roughly the same level in 1996 as in 1980. This development led to some convergence in total taxation. However, since the early 1990s the trends in this respect give little support to the convergence hypothesis. Moreover, contrary to what should be expected from the 'pressure' literature, convergence did occur in the form of a catch-up effect: Southern countries increased their taxation levels, while the Nordic countries did not decrease theirs. It is also worth noting that the cross-sectional inspection of country groupings suggests a differentiation of the Nordic from the Continental countries between 1985 and 1990, while Figure 10.1 suggests that some overall convergence took place. In other words, overall variation declined at the same time as there began to emerge evidence of some group-specific characteristics in total taxation. Separate calculations for different country groups (not shown here) also confirm that convergence occurred *within* the Nordic, Continental and Southern groups of countries.

Tax components

Before moving on to examine financing of social protection, it is useful to take a look at the development in the major tax components. Table 10.2 shows average taxation development in the EU countries by decomposing total taxation into three main tax aggregates (see note in Table 10.1): indirect taxes (taxes levied on production and imports), direct taxes (personal and corporate income) and social contributions (from employers, employees and self-employed). Looking first at the tax aggregates as percentage of GDP it is notable that the share of indirect taxes as percentage of GDP remains rather constant over the 15-year period. Direct taxes increase a little, while social contributions are 2 percentage units higher in 1996 than 1980. Both the employers' and employees' financing shares as percentage of GDP increase, although the relative increase for employees is more pronounced. Furthermore, examining the distribution within total taxation confirms that the share of social contributions of total taxation also grew. The trend was rather stable during the 1980s, the increase occurring during the 1990s. In light of the average figures no major restructuring of financing seems to have taken place in Europe.

It could be argued that even if at aggregate European level we fail to find any clear signs of restructuring finance, there may be more obvious changes at country level. Moreover, some cluster-specific adjustment routes might be detected on closer inspection, e.g. the Nordic countries could be adjusting in a uniform way. Eurostat statistics on general government accounts between 1980 and 1995 were used to investigate these suggestions (*The Government Sector in the European Union* 1997). Table 10.3 summarises the changes in the relative roles of different tax components for fourteen countries. It is evident that structures of taxation vary widely between the European countries. The Nordic nations stand apart from others in collecting a higher share of tax revenues from direct taxes and a lower share from social contributions. A country-by-country examination of the relative roles of the three most important revenue components confirms that no uniform shifts took place. In some countries direct taxes increased their importance in state finances, in others indirect taxes became more prominent, and in still others social contributions by the mid-1990s accounted for a larger part of overall financing than in 1980. The most common trend seems to be the decrease in the share of indirect taxes. Nor is it easy to detect any crystal-clear group-specific adjustment patterns. Within country groups we can find opposite trends. For instance, among the Nordic countries the relative role of direct taxes increased in Denmark,

Table 10.2 Development in main tax revenue components, European averages, 1980–96

Indirect taxes, direct taxes and social contributions as percentage of GDP, European averages, 1980–96

	1980	1985	1990	1996	Change 1980–96
Indirect taxes	13.5	13.5	13.1	13.6	0.1
Direct taxes	12.4	13.3	12.9	13.2	0.8
Social contributions, of which	13.4	14.1	13.7	15.3	1.9
Employers' social contributions	7.8	7.9	7.8	8.3	0.5
Employees' social contributions	4.3	4.7	4.5	5.1	0.8
Self- and non-employed social contributions	1.3	1.5	1.4	1.9	0.6

Indirect taxes, direct taxes and social contributions as percentage of total taxation, European averages, 1980–96

	1980	1985	1990	1996	Change 1980–96
Indirect taxes	34.4	33.0	32.9	32.5	−1.9
Direct taxes	31.5	32.5	32.5	31.2	−0.3
Social contributions	34.0	34.5	34.5	36.3	2.3

Source: Structures of the Taxation Systems in the European Union 1998.
Note:
As country-level information for all categories was not available, European averages include Luxembourg.

but decreased in Finland and Sweden. On the other hand the role of social contributions expanded in all Continental countries and the role of direct taxes in all Southern countries. In Ireland and the UK indirect taxes appear to have moved in the same direction.

With the help of yearly data on the relative shares of different tax components as percentage of total tax revenue we can calculate the coefficients of variation in order to examine convergence/divergence for each revenue component. The results presented in Figure 10.2, show some convergence in the role of indirect taxes, less clear convergence in the role of social contributions and *no* convergence in the role of direct taxes. This finding partly contradicts Greve's (1996: 362) account based on OECD data, according to which there is a trend towards a more common tax structure *in all areas*. According to the calculations presented here approximation of taxes thus occurred for taxes related to production and imports, such as VAT and excise

Table 10.3 Relative shares of main tax revenue components of total tax revenue, 1980–95, percentages

	Direct taxes as % of total tax revenue			*Indirect taxes as % of total tax revenue*			*Social contributions as % of total tax revenue*		
	1980	*1995*	*Change*	*1980*	*1995*	*Change*	*1980*	*1995*	*Change*
Denmark	58	62	5	40	34	–6	2	3	1
Finland	40	39	–1	36	29	–8	24	32	9
Sweden	44	43	–1	28	29	1	29	28	–1
Mean	*47*	*48*	*1*	*35*	*31*	*–4*	*18*	*21*	*3*
Austria	29	29	0	39	34	–5	32	37	5
Belgium	43	40	–3	26	25	–1	31	35	4
France	21	22	1	36	33	–3	44	45	1
Germany	31	27	–4	30	29	–1	39	44	6
Netherlands	35	30	–6	25	27	2	40	44	4
Mean	*32*	*30*	*–2*	*31*	*30*	*–2*	*37*	*41*	*4*
Italy	32	38	5	29	30	1	39	33	–6
Portugal	22	27	4	48	41	–7	30	33	3
Spain	27	34	6	26	29	3	47	37	–10
Mean	*27*	*33*	*5*	*34*	*33*	*–1*	*38*	*34*	*–4*
Ireland	38	42	5	47	42	–5	16	16	0
UK	40	40	0	42	40	–2	18	20	2
Mean	*39*	*41*	*2*	*44*	*41*	*–3*	*17*	*18*	*1*
Median	35	38	2	36	30	–6	31	33	2
Unweighted mean	35	36	1	35	32	–2	30	31	1

Source: The Government Sector in the European Union 1997.

Note:

Greece does not supply this kind of data to Eurostat and could not be included.

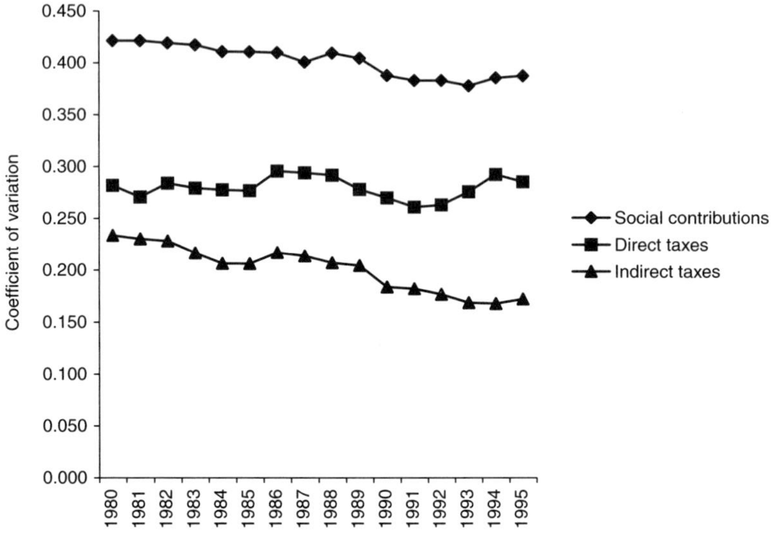

Source: Own calculations based on data from *The Government Sector in the European Union* 1997.

Figure 10.2 Convergence in the relative shares of main tax components, 1980–95

duties. This probably comes as no surprise given the efforts to remove tax barriers from free circulation of goods and services. The result is also in line with suggestions about ways to adjust to external pressures. In contrast, it is interesting to see that variation in direct taxes persisted for the fifteen years under study. This can be interpreted as showing that external pressures – in whatever form – did not lead to an approximation of taxes on income and wealth.

Financing social protection[11]

After this exposé on overall public finance, it is time to look closer at how social protection is financed in different countries. As a dynamic perspective on financing has by and large been missing from previous studies, a longitudinal perspective is also provided. Has there been a Nordic model of financing social protection? And if so, does it still exist? To answer these questions information on the *level* of financing of social protection and information on how financing is *shared* between different parties is needed. Social protection expenditure as a share of GDP serves as an indicator of total financing needed.[12]

The revenues for social policies in turn come from two main sources: social security contributions and taxes.[13] Social contributions can be collected from both employers and employees (and other insured persons).

With this information financing of social protection may be approached with a two-dimensional perspective (see Kangas 1994; Bonoli 1997). The strength of a two-dimensional classification, Bonoli argues, is its ability to reflect social policy developments in terms of both the expansion/contraction of state welfare and the convergence/divergence of European social policies. Thus Bonoli's idea is to gather data about the 'quantity of welfare' ('how much') that welfare states provide and about where they stand with respect to 'how' welfare is arranged (see Bonoli 1997: 360). Although Bonoli's interest is not in financing, these indicators are also the best information available on differences between the countries on how they finance their welfare schemes. But additionally, longitudinal data are needed[14] to answer questions about convergence. Following Bonoli and Kangas it is possible to draw a quadrant using data on social protection expenditure and on financing shares. This is done in Figures 10.3, 10.4 and 10.5, where countries are located depending on whether their social protection expenditure as percentage of GDP and general government contributions as percentage of total social protection financing were above or below the median.

Figure 10.3 presents the situation in 1980, when Spain, Italy and Portugal are revealed to have had low social spending and little government funding. Greece, the UK, Ireland, Finland and Norway were low spenders emphasising government tax financing, while France, the Netherlands, Germany and Belgium were high spenders with little government funding. Finally, Denmark and Sweden were high spenders with high government share in financing. In 1980 only the Continental countries occupied their 'own' separate quadrant. The Nordic countries were split into two quadrants; Norway and Finland as low spenders resembled the UK. Sweden and Denmark may be seen as outliers in the European scene.

In 1990 (Figure 10.4), the positions of countries seem to follow the conventional typology-wisdom. The Southern countries were now located in their own quadrant, while the UK and Ireland were alone in the quadrant of low spenders and tax financers. Finland and Norway had moved closer towards Denmark and Sweden and a Nordic cluster of financing social protection had started to take shape. Austria's financing pattern in 1990 resembled that of Finland, the country being located in the upper right quadrant together with

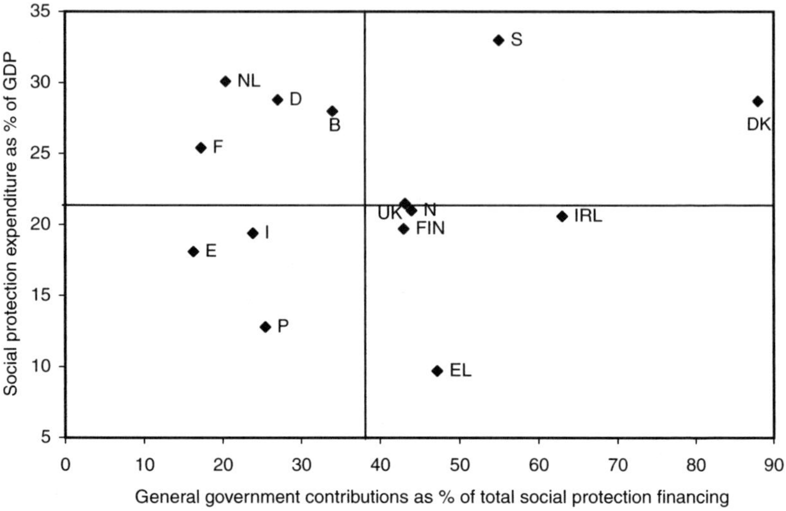

Source: Calculations based on *Social Protection Expenditure and Receipts* 1996.
Note: Data for Norway from *Yearbook of Nordic Statistics* 1983:18.

Figure 10.3 European welfare states two-dimensionally, 1980

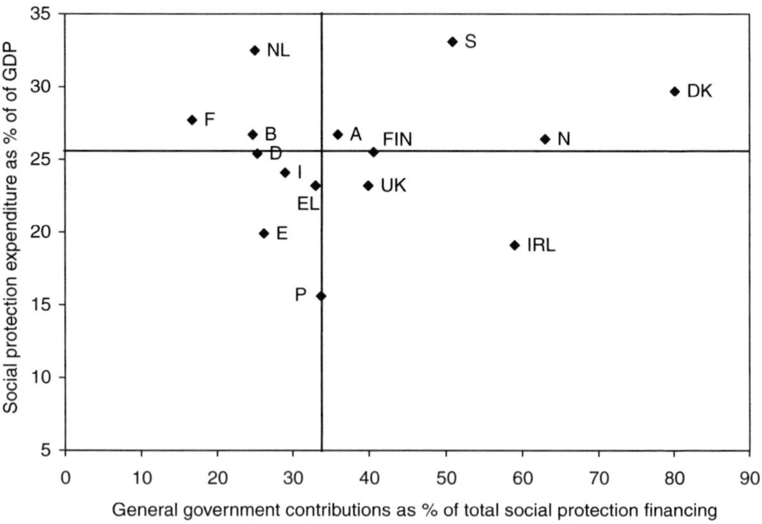

Source: Social Protection Expenditure and Receipts 2000: Table D 1.2.3 and Table B 1.1.

Figure 10.4 European welfare states two-dimensionally, 1990

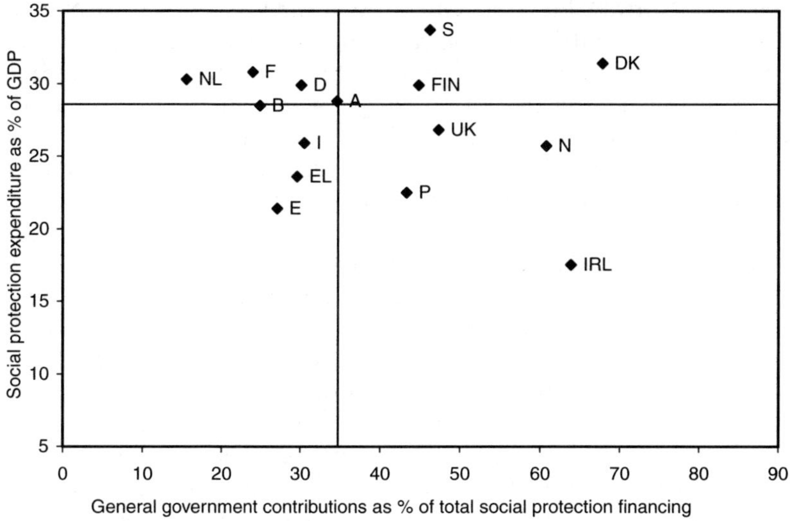

Source: Social Protection Expenditure and Receipts 2000: Table D 1.2.3 and Table B 1.1

Figure 10.5 European welfare states two-dimensionally, 1997

the Nordic countries. The Continental countries Belgium, Germany, the Netherlands and France remained in their original quadrant.

Figure 10.5 presents the situation in 1997. Finland is even closer to the two other Nordic countries Denmark and Sweden, but Norway has moved out of this grouping. Greece, Spain and Italy have become more similar to each other while Portugal is now located on the other side of the median line. The UK and Ireland remain in the quadrant of low spending and high share of tax financing. The Continental countries Belgium, the Netherlands, France and Germany seem to have consolidated their positions as countries with high spending and low tax financing. Austria is situated at the junction of the median lines, but is arguably closer to the Continental countries than to the other groupings.

Looking at development over time it is evident that the range of government financing narrowed, mainly due to changes in Denmark, although the median did not vary much. Also, the range of social protection expenditure became smaller; here the median increased over time. Weighing changes in countries' positions in the three quadrants presented, it is clear that major movement occurred in Finland,

Denmark, Norway, Portugal, Greece, Spain and Italy, i.e. in the Nordic and Southern countries. In contrast, only minor changes occurred in the Continental group of countries, and relative changes also appear minor in Ireland and the UK. Changes within the Nordic group of countries are worth noting; Finland and Sweden became very similar as a result of diverging trends, while Denmark and Norway also moved closer to each other after following very different development paths.

In conclusion, while at the beginning of the 1980s there are few grounds for justifying social protection financing clusters that would be identical to typologies, the evidence presented here suggests such clustering may have taken place towards the end of the period examined. In a long perspective the most stable cluster seems to be the Continental group of countries, formed by France, Belgium, the Netherlands and Germany. These countries were already located close to each other in 1980. Due to lack of data the position of Austria at that point is unclear, but at least towards the end of the period it could be counted in this group, too. Changes in the UK and Ireland also appear limited: low levels of social spending and high share of general government financing characterise these countries throughout the period. In contrast, the Southern countries (especially Greece and Portugal) and the Nordic countries (especially Finland) experienced more visible changes regarding their financing patterns. However, these changes could be explained by more sweeping social policy reforms, maturation of social policy schemes and/or by more pronounced fluctuation in the GDP and employment that have had consequences for the financing patterns, rather than by intentional reshuffling of financing arrangements. Whatever the reasons, a two-dimensional examination gives only feeble and partial support to consistency in the clustering of financing patterns.[15]

Sharing the burden of financing social protection

So far it can be concluded that governments did not retreat from their welfare responsibility. On the contrary, they collected more tax revenues (witnessed by an increase in total tax levels) and targeted more resources to welfare (witnessed by a growing share of social protection expenditure as percentage of GDP). In addition, according to Figures 10.3, 10.4 and 10.5 there existed no general European trend in terms of government responsibility. In fact, an equal number of decreases and increases in state responsibility in financing social protection seems to have taken place. Nor were there any 'cluster-specific' trends in this respect. The more pronounced decreases in government responsibility took place in Denmark and in the Netherlands. The government's share of financing especially increased in the UK and Portugal.

Turning now to the question of possible systematic patterns in the development of social protection financing responsibilities during the 1990s, one may ask whether shifts nevertheless occurred in the relative shares of financing social protection for the employers and/or for the insured.

In order to examine such changes two scatter diagrams (Figures 10.6 and 10.7) plotting the countries position in 1990 and 1997 are presented, one for each of the two remaining financers: employers and the insured (consisting of employees, self-employed, pensioners and others). The line across the diagram divides the countries into those

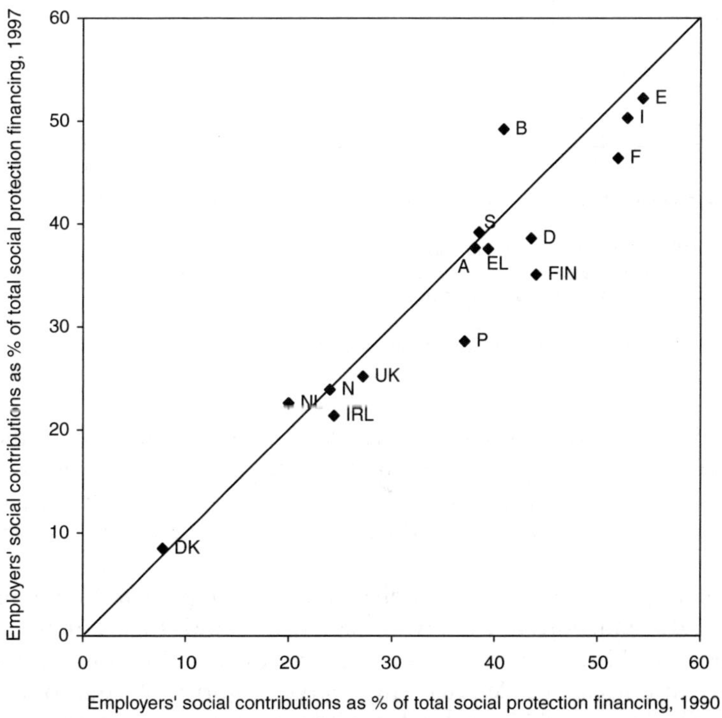

Source: Social Protection Expenditure and Receipts 2000.
Note: For Sweden data for 1993 instead of 1990 are used.

Figure 10.6 Social contributions from employers in 1990 and 1997

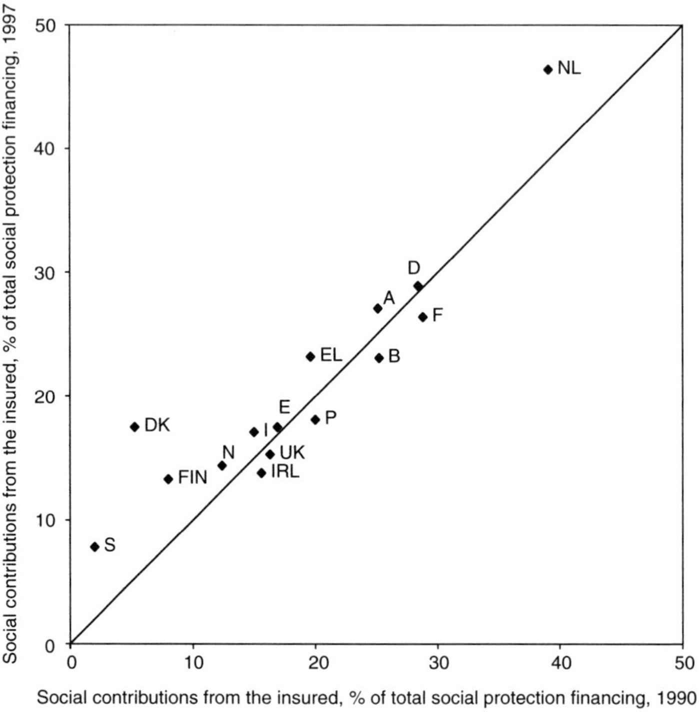

Source: Social Protection Expenditure and Receipts 2000: Table D 1.2.2.
Notes: For Sweden data for 1993 instead of 1990 are used. In Denmark labour market contributions have been included as insureds' social contributions since 1994.

Figure 10.7 Social contributions from the insured in 1990 and 1997

in which a relative increase or decrease in the 'burden of finance' occurred; a position above the line indicates an increase in financing responsibility from 1990 to 1997, and a position below the line the opposite. The distance to the dividing line shows how big a change took place.

According to the literature emphasising external pressures we should anticipate reductions in employers' financing shares. Figure 10.6 lends support to this proposition, as a relatively clear and uniform adjustment pattern can be detected. In a large majority of countries the employers' responsibility in total social protection financing decreased. The clearest shifts were in Finland and Portugal, but notable changes also occurred in Germany, France, Spain, Italy, Ireland and the UK. There are only three countries (Denmark, the Netherlands and

Belgium) showing an increase in the employers' financing responsibility. Of these, Denmark and the Netherlands have always had the two lowest shares for employers.

Finally, Figure 10.7 presents the shifts in the social contributions of the insured. As expected, the relative decrease in the employers' financing responsibility is partly compensated by an increase in the contributions from the insured. Most notably, contributions from the insured increased in *all* Nordic countries. Contributions from the insured decreased only in the UK, Ireland, Portugal, Belgium and France.

It may thus be concluded that some empirical support exists for the proposition of a shift in financing responsibilities, even within the short period between 1990 and 1997. It is hardly an accident that the employers' relative share of social protection financing (regardless of what it was in 1990) decreased in twelve of the fifteen countries examined in this chapter. To compensate for this decrease governments either opted for a larger public responsibility or introduced increases in the social contributions paid by insured persons.[16] In either case, it is the individual who felt the impact in his or her pocket.

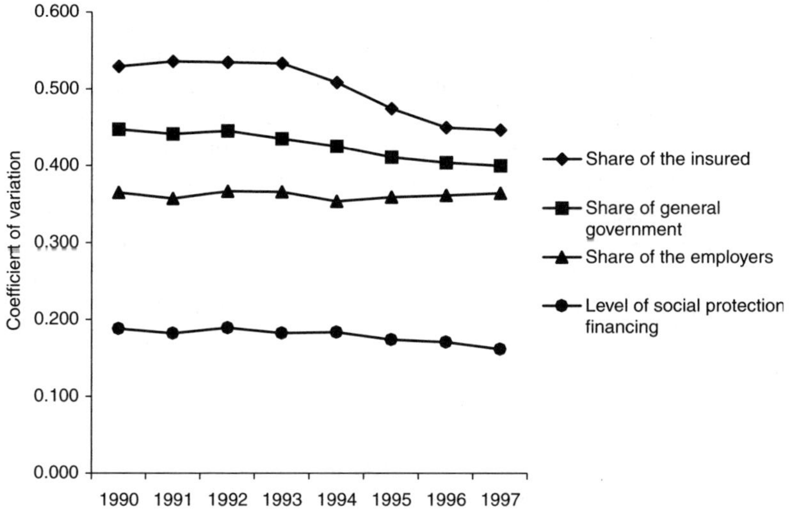

Sources: Own calculations based on data from *Social Protection Expenditure and Receipts* 2000: Tables B 1.1, D 1.2.1, D 1.2.2 and D 1.2.3.

Notes: Data for Sweden are missing for 1990–92; in convergence calculations data for 1993 are used for these years.

Figure 10.8 Convergence in financing social protection, 1990–97

To end the empirical part of this analysis it may be asked whether these changes led to convergence in financing social protection. As indicated earlier, due to the change in the methodology of the ESSPROS system revised data for different countries are only available for the 1990s. Besides, in older publications Austria, Finland, Sweden and Norway, respectively, are on different occasions missing from various publications. Due to these limitations coefficients of variation for the level of social protection financing and for the shares of different sources of financing are presented only for the period 1990–97 (Figure 10.8). The results show convergence in the level of financing,[17] in the share of general government financing and in the share of the insured. It is worth noting that as almost all countries reduced employers' shares, no convergence occurred in this indicator. It should be emphasised that despite the observed convergence in financing shares, the variation among the European countries was still considerable. However, there was much less variation in the overall level of financing social protection.

Conclusion

This chapter has addressed differences and changes in financing patterns in the context of external pressures from a comparative perspective. Although many see the state as powerless and obsolescent in the face of global capital and other external pressures, by many measures the state is in fact larger and more entrenched in social relations than ever before and some even argue that states have played an indispensable role in enabling the globalisation of capital (Scholte 1997). According to Hirst and Thompson (1996) this capacity is far from being lost, as there are no other regulatory alternatives yet in sight. Parallel to this one can argue that 'external pressures' have not resulted in the withdrawal of the welfare state. Levels of taxation and social spending have increased as costs for unemployment, ageing and other materialised social risks have to be met somehow, and it is the welfare state that still carries the overall responsibility. Judged by the data on total taxation countries became more similar regarding the overall financing of welfare states, as expected, but the variation declined not because of decreases in the Nordic or Continental countries but because the Southern countries increased their taxation.

The examination of the main tax aggregates revealed no major Western European shift in the balance between different tax components, unless the increase in the role of social contributions can be counted as such. Measured as a share of GDP, social contributions increased for both employers and employees. However, the increases were probably more determined by increases in need for social protection than by efforts to change the aggregate tax balance. Measuring convergence for different tax components revealed that this happened in indirect taxation, as could be expected. As a rule, countries with a high share of indirect taxation in total tax revenue decreased this share.

Signs of changes regarding financing of social protection also emerged. Rising costs of social protection have meant a growing tax burden and increased contributions. However, an examination of relative financing shares showed the increased burden of costs was accompanied by a shift in financing responsibilities. In particular, and according to views in the literature stressing external pressures, governments reacted in a way that decreased the employers' share. With few expectations this seems to have been a universal European trend between 1990 and 1997. Without such a shift the employers' contributions as percentage of GDP would have increased even more. There is more than one way to interpret this change. Some could consider this as a relatively straightforward reaction to external pressures: non-wage labour costs have been decreased to enhance the competitiveness of firms in the global markets. The reduction also accords with ideas stressing governments' need to reduce taxation for the most mobile production factors. But one could also interpret this as a welfare state's strategy to reduce unemployment by making hiring a more attractive alternative to the employer. In the Nordic countries reductions in employers' shares could also be related to the restructuring of social security schemes: simultaneous increases for contributions from the insured have certainly served as a compensatory source of revenue, but may also have been a response to increased demands for more private responsibility in social security schemes (see Svallfors 1996 for development of opinions in Sweden; Forma 1999 for Finland).

The grouping of countries into distinct financing clusters proved to be contingent upon time (see also Kangas 1994, 1999). Context may prove to be decisive. First, the financing pattern in a given period is affected by changes in the economy, unemployment and age group patterns. Second, observed differences may also reflect disparities in the relative importance of various schemes. For instance, depending on the financing rules of unemployment insurance schemes, changes in unemployment may have an effect on a country's financing pattern over a given period. Furthermore, reforms may affect the balance of financing duties. It could be that the growth in the share of the insured reflects the on-going shift from pay-as-you-go schemes towards funded pension schemes. This suggests the character of social protection financing is probably more affected by internal factors and actual needs for social protection rather than by externally imposed 'ceilings' to financing (see also Swank 1998).

The contingency in clustering of countries calls for some caution when considering equations between financing clusters and welfare state regimes. Typologies and financing clusters do not necessarily match. To interpret financing differences found between countries or groups of countries over a given period as merely reflecting differences in social policy systems is hazardous. Yet, a link between regime characteristics and financing patterns undoubtedly exists, although it is neither simple nor one that could be revealed with aggregate financing data used in this chapter.

The comparative focus in this chapter has repeatedly indicated some convergence within the Nordic group of countries. Back in the 1980s there were marked differences between the Nordic countries, both with regard to the levels of financing and how it was arranged. It is true that the major financing responsibility has been borne by the public authorities throughout the Nordic countries, but Denmark has clearly had a more tax-based system than the other three. Norway in turn has historically had higher contributions from the insured than the other three Nordic countries. This chapter has shown how in total taxation levels the Nordic countries converged in the late 1980s, how in the early 1990s they seemed to have the most similar social protection financing pattern in their history, and how during the 1990s (at least until 1997) they increased the financing shares of the insured. Still, even taking these changes into account it could be argued that Denmark remained an outlier and that the differences were big enough not to warrant the claim of a common Nordic financing pattern. Yet we may probably conclude that there is some evidence the Nordic countries became more like the other EU countries than they were in the early 1980s in terms of the shares of financing between different parties. Paradoxically, in an intra-Nordic comparison they were also more alike.

This highlights another issue that has been touched on in this chapter. Clustering of countries into distinct groups may occur simultaneously with an overall process of convergence. This is explained by the fact that convergence has not happened in a simple way as a process towards a common European average, as is often thought. It rather seems there might be more than one convergence process going on, as the above example of development in the Nordic countries testifies. While overall variation decreases, this does not rule out the possibility that countries within a cluster become more similar and that borders between clusters of countries become more visible.

This chapter has shown that there occurred convergence in total taxation, in the share of indirect taxes, in the level of social protection financing and in the relative shares of the insured and general government. Yet, despite this gradual convergence it may still be argued that there exists enduring diversity in the ways financing is arranged in Western Europe, and that changes appear both slow and limited. If there is 'path-dependency' in financing solutions (Schmidt 1999), the existing variation leaves space for further convergence and the question of convergence will probably remain on political agendas. Finally, if the patterns of financing social protection continue to converge, it is important in further research to consider whether this entails a convergence in policy design and welfare outcomes, too.

Notes

1 An earlier version of this chapter was presented at the Joint Economic and Social Research Seminar at the Swedish Institute for Social Research (SOFI) at the University of Stockholm in January 2000. I thank Johan Fritzell, Eero Carroll, Walter Korpi and Ingalill Järensjö Montanari for their helpful comments. I also wish to thank Bjørn Hvinden, Olli Kangas and Hannu Uusitalo for their careful reading and detailed comments, and the participants at the 'globalisation circle' at the University of Helsinki in March 2000.

2 On the other hand, this loss of policy sovereignty can be considered an important reason for the turn towards supranational bodies to compensate for these losses. Indeed, the creation of a European Monetary Union can be understood more in terms of creating an instrument to rescue the European nation–states from the evils of global money markets, rather than as an evil designed to force public budgets to become leaner.

3 Non-wage labour costs consist largely of employers' social contributions to the financing of social protection, payroll taxes, holiday pay, sickness leaves and other benefits. According to UNICE they add around 80 per cent to wage costs in the EU and represent almost all of the difference in labour costs between the EU and the USA (UNICE 1998).

4 Although there is no forced overall tax harmonisation taking place in the EU, there are still definite adjustments in taxation systems going on, as member states of the EU have to follow some common approaches concerning what to tax and how. There are both direct and indirect ways European integration affects financing of welfare states. For example, due to free movement of goods the Nordic countries have had to reconsider taxes on alcohol and tobacco and some taxes that were considered to be against the principle of the four freedoms have had to be abolished. Softer pressures for tax harmonisation also exist. For instance,

the European Commission's White Paper on 'Growth, Competitiveness and Employment' pointed to high labour taxation and social security contributions and recommended their reduction for making taxation systems more employment friendly. The recent 'strategy for modernising social protection' states as an objective that financing of social protection 'must take into account . . . the need to avoid the negative impact on employment arising from excessive charges and taxes on labour and the need for budgetary discipline' (COM (1999) 347 final: 13).

5 Decisions in tax matters have to be unanimous.

6 Article 130 in the Treaty on European Union states, 'The Community and Member States shall ensure that the conditions necessary for the competitiveness of the Community's industry exist.' Although promotion of social progress features in the Preamble of the Treaties on equal level with economic progress, it is well known that economic goals have been the priority in the policy-making of the European Union.

7 Already in 1958 Richard Titmuss showed that there are different ways to provide welfare, and that social welfare, occupational welfare and fiscal welfare may benefit different target groups (Titmuss 1958).

8 Unfortunately Norway is not included in Eurostat publications on government revenues and taxation structures and cannot be included in the analysis in this section for reasons of comparability.

9 The gross tax rate that is often used to express differences between countries may be misleading because some income transfers are taxed, some are not, some countries prefer using tax deductions rather than income transfers to facilitate the economic circumstances of households or firms in certain conditions, and there are differences between countries in these respects. Recently it has been shown how in comparisons based on net tax rates the differences between countries become smaller (see Adema *et al.* 1996). In this chapter the interest in financing patterns is limited to 'social welfare' due to lack of comparative data (see Greve 1994; Kvist and Sinfield 1996 for attempts to compare fiscal welfare).

10 Omitting the Southern countries Greece, Italy, Portugal and Spain from the calculations in fact shows that marked divergence took place among the ten remaining countries. Coefficients of variation increased from 0.093 in 1985 to 0.148 in 1996.

11 For financing of social protection there exist Eurostat data for Norway, which is thus included in the rest of the chapter.

12 It should be borne in mind that the share of social protection as a percentage of GDP is affected by the generosity of the system and the number of people in need of social protection. In addition, economic development should be considered. Thus apparently similar changes in this indicator may result from differing development within the social reality of countries.

13 To an economist the difference between taxes and social contributions may look artificial. Whether labour costs are financed by taxation or social contributions does not play a big role for a standard economist, as all costs are ultimately transferred into product prices. Nor is there a big difference between taxes and social insurance contributions from the point of view of an individual's disposable income formation. Both forms of payment are compulsory, and the benefits provided are usually not in proportion

to the payments. Nevertheless, the divide between these two revenue sources is considered an important one, at least among welfare state researchers, because in principle contributions are by nature ear-marked for a specific purpose (pension contributions are used to finance pensions, etc.), whereas tax money can be channelled more freely between different purposes. As pointed out by De Kam and Owens (1999) this is not always self-evident, either. Contributions are not always self-financing and the governments may need to top up from tax revenues.

14 Bonoli gives a cross-sectional picture by using averages for 1989–92, while Kangas shows a longer time period (1950–93). Using the most recent Eurostat data, which also include the Nordic countries, it is possible to examine the development between 1980 and 1997. The period used naturally affects interpretations concerning change.

15 As a sensitivity test, social expenditure as percentage of GDP was substituted first with data on social protection expenditure per head in PPS and second with social protection expenditure per head in ECU. The relative positions of countries in different periods followed roughly the same trajectories using these alternative indicators. The major difference is that using these alternative spending measures Norway appears much more 'generous' than Finland in 1997, qualifying Norway to join the company of Denmark and Sweden, while Finland falls close to the European average.

16 Or even, as is the case in the Nordic countries, introduced such social contributions for the insured in the first place.

17 Calculations based on older data and without data for Finland, Norway, Sweden and Austria also showed rapid convergence between 1980–89 in the level of social protection financing (a decline from 0.273 in 1980 to 0.190 in 1989).

11 Conclusion: Nordic welfare states in the European context

Mikko Kautto, Johan Fritzell, Bjørn Hvinden, Jon Kvist and Hannu Uusitalo

The issues

In this volume we have examined diversity and change among Western European welfare states over the past twenty years. The common key question addressed in all the chapters has been whether we can still conceive of a systematically different group of Nordic welfare states, or has their 'distinctiveness' evaporated over time. In short, is there still a distinct Nordic welfare model?

Theoretically, the empirical studies have largely been informed by the contrasting notions of welfare state models and convergence. First, after identifying some potential pitfalls in typology thinking, we made a distinction between ideal–typical models and their empirical equivalents. By an ideal–typical model we mean an analytical construct or theoretical standard against which empirical cases can be contrasted. A number of such standards have crystallised during recent decades of welfare state analysis and our studies have addressed some of the elementary ones that concern social policy and outcomes. Separate analyses have adopted different methods and focused on selected characteristics relevant to the particular field of interest, but all have aimed to answer two related questions, (1) whether the Nordic countries together still form a group; and (2) whether the Nordic countries' characteristics are closer in degree to the ideal–typical standard when compared with other countries.

Second, seeking to highlight processes of change we have also entered into a dialogue with some of the recent literature on convergence. This literature suggests that globalisation and European integration add to or reinforce the variety of 'pressure factors' that welfare states have had to face for some time, and could lead to less variation among them. In this sense globalisation and integration certainly stimulate new calls for adaptation and restructuring of the welfare state, if not outright dismantling and retrenchment. Yet even if such views are heard from different quarters it is not obvious that they have led to substantial changes in practice. Since they have nevertheless had some prominence in the recent ongoing debate about the welfare state we were interested to examine whether any clear trends towards convergence could be identified in the areas chosen for substantive analysis.

With these contrasting ideas as a backdrop we addressed some key issues for social policy from a framework emphasising the interrelationships between societal institutions – above all the welfare state, the market, the family and labour market. The inherent dynamics in these institutions and their inevitably changing interrelationships raise new challenges for the welfare states, which need to adapt to changing market conditions as well as to new family patterns and forms of labour market participation and operation. But welfare states do not only relate to these changes in a reactive manner, they may also – intentionally or unintentionally – stimulate changes in the other institutions and in the behaviour of individuals. In our framework we have regarded policy challenges as stemming from the complex interplay between the institutions, and the task for this volume has been to address various aspects of this interplay and some of its consequences for individual welfare and living conditions.

This conclusion considers the various findings reported in this volume on a more general level than is possible in the individual chapters. The discussion thus addresses more overall patterns and trends. Rather than offering a straightforward summary of the chapters we use our framework to gather together the results and key concerns of the different empirical studies. We first address variation in European social policy, second, we consider trends, and finally welfare state adaptation.

The Nordic welfare states still appear distinct, but not in all respects

An obvious general conclusion is that we cannot give a simple and straightforward 'yes' or 'no' answer to the question of Nordic distinctiveness. In a number of aspects we can find an empirical equivalent to the ideal–typical Nordic model, and in others not, while in some aspects only a few of the countries seem to resemble or approach the ideal–typical trait. Here, as is usually the case, reality displays much greater complexity and ambiguity than theoretical models. This being said, our second main conclusion is that the Nordic countries as a group tend to be different from other groups of Western European countries in key dimensions of policy and welfare.

Most clear of all is that a 'Nordic model' in welfare or living conditions seems to persist. Chapters 2, 4 and 5 reveal systematic similarities among the Nordic countries; they display a lower level of income inequality, and relative poverty rates among typically vulnerable groups still appear to be lower than in other countries. Regarding gender equality, a Nordic unity seems to exist, although on closer examination perhaps the contrast to the Netherlands or the UK is less than before in some respects. The paths towards greater gender equality were very similar among the Nordic countries, to the extent that it may be relevant today to speak of a Nordic gender equality model. The more detailed findings on earnings differentials between men and women and the degree of economic dependence among spouses support this conclusion. All four Nordic countries had the lowest gender gap in earnings, resulting from higher labour force participation rates and lower gender disparities in wages. If we look at the relative position of the sexes, women in the Nordic countries are less concentrated at the lowest end of the earnings distribution and less economically dependent on their husbands than elsewhere. Also, being a mother of small children has less impact on economic independence in the Nordic countries. Indeed, a systematic Nordic pattern of more pronounced gender equality was found in almost all aspects studied.

In terms of the interrelationship between the welfare state and welfare, it is obvious that not all of the credit for the positive findings on the distribution of welfare in the Nordic countries should go to the welfare state. But given that actual outcomes seem to be somewhat congruent with deliberate policy intentions, it would be unreasonable to assume that policies have had no role in achieving this result. The chapter on income inequalities argued strongly for substantial variation among the countries, not only when it came to income inequality but also with regard to the influence of welfare state provisions on the distribution of income and relative poverty rates. For instance, the redistributive effect of the welfare state was most pronounced in three of the Nordic countries. Norway was the exception in displaying a weaker redistributive effect, although this may just reflect a better overall employment situation rather than a difference in the emphasis of redistribution. Also, some would prefer to think that covariance between gender policies (principally those aimed at facilitating women's employment and participation in politics) and outcomes such as earnings developments support a conclusion along the lines of the 'politics matter' stance. Yet, in this case, too, there are conflicting examples that show policies are not the only causes of increased gender equality, and also that even when they are aimed at this goal the results may be disappointing. The role public policy has played thus remains unresolved, and as mentioned in Chapter 5, more pronounced gender equality may also have affected the shape that gender policies have taken. In terms of health inequalities, too, it is clear that several distinct processes underlie them. Differing policy practice is surely one, but to what extent among other determinants and to what degree in differing countries is another question. In short, the chapters have provided different answers to this problem area, and here we can merely confirm that the causal relationship between the welfare state and welfare is surely not one-way, and that outcomes are determined by multiple factors.

Regarding the distinctiveness of Nordic social policies, we also seem to have more evidence for similarity than dissimilarity (Chapters 4, 6, 7, 8, 9 and 10). The analysis of gender policy processes that have led to the currently prevailing gender approach shows almost identical development paths among the Nordic countries. The differences found were minor details when the overall process was compared to that occurring in the Netherlands and the UK. When one then adds the findings concerning different alternatives for arranging care for the elderly and children, the first inclination may be to interpret the results as lending little support to Nordic distinctiveness, at least when it comes to availability of services. Nevertheless, focusing on policy differentiation within a 'social' trajectory rather than within 'education' or 'health' trajectories reveals something distinct to the Nordic countries. Moreover, the Nordic countries appear to be continuing to solve care needs by providing publicly run care services. Therefore, and despite some signs of reductions in public provision, especially in Finland and Sweden, in the European comparison they still all qualify as service states, or to be more precise, as social service states.

Both chapters addressing the relationship between welfare and work again seem to confirm a Nordic similarity. As a group the Nordic countries spent most on 'active measures', while their spending on 'passive measures' also remained highest. On different criteria they came closest to the ideal-type regarding the approach towards activating labour market policies, although how distinct they were compared with the Continental group of countries is debatable. In turn, when analysing the degree of patterning in unemployment-related benefits and assistance, it was possible to identify a distinct overall configuration of policies in the Nordic countries, even if they scored somewhat differently on the separate dimensions. And when it comes to changes in financing policies we could again see all Nordic countries reacting in a uniform way: a similar pattern of increasing the shares of the insured in overall social protection financing was detected. Although these findings may not satisfy all those hoping for more proof of policy uniformity, they seem to suggest some overall similarity among the Nordic countries concerning the interplay between their different institutions.

On the other hand, while we have so far argued that the Nordic countries remain fairly distinct, we do not want to declare or imply that they are so in all respects. Indeed, we have a number of results underlining that we should not expect Nordic homogeneity in all areas. Above all, the responses of social security to changing family patterns did not follow any typology-specific routes. Here, in fact, the four Nordic countries could be located in three differing response groups, Finland appearing as most conservative alongside Germany, with Sweden and Norway as pragmatic, and Denmark together with the Netherlands as radical. This should be contrasted with the finding that arguably the severity of family challenges did follow group-specific lines, i.e. cohabitation as a phenomenon was most pronounced in the Nordic countries. Here one should thus emphasise that despite apparent similarities in existing policy configuration and 'severity' of pressure, country responses may still flow in differing directions. Also, the uniformity in social protection financing patterns is arguably less clear in the case of the Nordic countries than for some other groups, especially the Continental countries. Moreover, findings on one aspect of living conditions, i.e. health outcomes measured as health inequalities, showed substantial variation in Western Europe, and only partially confirmed a Nordic unity. What is more, against expectations the Nordic countries seemed to have larger relative inequalities in perceived health by education than other European countries, although not in terms of health inequalities by household income. Anyway, no clear Nordic model emerged regarding health inequalities. Such findings underline that the actual patterning of policies and living conditions is not necessarily consistent with specific models, and that there is a need to differentiate findings concerning group specificity depending on the dimension in question.

A major issue for future research is whether the Nordic countries – although still grouping together – are more remote from meeting the ideal–typical standards than they used to be. In other words, are the characteristics of the models or regimes identified by Titmuss,

Esping-Andersen and others in the second half of the twentieth century to be treated as everlasting and unchanging, or would it be fruitful at some stage to redefine them? Thinking of our premises, certainly full employment, or low level of unemployment, features less prominently in the Nordic countries than it used to. One could also consider whether the changes implemented, for instance, in access to or universality of various social protection schemes accompanied by the growing importance of private and occupational schemes, are requiring researchers to reconsider some of the characteristics of the 'Nordic social insurance system'. In the analysis of care services, too, it is questionable whether reductions in public service supply and increases in private and non-profit supply have meant a *de facto* change in the universality principle of the Nordic countries. It could be argued that the preconditions for policy-making have changed much since the early 1980s, and the magnitude of subsequent policy reforms would certainly legitimise a quest to critically revise the established features.

On the other hand, one could argue that at least in the areas and with the types of indicators applied in our research there have not been any remarkable changes in outcomes. Contrary to many warnings, we do not see signs of a backlash against gender equality – rather the opposite. Findings concerning poverty among less privileged groups and overall income inequality were favourable for the Nordic countries. However, one needs to highlight income development among different age groups in the Nordic countries; a striking and systematic similarity in all four was found in the development of relative incomes according to age, in the sense that the young appear to have experienced more negative development in their incomes compared to other age groups. Throughout our research project there are consistent findings indicating that the development in living conditions and welfare for the younger segments of the Nordic populations has been far less favourable than for other groups (see Chapter 2 and Fritzell 1999, Gustafsson *et al.* 1999, and Halleröd and Heikkilä 1999 in our earlier volume, *Nordic Social Policy*). To what extent this is related to starting to live on one's own at an earlier age and variation between countries in this phenomenon, to changing education patterns, or to changes in the way welfare states operate, remains unclear and awaits further research. At any rate, a closer targeted perspective to monitor welfare of the young as well as other population groups, and with different indicators and methods, could further substantiate the need to revise our understanding of the Nordic model regarding outcomes.

Some signs of convergence, mainly parallel trends and examples of outright divergence

In terms of the direction of policy trends and development in individual welfare one can in theory conceive of different dynamics. Basically, the options are between widening or narrowing differences, or more or less stability. As pointed out in the Introduction, many scholars and commentators envisage a trend towards narrower differences, and if this prediction is correct it would be important to know whether the trend is resulting from 'catch-up convergence' or rather stems from 'Europeanisation' of the Nordic welfare states.

Starting with the direction of trends, it can be argued that in the long run many aspects of social reality, such as labour markets, family patterns and social structures have indeed converged in Western Europe (e.g. Therborn 1995). But in the short- to medium-term perspective – as in the ten to twenty years covered by this book – and with regard to changes in social policy and outcomes, we do not find unequivocal evidence that countries have become more similar than before. The 'convergence thesis' simply does not receive much – and certainly not consistent – support in our empirical analysis. Although convergence does seem to be occurring in some areas of the welfare state, overall developments tend to be characterised more by parallel trends. Sometimes even outright divergence is apparent.

Considering income inequality first, no convergence of inequality in incomes was found despite repeated claims to the contrary. Indeed, the findings on income inequality actually suggest divergence among the set of countries compared. This is all the more important to stress as recent national studies have noted increasing inequality in incomes in the Nordic countries. Here we need to underline that this trend has occurred in Finland, Norway and Sweden in a similar manner: income inequality has increased since the economic turbulence of the early 1990s. In Finland and Sweden this has been accompanied by improvements in employment, growing importance of capital income and cuts in income transfers. The apparent outcome is that income inequality in recent years has been growing in the Nordic countries, as it has in so many others, albeit in slightly differing time frames. So, while trends in the different countries seem to be pointing in the same direction, it is fair to say that at least as yet there is no proof of a narrowing gap between the Nordic and European countries in this dimension.

Our studies also provide evidence of parallel trends. The differences in gender approaches arguably exhibit some convergence, although not to the extent of disqualifying separate models. It might even be claimed that as dividing lines between the Nordic and the other countries analysed seem to persist, one should perhaps rather speak of parallel trends. We also see parallel trends regarding developments in earnings differentials between men and women. While all countries moved towards closing the gender gap and all have been able to achieve more economic independence for women, the differences between the countries have not changed much. In terms of overall health and social service development one conclusion in Chapter 7 was that no policy convergence had occurred within the institutional avenues where policies develop. Furthermore, one could make the case that the findings regarding the linkage between work and welfare provide no consistent support for officially stated views, at least in so far as OECD and EU documents exemplify the current standpoints. The various indicators used provide quite a strong argument that no convergence in terms of increased policy emphasis on activation occurred during the 1990s. The trend was more of a parallel one in that all sixteen Western European countries seemed to enforce requirements of 'active job-search' and 'availability for work' more vigorously than before. And while all countries did place greater emphasis on work when designing or modifying their employment-related benefits, the end-result could still be interpreted as enduring diversity because of the differing speed and context of changes. Again, these overall trends did not lead to a re-alignment of country groupings. The combined evidence could be interpreted as support for the view that countries associated with different regimes follow roughly similar paths within certain limits.

Yet our studies have also generated findings supportive of convergence. Two rather safe conclusions can be drawn about the nature of these trends. First, against widespread anticipations, signs of 'Europeanisation of Nordic social policy'-type of convergence appear very limited, at least in the policy fields and with the kinds of indicators and methods applied in our studies. The only clear case of such convergence to emerge here was the change in the relative responsibility for financing social protection. In the light of available data the responsibilities of different parties for financing in the Nordic countries have become more like the picture in the rest of Western Europe. To what extent this implies convergence in the nature of social protection policies is another story, especially as it seems that no uniform Nordic pattern existed in the first place. Besides, the persistent diversity may well outweigh much of the gradual convergence that has taken place.

Second, there are good grounds to argue that when convergence has occurred, it has primarily been of the nature of 'catch-up convergence'. A number of non-Nordic countries are adopting policy measures similar to those in the Nordic countries. For example, the active promotion of employment and gender equality are more visible these days on the political agendas of many European governments and international organisations than they used to be, with potentially far-reaching consequences for the design of supportive policies in Western European countries. In terms of employment opportunities, especially for women, this may in turn result in a more active role for the public sector in guaranteeing child care and elderly care. Indeed, some signs of such a development are already in sight, the Netherlands and France and their child care policies being examples of this. Or, regarding financing trends, most indicators show it is the Southern European countries which, by investing more in social programmes, have narrowed the gap to the EU member states that used to have higher taxation and social spending levels. Active labour market policies also provide good grounds for arguing that catch-up convergence could be taking place. Nordic countries, especially Sweden as an activation pioneer, have been used as examples of good practice for the other EU member states. Non-Nordic countries like France, Ireland, Italy and the Netherlands did indeed become more activist in the last decade. As we have seen, the concern to get more people to work more rather than less appears to be dominant in most Western European countries, and in so far as this may translate into changing social and employment policies, it may further the tendency towards catch-up convergence. But even so, it is unlikely that in the foreseeable future other countries would adopt exactly the same type and scope of policies prevalent in the Nordic countries, and so some version of the Nordic welfare model could well continue to be distinct.

Finally, the empirical studies have certainly demonstrated that a variety of policy responses to 'common pressures' exists, as hypothesised in the Introduction. Instead of complying with the slogan 'common pressures, common responses' the reality seems rather to be along the lines of 'common pressures, different responses'. For example, the shared call for greater gender equality and better reconciliation of family and working life in the countries studied has been addressed in different ways that can be broadly said to follow model-specific routes or reflect path dependency. In the Netherlands and Germany, for instance, women with caring responsibilities are credited points for social rights in line with ordinary employment, whereas in the Nordic countries the answer has been more of a move towards the individualisation of social security and an expansion of care services and specific care allowances (see Chapters 4, 6 and 7). Thus institutions still matter by setting limits for the available options when solutions for new responses are being sought.

But the path-dependency argument does not provide answers in all instances, as countries presumed to be following similar paths have sometimes opted for different policy solutions. For instance, no common and particular Nordic path could be located in activation policies, while in changes regarding financing we saw differences across Europe and sometimes within the Nordic countries: no cluster-specific adjustments emerged in changes in the relative balance of different taxes or government responsibility for financing social protection. This emphasises that the politics of and within nation–states still matter – even to the extent of allowing break-away from path-dependencies and from association with certain typologies.

The dynamics of welfare states and their capacity to adapt

Although European welfare states may not be converging, they are all in a state of flux. However, some national welfare states change faster and perhaps more profoundly than others. This study has given us the opportunity to reflect on the nature of welfare reform in the Nordic countries in light of the European experience, and also in view of the conclusions stressing stability in our previous volume *Nordic Social Policy*.

In the past twenty years the Nordic welfare states have overcome a sea of changes in family structures and labour markets, and even demonstrated a remarkable ability to survive through periods of dramatic economic turmoil as witnessed in Denmark in the 1980s and in Sweden and Finland a decade later. Thus, so far, the Nordic welfare states seem to have been able to cope with globalisation, eroding family structures and so forth – challenges frequently characterised as profound and even insurmountable.

There may be a multitude of reasons for this. Interestingly, some of the study findings in this volume hint that the Nordic welfare states may, after all, have a greater capacity to adjust than other countries. It emerged, for example, that in health care and social care services they have been faster to adjust than the Continental countries. It was argued that tax-financed schemes that do not give the individual strictly legal rights to services may after all be easier to adjust than schemes based on contribution-financing, as the latter tend to establish a more strict legal entitlement to services (Chapter 7). Also, in Chapter 9 the authors maintain that activation strategies have been easier to implement in the Nordic countries than in Germany and the UK. Germany was identified as the country where such changes have been most difficult to enact. Moreover, according to the statistical analysis in Chapter 10 the Continental financing pattern has been the most stable over time, both in terms of the level of total financing and of the sharing of financing responsibilities between different parties. The UK also appeared rather resistant to change in these respects (although not so in many other areas), whereas the Nordic financing patterns seem to have evolved more. Certainly there have been many changes in all countries, and more information would be welcomed, both on attempts at reforms and on their success in different countries, in order to help deepen our understanding of the subject.

The capacity of welfare states to adjust while still retaining their central characteristics has not been our prime focus, and more work is surely needed on this topic. Nevertheless, a possible paradox may be worth noting at this point. Whereas large and institutionalised welfare states have often been criticised for rigidity and lack of dynamism, the Nordic experience of the 1990s suggests that in many respects they may be in a better position, and perhaps even more eager, to implement changes in response to new challenges. To the extent that further analysis substantiates this claim, there are important implications. Policy makers in the Nordic countries may find it easier to implement changes in national social policy and revenue programmes than many of their European counterparts. Decisions concerning tax-funded public sector programmes are made in one place with majority decisions, while in countries that have followed occupational welfare strategies the reforms need to be implemented in consultation with a multitude of partners and interest groups, and seem to meet harder resistance. Partly on the basis of this strength, it also seems fair to claim that the relatively generous and comprehensive Nordic welfare states do not appear economically unsustainable, nor likely to face imminent death or dismantling as somctimes prophesised by the most extreme adherents of the convergence thesis.

References

Aaberge, R., Björklund, A., Jäntti, M., Palme, M., Pedersen, P. J., Smith, N. and Wennemo, T. (1999) 'Income inequality and income mobility in the Scandinavian vountries compared to the United States', mimeo, Statistics Norway *et al.*

Aaberge, R., Björklund, A., Jäntti, M., Pedersen, P. J., Smith, N. and Wennemo, T. (2000) 'Unemployment shocks and income distribution: how did the Nordic countries fare during their crises?', *Scandinavian Journal of Economics* 102: 77–99.

Abrahamson, P. (1998) 'Efter velfærdsstaten: Ret og pligt til aktivering' (After the welfare state: right and duty for activation), *Nordisk social arbeid* 18(3): 133–43.

Abrahamson, P. (1999) 'The welfare modelling business', *Social Policy & Administration* 33(4): 349–415.

Adema, W., Einerhand, M., Eklind, B., Lotz, J. and Pearson, M. (1996) *Net Public Social Expenditure*, Labour Market and Social Policy Occasional Papers No. 19, Paris: OECD.

Agell, A. (1980) 'Cohabitation without marriage in Swedish Law', in J. M. Eekalar and S. M. Katz (eds), *Marriage and Cohabitation in Contemporary Societies: Areas of Legal, Social and Ethical Change*, London: Butterworths, 245–57.

Alban, A. and Christiansen, T. (eds) (1995) *The Nordic Lights: New Initiatives in Health Care Systems*, Odense: Odense University Press.

Alber, J. (1981) 'Government responses to the challenge of unemployment: the development of unemployment insurance in Western Europe'. See Flora and Heidenheimer (1981), 151–86.

Alber, J. (1988) 'Is there a crisis of the welfare state? Cross-national evidence from Europe, North America and Japan', *European Sociological Review* 4(3): 181–207.

Alber, J. (1994) 'A framework for the comparative study of social services departing from Stein Rokkan's approach to the study of European political development', paper originally given as the Stein Rokkan Memorial Lecture at the University of Bergen.

Alber, J. and Standing, G. (eds) (2000) 'Europe in a comparative global context', *Journal of European Social Policy* (special issue): 10(2), 99–119.

Alestalo, M. and Flora, P. (1994) 'Scandinavia: welfare states in the periphery – peripheral welfare states?', in M. Alestalo, E. Allardt, A. Rychard and W. Wesolowski (eds) *The Transformation of Europe. Social Conditions and Consequences*, Warsaw: IFIS Publishers, 53–73.

Alestalo, M. and Uusitalo, H. (1986) 'Finland', in P. Flora (ed.) *Growth to Limits, Vol. 1*, Berlin: Walter de Gruyter, 197–292.

Allardt, E. (1975) *Att ha, att älska, att vara. Om välfärden i Norden (Having, Loving, Being. On Welfare in the Nordic Countries)*, Lund: Argos.

Allardt, E. (1999) 'Filosofinen ja sosiologinen hyvää elämää koskeva keskustelu terveystutkimuksen kannalta' (Philosophical and sociological debate on good life and its relevance to health research), *Sosiaalilääketieteellinen Aikakauslehti* 36: 203–12.

Andenæs, A. (1998) 'Faglige premisser i politiske diskusjoner: Fra kontanstøttedebatten 1997–1998' (Professional arguments in political debates: debate on cash benefits for families with small children 1997–1998), *Kvinneforskning*, Vol. 2, Norges Forskningsråd, Oslo, 12–26.

Anker, R. (1998) *Gender and Jobs: Sex Segregation of Occupations in the World*, Geneva: International Labour Office (ILO).

Anttonen, A. and Sipilä, J. (1996) 'European social care services: is it possible to identify models?', *Journal of European Social Policy* 6(2): 87–100.

Ashton, J. (1999) '1997 Chadwick Lecture – Is a healthy North West Region achievable in the 21st century?', *Journal of Epidemiology and Community Health* 53: 370–82.

Asplund, R., Barth, E., Schmidt, N. and Wadensjö, E. (1996) 'The male-female wage gap in the Nordic countries', in E. Wadensjö (ed.) *The Nordic Labour Markets in the 1990's*, North Holland: Elsevier Science, 57–82.

Atkinson, A. B. (2000) 'Is rising income inequality inevitable? A critique of the transatlantic consensus', 1999 WIDER Annual Lecture, Helsinki: UNU/WIDER.

Atkinson, A. B., Rainwater, L. and Smeeding, T. M. (1995) *Income Distribution in OECD Countries*, OECD Social Policy Studies No. 18, Paris: OECD.

Baldersheim, H. and Ståhlberg, K. (eds) (1999) *Nordic Region-Building in a European Perspective*, Aldershot: Ashgate.

Baldwin, P. (1990) *The Politics of Solidarity: Class Bases in the European Welfare State, 1875–1975*, Cambridge: Cambridge University Press.

Barne-og Familiedepartementet (1998) *Småbarnsforeldres rettigheter (The Rights of the Parents of Small Children)*, ODIN presentation on Internet.

Beck, U. (1992) *Risk Society*, London: Sage.

Beck, W., van der Maesen, L. and Walker, A. (1997) *The Social Quality of Europe*, The Hague: Kluwer Law International.

Becker, G. S. (1981) *A Treatise on the Family*, Cambridge, MA: Harvard University Press.

Bergqvist, C. *et al.* (eds) (1999) *Likestilte demokratier? Kjønn og politikk i Norden* (Equal democracies? Gender and politics in the Nordic countries), Oslo: Universitetsforlaget/Nordic Council of Ministers.

Bianchi, S. M., Casper, L. M. and Peltola, P. K. (1996) *A Cross-national Look at Married Women's Earnings Dependency*, Luxembourg Income Study, Working Paper Series No. 143, Luxembourg.

Birch Sørensen, P. (ed.) (1998) *Tax Policy in the Nordic Countries*, London: Macmillan Press.

Blau, F. D. and Kahn, L. M. (1992) 'The gender earnings gap: learning from international evidence', *American Economic Review* 82(2): 533–8.

Blaxter, M. (1989) 'A comparison of measures of inequality in morbidity', in A. J. Fox (ed.) *Health Inequalities in European Countries*, Aldershot: Gower, 100–230.

Blöndahl, S. and Pearson, M. (1995) 'Unemployment and other non-employment benefits', *Oxford Review of Economic Policy* 11(1): 136–69.

Blossfeld, H.-P. (1995) *The New Role of Women. Family Formation in Modern Societies*, Boulder, CO: Westview Press.

Blossfeld, H.-P. and Hakim, C. (1997) *Between Equalization and Marginalization . Women Working Part-time in Europe and the United States of America*, Oxford: Oxford University Press.

Blossfeld, H.-P., Manting, D. and Rohwer, G. (1994) 'Patterns of change in family formation in the FRG and the NL: some consequences for solidarity between generations', in H. Becker and P.L.J Hermkens (eds) *Demographic, Economic and Social Change, and its Consequences*, Amsterdam: Thesis Publisher, 175–96.

Bonoli, G. (1997) 'Classifying welfare states: a two-dimension approach', *Journal of Social Policy* 26(3): 351–72.

Bonoli, G., George, V. and Taylor-Gooby, P. (2000) *European Welfare Futures*, Cambridge: Polity Press.

Borgan, J.-K. (1996) 'Socio-economic trends in differential mortality among middle-aged males in Norway 1960–1990', Helsinki: *Yearbook of Population Research in Finland*, vol. 33: 73–81.

Bosco, A. and Chassard, Y. (1999) 'Shift in the paradigm: surveying the European Union discourse on welfare and work'. See M. Heikkilä (1999), 43–58.

Bouget, D. and Palier, B. (eds) (1999) *Comparing Social Welfare Systems in Nordic Europe and France*, Paris: MIRE-DREES.

Bowling, A. (1991) *Measuring Health. A Review of Quality of Life Measurement Scales*, Buckingham: Open University Press.

Bowling, A. (1995) *Measuring Disease. A Review of Disease-specific Quality of Life Measurement Scales*, Buckingham: Open University Press.

Bradbury, B. and Jäntti, M. (1999) *Child Poverty across Industrialized Nations*, Innocenti Occasional Papers, Economic and Social Policy Series, No. 71, Florence: UNICEF.

Branth, B. and Øverli, B. (1998) *Omsorgspermisjon med 'kjærlig tvang'. En kartlegging av fedrekvoten (Care Leave through 'Gentle Coercion': A Study on the Fathers' Quota Scheme)*, Trondheim: Allforsk.

Breuil-Genier, P. (1999) 'A wide range of forms of care for elderly dependent persons'. See Bouget and Palier (1999), 363–84.

Buhmann, B., Rainwater, L., Schmaus, G. and Smeeding, T. (1988) 'Equivalence scales, well-being, inequality and poverty: sensitivity estimates across ten countries using the Luxembourg income study database', *Review of Income and Wealth* 34: 115–42.

Bull, K. S. (1990), *Ugift Samliv (Cohabitation)*, Oslo: Tano.

Bussemaker, J. (1998) 'Rationales of care in contemporary welfare states: the case of childcare in the Netherlands', *Social Politics: International Studies in Gender, State and Society* 5: 70–96.

Bussemaker, J. and van Kersbergen, K. (1994) 'Gender and welfare state: some theoretical reflections', in D. Sainsbury (ed.) *Gendering Welfare States*, London: Sage, 8–25.

Cameron, D. (1978) 'The expansion of the public economy: a comparative analysis', *The American Political Science Review* 72(4): 1243–61.

Carroll, E. (1999) *Emergence and Structuring of Social Insurance Institutions: Comparative Studies on Social Policy and Unemployment Insurance*, Stockholm: SOFI.

Castles, F.G. (1998) *Comparative Public Policy: Patterns of Post-war Transformation*, Cheltenham: Edward Elgar.

Castles, F.G. and Mitchell, D. (1990) *Three Worlds of Welfare Capitalism or Four?* Australian National University Discussion Paper 21, Canberra: ANU.

Cavelaars, A. (1998) 'Cross-national comparisons of socio-economic differences in health indicators', thesis, Department of Public Health, Erasmus University Rotterdam, Rotterdam.

Cavelaars, A., Kunst, A., Geurts, J., Crialesi, R., Grötvedt, L., Helmert, U., Lahelma, E., *et al.* (1998a) 'Differences in self reported morbidity by educational level: a comparison of 11 Western European countries', *Journal of Epidemiology and Community Health* 52: 219–27.

Cavelaars, A., Kunst, A., Geurts, J., Helmert, U., Lahelma, E., Lundberg, O., Matheson, J., *et al.* (1998b) 'Differences in self-reported morbidity by income level in six European countries'. See Cavelaars (1998), 49–66.

Cavelaars, A., Kunst, A., Geurts, J., Crialesi, R., Grötvedt, L., Helmert, U., Lahelma, E., *et al.* (2000) 'Educational differences in smoking: an international comparison', *British Medical Journal* 320: 1102–7.

Cavelaars, A., Kunst, A., Geurts, J., Helmert, U., Lundberg, O., Matheson, J., Mielck, *et al.* (1998c) 'Morbidity differences by occupational class among men in seven European countries: an application of the Erikson-Goldthorpe social class scheme', see Cavelaars (1998) 33–47.

Chafetz, J. S. (1990) *Gender Equity: An Integrated Theory of Stability and Change*, Newbury Park, CA: Sage Publications.

Chamberlayne, P. (1993) 'Women and the state: changes in roles and rights in France, West Germany, Italy and Britain, 1970–1990', in J. Lewis (ed.) *Women and Social Policies in Europe: Work, Family and the State*, Aldershot: Edward Elgar Publications, 170–93.

Christensen, A. D. (1999) 'Kvinder i de politiske partier' (Women in political parties), in C. Bergquist *et al.* (eds) *Likestilte demokratier? Kjønn og politikk i Norden,* Oslo: Scandinavian University Press/Nordic Council of Ministers, 62–82.

Clasen, J. (ed.) (1997) *Social Insurance in Europe*, Bristol: Policy Press.

Clasen, J. (2000) 'Motives, means and opportunities: reforming unemployment compensation in the 1990s', *West European Politics*, special issue on 'Recasting European Welfare States', M. Ferrera and M. Rhodes (eds) 23(2): 89–112.

Clayton, R. and Pontussen, J. (2000) 'Welfare state retrenchment revisited', in C. Pierson and F. G. Castles (eds) *The Welfare State Reader*, Oxford: Polity Press, 320–34.

COM (1999) 347 final, Communication from the Commission: A concerted strategy for modernising social protection, Bruxelles: Commission of the European Communities.

Cowell, F. A. (1984) 'The structure of American income inequality', *Review of Income and Wealth* 30: 351–75.

Dahl, E. and Birkelund, G. E. (1999) 'Sysselsettning, klasse och helse 1980–1995: en analyse av fem norske levekårsundersökelser' (Employment, class and health 1980–1995: an analysis of five Norwegian level of living studies), *Tidskrift for samfunnsforskning* 40: 3–23.

Dahlerup, D. (1987) 'Confusing concepts – confusing reality: a theoretical discussion of the patriarchal state', in A. Showstack Sassoon (ed.) *Women and the State: The Shifting Boundaries of Public and Private*, London: Unwin Hyman Ltd, 93–127.

Daly, M. (1997) 'Welfare states under pressure: cash benefits in European welfare states', *Journal of European Social Policy* 7(2): 129–146.

Davey Smith, G., Bartley, M. and Blane, D. (1990) 'The Black Report on socioeconomic inequalities in health 10 years on', *British Medical Journal* 301: 373–7.

Davey Smith, G., Blane, D. and Bartley, M. (1994) 'Explanations for socioeconomic differentials in mortality', *European Journal of Public Health* 4: 131–44.

Deacon, A. (1997) 'Benefit sanctions for the jobless: "tough love" or rough treatment?', *Employment Policy Institute Economic Report*, 11, 7.

Deacon, A. (1998) 'The Green Paper on Welfare Reform: a case for enlightened self interest?', *Political Quarterly* 69: 306–11.

Deacon, B. (1998) *Global Social Policy: International Organizations and the Future of the Welfare*, London: Sage.

Deacon, B. (1999) 'Social policy in a global context', in A. Hurrell and N. Woods (eds) *Inequality, Globalization, and World Politics*, Oxford: Oxford University Press, 211–47.

De Bruin, A., Pichavet, H. S. J. and Nossikov, A. (1996) *Health Interview Surveys: Towards International Harmonisation of Methods and Instruments*, Copenhagen: WHO Regional Publications.

De Kam, F. and Owens, J. (1999) 'Financing social protection in the 21st century', in *Financing Social Protection in Europe* (1999) Ministry of Social Affairs and Health Publications, 1999: 21, Helsinki: Ministry of Social Affairs and Health.

Department of Social Security (1998) *New Ambitions for Our Country: A New Contract for Welfare*, Cm 3805, London: The Stationery Office.

Dickerson, J. W. (1998) 'Historical perspectives on health: aspects of public health up to Chadwick', *Journal of the Royal Society of Health* 118: 182–5.

van Dijk, L. (1996) 'The division of child care among mothers, fathers, and nonparental care providers in Dutch two-parent families', *Journal of Marriage and the Family* 58: 34–51.

Ditch, J. (1999) 'The structure and dynamics of social assistance in the European Union'. See Heikkilä (1999), 59–70.

Dodge, D. A. (1975) 'Impact of tax, transfer, and expenditure policies of government on the distribution of personal income in Canada', *Review of Income and Wealth* 21: 1–52.

van Doorslaer, E., Wagstaff, A., Bleichrodt, H., Calonge, S., Gerdtham, U. G., Gerfin, M., Geurts, J., *et al.* (1997) 'Income-related inequalities in health: some international comparisons', *Journal of Health Economics* 16(1): 93–112.

Dowrick, S. and Ngyuyen, D. T. (1989) 'OECD comparative economic growth 1950–85: catch-up and convergence', *American Economic Review* 79: 1010–31.

Drøpping, J. A., Hvinden, B. and Vik, K. (1999) 'Activation policies in the Nordic countries'. See Kautto *et al.* (1999), 133–58.

Dunning, J. H. (ed.) (1997) *Governments, Globalization and International Business*, Oxford: Oxford University Press.

Eardley, T., Bradshaw, J., Ditch, J., Gough, I. and Whiteford, P. (1996) *Social Assistance in OECD Countries: Synthesis Report*, London: HMSO.

EC (1997a) *1998 Guidelines for Member States Employment Policies*, Brussels: The European Commission.

EC (1997b) *Social Action Programme 1998–2000*, Communication, Brussels: The European Commission.

EC (1997c) *Modernising and Improving Social Protection in the European Union*, COM (97) 102, Brussels: The European Commission

EC (1998a) *1999 Employment Guidelines*, Brussels: The European Commission.

EC (1998b) *From Guidelines to Action: The 1998 National Action Plans for Employment: Overall Assessment*, Brussels: The European Commission.

EC (1998c) *Social Protection in Europe 1997*, Luxembourg: Office for Official Publications of the European Communities.

EC (1999a) *A Concerted Strategy for Modernising Social Protection*, document drawn up on the basis of COM (99) 347 final, Brussels: The European Commission.

EC (1999b) *Joint Employment Report 1999 Part I, The European Union*, draft document, Brussels: The European Commission.

EC (1999c) *2000 Employment Guidelines*, Brussels: The European Commission.

Economic Commission for Europe (1995) Women and Men in Europe and North America 1995, ECE/ UN/SCB/ Eurostat, Geneva

Erikson, R. (1992) 'Social policy and inequality in health: considerations from the Swedish experience', *International Journal of Health Sciences* 3: 215–22.

Erikson, R., Hansen, E. J., Ringen, S. and Uusitalo, H. (eds) (1987) *The Scandinavian Model: Welfare States and Welfare Research*, Armonk, NY: M.E. Sharpe.

Erikson, R. and Uusitalo, H. (1987) 'The Scandinavian approach to welfare research'. See Erikson *et al.* (1987), 177–93.

Esping-Andersen, G. (1990) *The Three Worlds of Welfare Capitalism*, Oxford: Polity Press.

Esping-Andersen, G. (1996) 'Positive-sum solutions in a world of trade-offs?', in G. Esping-Andersen (ed.), *Welfare States in Transition*, London: Sage, 256–67.

Esping-Andersen, G. (1999) *Social Foundations of Postindustrial Economies*, Oxford: Oxford University Press.

Esping-Andersen, G. and Korpi, W. (1987) 'From poor relief to institutional welfare states: the development of Scandinavian social policy'. See Erikson *et al.* (1987), 39–74.

EU (1992) Council Recommendation 92/442/EEC of 27 July 1992

EU (1997a) *Presidency Conclusions*, Extraordinary European Council Meeting on Employment, Luxembourg November 1997 (http://europa.eu.int/)

EU (1997b) *What Does the Amsterdam Treaty Mean for Employment?* (http://europa.eu.int/)

European Commission Network on Childcare (1996) *A Review of Services for Young Children in the European Union 1990–1995*, Brussels: DGV.

European Foundation for the Improvement of Living and Working Conditions (1999) *Linking Welfare and Work*, Dublin: European Foundation.

Eurostat (1995) *Women and Men in the European Union: A Statistical Portrait*, Luxembourg: Office for Official Publications of the European Communities.

Eurostat (1997) *Yearbook*, Luxembourg: Office for Official Publications of the European Communities.

Eurostat (1998/99) *Yearbook*, Luxembourg: Office for Official Publications of the European Communities.

Eurostat (2000) *Social Protection, Expenditure and Receipts: European Union, Iceland and Norway, Data 1980–97*, Luxembourg: Office for Official Publications of the European Communities.

Everaers, P., van der Laan, P. and McDonald, M. K. (2000) 'Conceptual overview', paper presented at the Canberra Group Meeting in Luxembourg, May 2000, Statistics Netherlands and Australian Bureau of Statistics.

Ferge, Z. (1997) 'A Central European perspective on the social quality of Europe', in W. Beck, L. van der Maesen and A. Walker (eds) *The Social Quality of Europe*, The Hague: Kluwer Law International, 165–79.

Ferlie, E., Pettigrew, A., Ashburner, L. and Fitzgerald, L. (1996) *The New Public Management in Action*, Oxford: Oxford University Press.

Ferrera, M. (1993) *Modelli di solidarieta*, Bologna: Il Mulino.

Ferrera, M., Hemerijk, A. and Rhodes, M. (2000) *The Future of Social Europe: Recasting Work and Welfare in the New Economy*, report for the Portuguese Presidency of the European Union, Lisbon, April 2000.

Financing Social Protection in Europe (1999) Ministry of Social Affairs and Health Publications, 1999: 21, Helsinki: Ministry of Social Affairs and Health.

Finer, C. J. (1999) 'Trends and developments in welfare states', in J. Clasen (ed.) *Comparative Social Policy*, Oxford: Blackwell, 15–33.

Finn, D. (1997) 'The stricter benefit regime and the New Deal for the unemployed', paper presented at the Social Policy Association, 31st Annual Conference, University of Lincolnshire and Humberside, 15–17 June.

Flora, P. and Alber, J. (1981) 'Modernization, democratization, and the development of welfare states in Western Europe', see Flora and Heidenheimer (1981), 37–80.

Flora, P. and Heidenheimer, A. J. (eds) (1981) *The Development of Welfare States in Europe and America*, New Brunswick: Transaction Books.

Forma, P. (1999) *Interests, Institutions and the Welfare State: Studies on Public Opinion Towards the Welfare State*, Stakes Research Report 102, Jyväskylä: Stakes.

Fox, J. (ed.) (1989) *Health Inequalities in European Countries*, Aldershot: Gower.

Fritzell, J. (1990) 'The dynamics of income distribution: economic mobility in Sweden in comparison with the United States', *Social Science Research* 19: 17–46.

Fritzell, J. (1991) 'The gap between market rewards and economic well-being in modern societies', *European Sociological Review* 7: 19–33.

Fritzell, J. (1992) 'Ojämlikhets- och fattigdomsutveckling under 1980–talet: Sverige i internationell belysning' (Development of inequality and poverty in the 1980s: Sweden in international comparison), in A. Björklund and J. Fritzell (eds) *Inkomstfördelningens utveckling*, Stockholm: Allmänna Förlaget.

Fritzell, J. (1993) 'Income inequality trends in the 1980s: a five-country comparison', *Acta Sociologica* 36: 47–62.

Fritzell, J. (1999) 'Changes in the social patterning of living conditions', see Kautto *et al.* (1999), 159–84.

Gallie, D. and Paugam, S. (eds) (2000) *Welfare Regimes and the Experience of Unemployment in Europe*, Oxford: Oxford University Press.

Garrett, G. (1998) *Partisan Politics in the Global Economy*, Cambridge: Cambridge University Press.

Garrett, G. and Mitchell, D. (1995) 'Globalization and the welfare state: income transfers in the industrial democracies 1965–1990', paper presented at the conference 'Comparative Research on Welfare State Reforms', Pavia, 14–17 September 1995.

George, V. and Taylor-Gooby, P. (1996) *European Welfare Policy: Squaring the Welfare Circle*, London: Macmillan Press.

Giddens, A. (1999) *Runaway World*, London: Profile Books.

Goldthorpe, J. (1984) 'The end of convergence: corporatist and dualist tendencies in modern Western societies', in J. Goldthorpe (ed.) *Order and Conflict in Contemporary Capitalism*, Oxford: Clarendon Press, 315–43.

Gornick, J. C. and Jacobs, J. A. (1997) *Gender, the Welfare State, and Public Employment: A Comparative Study of Seven Industrialized Countries*, Luxembourg Income Study, Working Paper No. 168, Luxembourg.

Gottschalk, P. and Smeeding, T. M. (1997) 'Cross-national comparisons of levels and trends in inequality', *Journal of Economic Literature* XXXV: 633–87.

Gottschalk, P. and Smeeding, T. M. (2000) 'Empirical evidence on income inequality in industrialized countries', in A. B. Atkinson and F. E. Bourguignon (eds) *Handbook of Income Distribution*, North Holland: Elsevier, 261–307.

Gough, I. (1999) 'The needs of the capital and the needs of people: can the welfare state reconcile the two?', inaugural lecture at the University of Bath, 21 January 1999 (http://www.bath.ac.uk/~hssirg/inaug.htm).

Goul Andersen, J., Pettersen, P. A., Svallfors, S. and Uusitalo, H. (1999) 'The legitimacy of the Nordic welfare states: trends, variations and cleavages', see Kautto *et al.* (1999), 235–61.

Greenberg, S. J. (1997) 'The "Dreadful Visitation": public health and public awareness in seventeenth-century London', *Bulletin of the Medical Library Association* 85: 391–401.

Greve, B. (1994) 'The hidden welfare state, tax expenditure and social policy', *Scandinavian Journal of Social Welfare* 3(4): 203–11.

Greve, B. (1996) 'Indications of social policy convergence in Europe', *Social Policy & Administration* 30(4): 348–67.

Group of National Experts (1995) *Unemployment Benefits and Social Assistance in Seven European Countries – A Comparative Study*, Werkdocumenten No. 10, Den Haag: Ministerie van Soziale Zaken en Werkgelegenheid.

Group of National Experts (1998) 'Income benefits for early exit from the labour market in eight European countries – a comparative study', *European Economy*, Reports and Studies No. 3, European Commission: Directorate-General for Economic and Financial Affairs.

Guillén, A. (1999) 'Improving efficiency and containing costs: health care reform in Southern Europe', paper presented at a conference 'Beyond the Health Care State', Florence, 26–27 February.

Gustafsson, B., Aaberge, R., Cappelen, Å., Pedersen, P. J., Smith, N. and Uusitalo, H. (1999) 'The distribution of income in the Nordic countries', see Kautto *et al.* (1999), 215–34.

Hagen, K. (1999) 'Towards an Europeanisation of social policies? A Scandinavian perspective', see Bouget and Palier (1999), 661–90.

Halvorsen, K. (1990) *Innføring i sosialpolitikk (An Introduction to Social Policy)*, Oslo: Tano.

Halvorsen, K. (1996) *Grunnbok i helse- og sosialpolitikk (The Basics of Health and Social Policies)*. Otta: Tano-Aschehoug.

Halvorsen, K., Bakken, O. and Fugelli, P. (1986) *Arbeidsløs i velferdsstaten (Out of Work in the Welfare State)*, Oslo: Universitetsforlaget.

Hanesch, W. (1999) 'The debate on reforms of social assistance in Western Europe', see Heikkilä (1999), 71–86.

Hannan, M. and Tuma, N. B. (1978) 'Income and independence effects on marital dissolution: results from the Seattle and Denver income maintenance experiments', *American Journal of Sociology* 84: 611–33.

Hansen, E. J., Ringen, S., Uusitalo, H. and Erikson, R. (eds) (1993) *Welfare Trends in the Scandinavian Countries*, Armonk, NY: M.E. Sharpe.

Hansen, F. K. (1995) 'Velfærd og fordeling' (Welfare and distribution), *Samfundsøkonomen* 6: 9–14.

Hansen, H. (1999) *Elements of Social Security*, Copenhagen: The Danish National Institute of Social Research.

Hassenteufel, P. (1999) 'How do health insurance systems change? France and Germany in the 1990's', paper presented at a conference 'Beyond the Health Care State', Florence, 26–27 February.

Hatland, A. (1994a) 'Ny profil på trygdepolitikken' (A new profile of social insurance policy), in A. Hatland, S. Kuhnle and T.I. Romøren (eds) *Den norske velferdsstaten (The Norwegian Welfare State)*, Oslo: Ad Notam Gyldendal, 216–33.

Hatland, A. (1994b) 'Trygd og arbeid', in A. Hatland, S. Kuhnle, and T. I. Romøren (eds) *Den norske velferdsstaten (The Norwegian Welfare State)*, Oslo: Ad Notam Gyldendal, 187–215.

Heikkilä, M. (ed.) (1999) *Linking Welfare and Work*, Luxembourg: Office for Official Publications of the European Communities.

Heikkilä, M. and Uusitalo, H. (1997) *The Cost of Cuts: Studies on Cutbacks in Social Security and their Effects in the Finland of the 1990s*, Stakes, Saarijärvi: Stakes.

Heliövaara, M., Aromaa, A., Klaukka, T., Knekt, P., Joukamaa, M. and Impivaara, O. (1993) 'Reliability and validity of interview data on chronic diseases: the mini-Finland Health Survey', *Journal of Clinical Epidemiology* 46: 181–91.

Hernes, H. (1987a) *Welfare State and Woman Power: Essays in State Feminism*, Oslo: Norwegian University Press.
Hernes, H. (1987b) 'Women and the welfare state: the transition from private to public dependence', in A. Showstack Sassoon (ed.) *Women and the State: The Shifting Boundaries of Public and Private*, London: Unwin Hyman, 72–92.
Hirst, P. and Thompson, G. (1996) *Globalization in Question: The International Economy and the Possibilities of Governance*, Cambridge: Polity Press.
Hirst, P. and Thompson, G. (2000) 'Global myths and national policies', in B. Holden (ed.) *Global Democracy: Key Debates*, London: Routledge, 47–59.
Hout, W. (1998) 'Globalisation and national policy autonomy: the case of the Netherlands', in P. Kongshøj Madsen (ed.) *Work and Welfare*, Proceedings of the workshop of the COST A7 final conference in London, 12 and 13 December 1997, Luxembourg: European Commission.
Howell, J. (1998) 'Gender, civil society and the state in China', see Randall and Waylen (1998), 166–84.
Huber, E., Ragin, C. and Stephens, J. D. (1993) 'Social Democracy, Christian Democracy, constitutional structure, and the welfare state', *American Journal of Sociology* 99: 3.
Hutten, J. and Kerkstra, A. (1996) *Home Care in Europe: NIVEL*, Utrecht: Arena.
Hvinden, B. (1994) *Divided Against Itself*, Oslo: Scandinavian University Press.
Hvinden, B. (1999) 'Activation: a Nordic perspective', see Heikkilä (1999), 27–42.
Idler, E. and Benyamini, Y. (1997) 'Self-rated health and mortality: a review of twenty-seven studies', *Journal of Health and Social Behavior* 38: 21–37.
Illsley, R. and Svensson, P.-G. (eds) (1990) 'Health inequities in Europe', *Social Science & Medicine* (special issue) 27(3): 223–430.
ILO (1995) *World Employment*, Geneva: International Labour Organisation.
Independent Inquiry into Inequalities in Health (1999), London: The Stationery Office.
Jaco, G. (ed.) (1958) *Patients, Physicians and Illness: Source Book in Behavioral Science and Medicine*, New York: Free Press.
Jamieson, A. (ed.) (1991) *Home Care for Older People in Europe: A Comparison of Policies and Practices*, Oxford: Oxford University Press.
Janoski, T. (1998) *Citizenship and Civil Society: A Framework of Rights and Obligations in Liberal, Traditional, and Social Democratic Regimes*, Cambridge: Cambridge University Press.
Jäntti, M. and Danziger, S. (2000) 'Income poverty in advanced countries', in A. B. Atkinson and F. E. Bourguignon (eds) *Handbook on Income Distribution*, North Holland: Elsevier, 309–378.
Järensjö Montanari, I. (1995) 'Harmonization of social policies and social regulation in the European Community', *European Journal of Political Research* 27(1): 21–45.
Jenkins, S. P. (1999) *Trends in the UK Income Distribution*, Working Paper 99–22, Colchester: Institute for Social and Economic Research.

Jensen, U. J. (1985) *Sjukdomsbegrepp i praktiken. Det kliniska arbetets filosofi och vetenskapsteori.* Stockholm: Esselte Studium.

Johansson, S. (1970) *Om levnadsnivåundersökningen* (On level of living studies), Stockholm: Allmänna förlaget.

Johansson S. (1979) *Mot en teori för social rapportering* (Towards a theory of social reporting), Rapport nr 2 från levnadsnivåprojektet. Stockholm: Institutet för Social Forskning.

Jonung, C. (1979) 'Könsuppdelningen på arbetsmarknaden' (Gender segregation in the labour market), in *Kvinners levekår, en seminarrapport,* NAVFs sekretariat for kvinneforskning, Oslo: NAVF.

Kadushin, C. (1966) 'Social class and the experience of ill health', in R. Bendix and S. M. Lipset (eds) *Class, Status, and Power*, New York: The Free Press.

Kamerman, S. and Kahn, A. (eds) (1991) *Child Care, Parental Leave and the Under 3s – Policy Innovation in Europe*, New York: Auburn House.

Kangas, O. (1993) 'The Finnish welfare state – a Scandinavian welfare state?', in P. Kosonen (ed.) *The Nordic Welfare States as Myth and as Reality*, Helsinki: University of Helsinki.

Kangas, O. (1994) 'The merging of welfare state models? Past and present trends in Finnish and Swedish social policy', *Journal of European Social Policy* 4(2): 79–94.

Kangas, O. (1999) 'Past and present trends in the financing of social protection', in CD-Rom titled 'Conference on Financing Social Protection in Europe', 22–23 November, 1999, Helsinki, Ministry of Social Affairs and Health, Finland and the European Commission.

Kangas, O. and Palme, J. (forthcoming). 'Does social policy matter? Poverty cycles in OECD countries', *International Journal of Health Services.*

Kangas, O. and Ritakallio, V.-M. (1999) 'Social policy or structure? Income transfers, socio-demographic factors and poverty in the Nordic countries and in France', see Bouget and Palier (1999), 513–40.

Karisto, A. (1984) *Hyvinvointi ja sairauden ongelma. Suomea ja muita Pohjoismaita vertaileva tutkimus sairastavuuden väestöryhmittäisistä eroista ja sairastavuudesta hyvinvoinnin vajeena (Welfare and the problem of illness)*, Kansaneläkelaitoksen julkaisuja M:46.

Karisto, A., Notkola, V. and Valkonen, T. (1978) 'Socio-economic status and health in Finland and the other Scandinavian countries', *Social Science & Medicine* 12C: 83–8.

Katzenstein, P. J. (1985) *Small States in World Markets. Industrial Policy in Europe*, Ithaca, NY and London: Cornell University Press.

Kautto, M., Heikkilä, M., Hvinden, B., Marklund, S. and Ploug, N. (eds) (1999) *Nordic Social Policy: Changing Welfare States*, London: Routledge.

Keen, M. (1996) 'The welfare economics of tax coordination in the European Community', in M. P. Devereux (ed.) *The Economics of Tax Policy*, Oxford: Oxford University Press, 189–214 (first published in *Fiscal Studies* (1993) 14(12): 15–36).

KELA (1999) *Kansaneläkelaitoksen tilastollinen vuosikirja 1998 (Statistical Yearbook 1998 of the Social Insurance Institution)*, Helsinki: KELA.

Kerr, C., Dunlop, J. T., Harbison, F.H. and Myers, C. A. (1960) *Industrialism and Industrial Man*, Cambridge, Mass.: Harvard University Press.

Keskimäki, I. (1997) *Social Equity in the Use of Hospital Inpatient Care in Finland*, Stakes Research Reports 84, Jyväskylä, Stakes.

Keuzenkamp, S. (1998) *Statistics of Occupational and Pay Differences between Men and Eomen in the Netherlands*, Working Paper No. 4, Joint ECE/INSTRAW/UNSD Work session on Gender Statistics, Geneva, April.

Kiernan, K. E. (1996) 'Partnership behaviour in Europe: recent trends and issues', in D. Coleman (ed.) *Europe's Population*, Oxford: Oxford University Press.

Kiernan, K. E. (1999) 'Cohabitation in Western Europe', in *Population Trends* (Summer), London: Office for National Statistics.

Kjeldstad, R. and Lyngstad, J. (1993) *Arbeid, lønn og likestilling belyst ved statistikk og forskning (Employment, Wages and Gender Equality in the Light of Statistics and Research)*, Oslo: Universitetsforlaget.

Klausen, K. and Stahlberg, K. (1998) *New Public Management i Norden. Nye organisations- og ledelseformer i den decentrale velfærdsstat*, Odense: Odense University Press.

Knijn, T. (1994) 'Fish without bikes: revision of the Dutch welfare state and its consequences for the (in)dependence of single mothers', *Social Politics. International Studies in Gender, State and Society* 1: 83–105.

Knijn, T. (1998) 'Social care in the Netherlands', see Lewis (1998), 85–109.

Knudsen, R. (1987) *Sociale kontantydelser 1976–1987 (Social Security Benefits)*, Copenhagen: The Danish National Institute of Social Research.

Kohl, J. (1981) 'Trends and problems in postwar public expenditure development in Western Europe and North America', see Flora and Heidenheimer (1981), 307–44.

Kolberg, J. E. (ed.) (1991) *The Welfare State as Employer*, Armonk, NY: M.E. Sharpe.

Korpi, W. (1983) *The Democratic Class Struggle*, London: Routledge.

Korpi, W. and Palme, J. (1998) 'The paradox of redistribution and strategies of equality: welfare state institutions, inequality, and poverty in the Western countries', *American Sociological Review* 63: 661–87.

Kosonen, P. (1994) *European Integration – A Welfare State Perspective*, University of Helsinki, Sociology of Law Series No. 8, Helsinki.

Kosonen, P. (1998) 'Globalization, Europeanization and small welfare states', in P. Kongshøj Madsen (ed.) *Work and Welfare*, proceedings of the workshop of the COST A7 final conference in London, 12 and 13 December 1997, Luxembourg: European Commission.

Kuh, D., Power, C., Blane, D. and Bartley, M. (1997) 'Social pathways between childhood and adult health', in D. Kuh and J. Ben-Shlomo (eds) *A Life Course Approach to Chronic Disease Epidemiology*, Oxford: Oxford University Press, 169–98.

Kuhnle, S. (2000) 'European welfare lessons of the 1990s', in S. Kuhnle (ed.) *Survival of the European Welfare State*, London: Routledge, 234–7.

Kunst, A. (1997) *Cross-national Comparisons of Socio-economic Differences in Mortality*, Rotterdam: Erasmus University.

Kunst, A., Cavelaars, A., Groenhof, F., Geurts, J., Mackenbach, J. and EU Working Group on Socio-economic Inequalities in Health (1996) *Socio-economic Inequalities in Morbidity and Mortality in Europe: A Comparative Study. Main Reports, Vol. 1–4*. Department of Public Health, Rotterdam: Erasmus University.

Kunst, A. and Mackenbach, J. (1994) *Measuring Socioeconomic Inequalities in Health*, Copenhagen: WHO, Regional Office for Europe.

Kuznets, S. (1955) 'Economic growth and income inequality', *American Economic Review* 45: 1–28.

Kuznets, S. (1963) 'Distribution of income by size', *Economic Development and Cultural Change* 11: 1–80.

Kvist, J. (1998) 'Complexities in assessing unemployment benefits and policies', *International Social Security Review* 51(4): 33–55.

Kvist, J. (1999) 'Welfare reform in the Nordic countries in the 1990s: using fuzzy set theory to assess conformity to ideal types', *Journal of European Social Policy* 9(3): 231–52.

Kvist, J. and Sinfield, A. (1996) *Comparing Tax Routes in Denmark and the United Kingdom,* Copenhagen: The Danish National Institute of Social Research, 96 (7).

Kvist, J. and Torfing, J. (1996) *Changing Welfare State Models*, CWR Working Paper 5, Copenhagen: Centre for Welfare State Research.

Lahelma, E. and Arber, S. (1994) 'Health inequalities among men and women in contrasting welfare states: Britain and three Nordic countries compared', *European Journal of Public Health* 4: 227–40.

Lahelma, E., Arber, S., Rahkonen, O., Silventoinen, K. (2000) 'Widening or narrowing inequalities on health? Comparing Britain and Finland from the 1980s to 1990s', *Sociology of Health and Illness* 22: 110–36.

Lahelma, E., Karisto, A., Manderbacka, K., Rahkonen, O. (1994) 'Comparisons of inequalities in health: evidence from national surveys in Finland, Norway and Sweden', *Social Science & Medicine* 38: 517–24.

Lahelma, E., Manderbacka, K., Rahkonen, O., Sihvonen, A.-P. (1993) *Ill-health and its Social Patterning in Finland, Norway and Sweden*, Stakes Research Reports 27, Helsinki.

Lahelma, E. and Rahkonen, O. (eds) (1997) 'Health inequalities in modern societies and beyond', *Social Science & Medicine* (special issue) 44(6): 721–910.

Langager, K. (1997) *Indsatsen over for de forsikrede ledige (Measures for the Insured Unemployed)*, Copenhagen: The Danish National Institute of Social Research.

Lappegård, T. (1998) 'Større ulikhet i barnetall' (Greater inequality in the number of children), *Samfunnsspeilet* 12(5): 42–8.

Lappegård, T. (1999) 'Akademikere får også barn' (University graduates also get children), *Samfunnsspeilet* 13(5): 7–14.

Larsen, M. and Langager, K. (1998) *Arbejdsmarkedsreformen og arbejdsmarkedet (The labour-market reform and the labour market)*, Copenhagen: The Danish National Institute of Social Research.

Lehto, J. (1997) 'Policy responses to the financial problems facing social services in Europe', in M. Kautto (ed.) *European Social Services – Policies and Priorities to the Year 2000*, Saarijärvi: Stakes.

Lehto, J. (forthcoming) *Changing Nature of Employment and Job Creation in Social Public Services in the Context of Public Service Reforms*, European Foundation for the Improvement of Working and Living Conditions.

Lehto, J., Moss, N. and Rostgaard, T. (1999) 'Universal public social care and health services?', see Kautto *et al.* (1999), 104–32.

Leibfried, S. (1992) 'Towards a European welfare state? On integrating poverty regimes into the European Community', in Z. Ferge and J. E. Kolberg (eds) *Social Policy in a Changing Europe*, European Centre for Social Welfare Policy and Research, Frankfurt: Campus/Verlag, 245–80.

Leibfried, S. and Pierson, P. (2000) 'Social policy: left to courts and markets?', in H. Wallace and W. Wallace (eds) *Policy-making in the European Union*, 4th edn, Oxford: Oxford University Press, 267–93.

Leira, A. (1998) 'Caring as social right: cash for child care and daddy leave', *Social Politics: International Studies in Gender, State and Society* 5: 362–78.

Lewis, J. (1993) *Women and Social Policies in Europe*, Aldershot: Edward Elgar.

Lewis, J. (ed.) (1997) *Lone Mothers in European Welfare Regimes*, London: Jessica Kingsley.

Lewis, J. (1998a) 'Feminist perspectives', in P. Alcock, A. Erskine and M. May (eds) *The Students Companion to Social Policy*, Oxford: Blackwell, 85–90.

Lewis, J. (ed.) (1998b) *Gender, Social Care and Welfare State Restructuring in Europe*, Aldershot: Ashgate.

Levy, F. and Murnane, R. J. (1992) 'U.S. earnings levels and earnings inequality: a review of recent trends and proposed explanations', *Journal of Economic Literature* XXX: 1333–81.

Likestillingssenteret (1998): *Likt og Ulikt (Equal and Unequal)* nr. 23, Oslo.

Lilja, R. and Savaja, E. (1999) 'En översikt av systemet för arbetslöshedsskydd i Finland' (An overview of the unemployment security system in Finland), Discussion papers, No. 680, Helsinki: Elinkeinoelämän Tutkimuslaitos.

Lindqvist, R. and Marklund, S. (1995) 'Forced to work and liberated from work, historical perspective on work and welfare in Sweden', *Scandinavian Journal of Social Welfare* 4: 224–37.

Lister, R. (1990) 'Women, economic dependency and citizenship', *Journal of Social Policy* 19: 445–67.

Lister, R (1995) 'Dilemmas in engendering citizenship', *Economy and Society* 24: 1–40.

Ljones, O. (1979) *Kvinners yrkesdeltaking i Norge (Women's Labour Market Participation in Norway)*, Samfunnsøkonomiske studier 39, Statistics Oslo: Norway.

Lødemel, I. and Trickey, H. (eds) (2000) *'An offer you can't refuse': Workfare in International Perspective*, Bristol: Policy Press.

Lundberg, O. (1986) 'Class and health: comparing Britain and Sweden', *Social Science & Medicine* 26: 511–17.

Lundberg, O. (1991a) 'Childhood living conditions, health status, and social mobility: a contribution to the health selection debate', *European Sociological Review* 7: 149–162.

Lundberg, O. (1991b) 'Causal explanations for class inequality in health: an empirical analysis', *Social Science & Medicine* 32: 385–93.

Lundberg, O. (1993) 'The impact of childhood living conditions on illness and mortality in adulthood', *Social Science & Medicine* 36: 1047–52.

Lundberg, O. (1998) '*". . . däruti få af de förmögnare sjukna"* – Om ohälsans ojämlika fördelning i dagens Sverige' (On unequal distribution of health in today's Sweden) in *En god hälsa ett socialt privilegium?*, Stockholm: Nationella folkhälsokommittén, 7–46.

Lundberg, O., Diderichsen, F. and Åberg, Y. (2001) 'Changing health inequalities in a changing society: Sweden in the mid-1980s and the mid-1990s', *Scandinavian Journal of Public Health* (forthcoming).

Lundberg, O. and Fritzell, J. (1994) 'Income distribution, income change, and health: on the importance of absolute and relative income for health status in Sweden', in L. S. Levin, L. McMahon and E. Ziglio (eds) *Economic Change, Social Welfare and Health in Europe,* WHO Regional Publications European Series, No. 54, Copenhagen: WHO.

Lundberg, O. and Manderbacka, K. (1996) 'Assessing the reliability of a measure of self-rated health', *Scandinavian Journal of Social Medicine* 24: 218–24.

Lynch, J., Kaplan, G. and Salonen, J. T. (1997) 'Why do poor people behave poorly? Variations in adult health behaviours and psychosocial characteristics by stage of the socioeconomic lifecourse', *Social Science & Medicine* 44: 809–19.

Mabbett, D. and Bolderson, H. (1999) 'Theories and methods in comparative social policy', in J. Clasen (ed.) *Comparative Social Policy*, Oxford: Blackwell.

Macintyre, S. (1986) 'Health and illness', in R. G. Burgess (ed.) *Key Variables in Social Investigation*, London: Routledge & Kegan Paul, 76–98.

Macintyre, S. (1997) 'The Black Report and beyond: what are the issues?', *Social Science & Medicine* 44: 723–45.

Mackenbach, J., Kunst, A., Cavelaars, A., Groenhof, F., Geurts, J. and the EU Working Group on Socio-economic Inequalities in Health (1997) 'Socioeconomic inequalities in morbidity and mortality in Western Europe', *Lancet* 349: 1655–9.

Madsen, P. K. (1999) *Denmark: Flexibility, Security, and Labour Market Success*, Employment and Training Papers, Geneva: International Labour Organization.

Madsen, P. K. and Loftager, J. (1997) 'Denmark', in H. Compston (ed.) *The New Politics of Unemployment: Radical Policy Initiatives in Western Europe*, London: Routledge, 123–45.

Manderbacka, K., Lahelma, E. and Martikainen, P. (1998) 'Examining the continuity of self-rated health', *International Journal of Epidemiology* 27: 208–13.

Manderbacka, K., Lahelma, E. and Rahkonen, O. (2001) 'Structural changes and social inequalities in health in Finland 1986–1994', *Scandinavian Journal of Public Health* (forthcoming).

Manniche, E. (1991) 'Marriage and non-marital cohabitation in Denmark', in *Family Reports*, Sweden: Uppsala University.

Manting, D. (1996) 'The changing meaning of cohabitation and marriage', *European Sociological Review*, May 1996: 53–65.

Marklund, S. (1988) *Paradise Lost?*, Lund: Arkiv.

Marklund, S. (1997) 'Svensk socialpolitik i förändring (Swedish social policy in transition)', in *Välfärd och öjamlikhet i 20–årspespektiv 1975–1995 (Welfare and Inequality 1975–1995)*, Stockholm: SCB, Statistiska centralbyrån, 565–74.

Marklund, S. and Nordlund, A. (1999) 'Economic problems, welfare convergence and political instability', see Kautto *et al.* (1999), 19–53.

Marmot, M. and Dowall, M. (1986) 'Mortality decline and widening social inequalities', *Lancet* 2: 274–76.

Martikainen, P., Aromaa, A., Heliövaara, M., Klaukka, T., Knekt, P., Maatela, J. and Lahelma, E. (1999) 'Reliability of perceived health by sex and age', *Social Science & Medicine* 48: 1117–22.

Martikainen, P. and Valkonen, T. (1995) 'Lama ja ennenaikainen kuolleisuus' (Recession and premature mortality), Helsinki: Statistics Finland, *Population 1995* (11).

Martin, A. (1996) *What Does Globalization Have to do with the Erosion of Welfare States? Sorting out the Issues, Arena Working Paper* No. 17, Oslo: University of Oslo Printing Office.

Martin, C., Math, A. and Renaudat, E. (1998) 'Caring for very young children and dependent elderly people in France: towards a commodification of social care?', see Lewis (1998).

Martin, J. P. (1998) *What Works among Active Labour Market Policies: Evidence from OECD Countries' Experiences*, OECD Labour Market and Social Policy, Occasional Papers, No. 35, October 1998.

McKeown, T. (1976) *The Role of Medicine*, London: Nuffield Provincial Hospitals Trust.

van den Meer, J. (1998) 'Equal care, equal cure?', thesis, Amsterdam.

Melkas, H. and Anker, R. (1998) *Gender Equality and Occupational Segregation in Nordic Labour Markets*, Geneva: International Labour Office (ILO).

Merton, R. K. (1968) 'Manifest and latent functions', in *Social Theory and Social Structure*, New York: The Free Press, 73–138.

Millar, J. (1998) 'Social policy and family policy', in P. Alcock, A. Erskine and M. May (eds) *The Students Companion to Social Policy*, Oxford: Blackwell, 121–7.

Millar, J. and Warman, A. (1996) *Family Obligations in Europe: Family and Parenthood, Policy and Practice*, London: Family Policy Studies Centre, November.

Minister for Women (1999) *Fourth Report of the United Kingdom of Great Britain and the Northern Ireland: United Nations Convention on the Elimination of All Forms of Discrimination against Women (CEDAW).*

Ministry of Children and Family Affairs (1992) *Stortingsmeldning nr. 70, 1991–92: Likestillingspolitikk for 1990–åra (White Paper on Equality Policies for the 1990s)*, Oslo.

Ministry of Children and Family Affairs (1994) *Gender Equality in Norway. The National Report to the Fourth UN Conference on Women in Beijing 1995.*

Ministry of Health and Social Affairs, Norway (1999) *Utjamningsmeldinga, om fordeling av inntekt og levekår i Norge (Distribution of Income and Living Conditions in Norway)*, St. meld. nr 50, Oslo.

Mishra, R. (1977) *Society and Social Policy*, London: Macmillan

Mishra, R. (1993) 'Social policy in the post-modern world: the welfare state in Europe by comparison with North America', in C. Jones (ed.) *New Perspectives on the Welfare State in Europe*, London: Routledge, 18–40.

Mishra, R. (1999) *Globalization and the Welfare State*, Cheltenham: Edward Elgar.

Mjøset, L. (ed.) (1986) *Norden dagen derpå. De nordiske ekonomisk-politiske modellene og deres problemer på 70–80–tallet*, Oslo.

Montanari, I. (2000) 'Are social policies becoming more similar, again?: Virtual and empirical reality behind old and new convergence theorizing', mimeo, Stockholm: Swedish Institute for Social Research.

Morissens, A. (1999) *Solo Mothers and Poverty: Do Politics Matter? A Comparative Case Study of Sweden and Belgium*, LIS Working Paper Series No. 210, Luxembourg.

NEAP-S (1998) *National Employment Action Plan 1998,* Stockholm: The Swedish Government.

Nermo, M. (1999) 'Structured by gender. Patterns of sex segregation in the Swedish labour market. Historical and cross-national comparisons', doctoral dissertation. Department of Sociology, Stockholm University/Swedish Institute for Social Research.

Noack, T. (1997) 'Ekteskapelig status-statusvariabel på avveie?' (Marital status – a status variable gone astray?), *Sosiologisk Tidsskrift*: 285–99.

Nordic Council of Ministers (1994) *Women and Men in the Nordic Countries. Facts and Figures 1994*. Nord 1994:3, Copenhagen.

Nordic Council of Ministers (1995) *Gender Equality – the Nordic Model*, Copenhagen.

Nordic Council of Ministers (1999) *Women and Men in the Nordic Countries 1999. Facts and Figures*. Tema Nord 1999:514, Copenhagen.

NOSOSCO (1999) *Social tryghed i de nordiske lande 1997. Omfang, udgifter og finansiering 1997*, Nordisk Socialstatistisk Komité 99:11, Copenhagen.

O'Connor, J. (1973) *The Fiscal Crisis of the Welfare State*, New York: St. James Press.

OECD (1980–1998) *Labour Force Statistics*, Statistics directorate, Paris: OECD.

OECD (1993) *OECD Health Systems: Facts and Trends 1960–1991*, Paris: OECD.

OECD (1994) *Employment Outlook*, Paris: OECD.

OECD (1998a) *Income Distribution and Poverty in Selected OECD Countries*, Economic Department Working Papers No. 189, Paris: OECD.

OECD (1998b) *New Challenges: Policies for Low-paid Workers and Unskilled Job Seekers* (www.oecd.org).

OECD (1998c) *Background Documents – The Caring World: An Analysis*, Meeting of the Employment, Labour and Social Affairs committee at ministerial level on social policy, Paris, June 1998 (www.oecd.org).

OECD (1998d) *Benefit Systems and Work Incentives*, Paris: OECD.

OECD (1998e) *The OECD Jobs Strategy: Progress Report on Implementation of Country-Specific Recommendations*, Economic Department Working Papers No. 196, Paris: OECD.

OECD (1998f) *Employment Outlook*, Paris: OECD.

OECD (1998g) *OECD Economic Outlook December*, Paris: OECD.

OECD (1999a) *Employment Outlook*, Paris: OECD.

OECD (1999b) *Implementing the OECD Jobs Strategy: Assessing Performance and Policy*, Paris: OECD.

OECD (1999c) *A Caring World. The New Social Policy Agenda*, Paris: OECD.

OECD (1999d) *Economic Outlook December*, Paris: OECD.

OECD *Health Data* (1998) An electronic data base, Paris: OECD.

OECD *Social Expenditure Data* (1998). *An Electronic Data Base*, Paris: OECD.

Oppenheimer, V. K. (1997) 'Women's employment and the gain to marriage: the specialization and trading model', *Annual Review of Sociology* 23: 431–53.

Oppenheimer, V. K. and Lew, V. (1995) 'American marriage formation in the eighties: how important was women's economic independence?', in K. O. Mason and A. M. Jensen (eds) *Gender and Family Change in Industrialized Countries*, Oxford: Clarendon, 105–38.

Orloff, A. S. (1993) 'Gender and the social rights of citizenship: the comparative analysis of gender relations and welfare states', *American Sociological Review* 58: 303–28.

Österle, A. (1999) 'Equity in the provision of long-term care. A comparison of Austria, Italy, The Netherlands and the United Kingdom'. Paper presented at a conference 'Beyond the Health Care State', Florence, 26–27 February.

Palme, J. (1990) *Pension Rights in Welfare Capitalism*, Stockholm: Swedish Institute for Social Research.
Palme, J. and Wennemo, I. (1998) *Swedish Social Security in the 1990s: Reform and Retrenchment*, Stockholm: Välfärdsprojektet (the printing works of the cabinet office and ministries).
Parsons, T. (1949) 'The social structure of the family', in R. Anshen (ed.) *The Family: Its Functions and Destiny*, New York: Harper and Brothers, 173–201.
Pen, J. (1971) *Income Distribution*, London: Allen Lane.
Perraton, J. (2000) 'Hirst and Thompson's "Global myths and national policies"', in B. Holden (ed.) *Global Democracy: Key Debates*, London: Routledge, 60–72.
Piekkola, H. (1996) *Taxation under Economic Integration*, Working Papers 127, Helsinki: Labour Institute for Economic Research.
Pierson, P. (1994) *Dismantling the Welfare State*, Cambridge: Cambridge University Press.
Pierson, P. (1996) 'The new politics of the welfare state', *World Politics* 48(2): 143–79.
Pierson, P. (1998) 'Irresistible forces, immovable objects: post-industrial welfare states confront permanent austerity', *Journal of European Public Policy* 4(4): 539–60.
Ploug, N. and Kvist, J. (1996) *Social Security in Europe: Development or Dismantlement?*, The Hague: Kluwer Law International.
Pochet, P. and Vanhercke, B. (eds) (1998) *Social Challenges of Economic and Monetary Union*, Brussels: European Interuniversity Press.
Pochet, P. and Vanhercke, B. (1999) 'The challenges of economic and monetary union to social protection', in *Financing Social Protection in Europe*, 21, Helsinki: Ministry of Social Affairs and Health.
Pruzan, V. B. (1997) 'Familier i Europa' (Families in Europe), in *Børn, Familie Samfund (Children, Family, Society)*, Marts 1997, Copenhagen: Socialforskningsinstituttet.
Raaum, N. C. (1995) 'Politisk representasjon' (Political representation), in N. C. Raaum (ed.) *Kjønn og Politikk (Gender and Politics)*, Bergen: TANO, 88–112.
Raaum, N. C. (1999): 'Kvinner i offisiell politikk: historiske utviklingslinjer' (Women in official politics: historical developments), in C. Bergquist *et al.* (eds) *Likestilte demokratier? Kjønn og politikk i Norden (Egalitarian Democracies? Gender and Politics in the Nordic Countries)*, Oslo: Universitetsforlaget/Nordic Council of Ministers, 27–45.
Rahkonen, O., Arber, S. and Lahelma, E. (1997a) 'Health and social mobility in Britain and Finland', *Scandinavian Journal of Social Medicine* 25: 83–92.
Rahkonen, O., Lahelma, E. and Huuhka, M. (1997b) 'Past or present? Childhood living conditions and current socioeconomic status as determinants of adult health', *Social Science & Medicine* 44: 327–36.

Rahkonen, O., Lundberg, O., Huuhka, M. and Lahelma, E. (1998) 'Body mass and social class: a comparison of Finland and Sweden in the 1990s', *Journal of Public Health Policy* 18: 88–105.

Rainwater, L. and Smeeding, T. M. (1995) *Doing Poorly: The Real Income of American Children in a Comparative Perspective*, LIS Working Paper Series No. 127, Luxembourg.

Randall, V. (1998) 'Gender and power: women engage the state', see Randall and Waylen (1998), 185–205.

Randall, V. and Waylen, G. (eds) (1998) *Gender, Politics and the State*, London: Routledge.

Rehn, G. (1988) *Full sysselsättning utan inflation* (Full employment without inflation), Stockholm: Tidens förlag.

Reskin, B. and Padavic, I. (1994) *Women and Men at Work*, Thousand Oaks, CA: Pine Forge Press.

Rhodes, M. (1995) '"Subversive liberalism": market integration, globalization and the European welfare state', *Journal of European Public Policy* 2(3): 384–406.

Rhodes, M. (1996) 'Globalization and West European welfare states: a critical review of recent debates', *Journal of European Social Policy* 6(4): 305–27.

Ringen, S. (1991) 'Do welfare states come in types', in P. Saunders and D. Encel (eds) *Social Policy in Australia: Options for the 1990s*, University of New South Wales: Social Policy Research Centre, Reports and Proceedings, No. 96.

Ritsatakis, A., Barnes, R., Dekker, E., Harrington, P., Kokko, S. and Makara, P. (2000) *Exploring Health Policy Development in Europe*, WHO Regional Publications, European Series, No. 86, Copenhagen: WHO.

Rostgaard, T. and Fridberg, T. (1998) *Caring for Children and Older People: A Comparison of European Policies and Practices*, Social Security in Europe 6, Copenhagen: The Danish National Institute of Social Research 98: 20.

Rowntree, B. S. (1901) *Poverty: A Study of Town Life*, London: Macmillan.

Sainsbury, D. (1994) 'Women's and men's social rights: gendering dimensions of welfare states', in D. Sainsbury (ed.) *Gendering Welfare States*, London: Sage, 150–69.

Sainsbury, D. (1998): 'Gender and the making of the Norwegian and Swedish welfare states', paper presented at the Nordic/MIRE conference: 'Comparing social welfare systems in Nordic countries and France', Gilleleje, September.

Salter, B. (1998) *The Politics of Change in the Health Service*, Hong Kong: Macmillan.

Saltman, R. and Figueras, J. (1997) *European Health Care Reform: Analysis of Current Strategies*, Copenhagen: WHO.

Saltman, R., Figueras, J. and Sakellarides, C. (eds) (1998) *Critical Challenges for Health Care Reform in Europe*, Buckingham: Open University Press.

Scharpf, F. (1991) *Crisis and Choice in European Social Democracy*, Ithaca, NY and London: Cornell University Press.

Scharpf, F. (1997) 'Economic integration, democracy and the welfare state', *Journal of European Public Policy* 4: 1.

Scharpf, F. (1999) *Governing in Europe: Effective and Democratic?*, Oxford: Oxford University Press.

Schmidt, M. G. (1999) 'Why financing social protection differs? Cross-national comparisons of EU-Member States and industrial countries outside the European Union', in CD-Rom titled 'Conference on Financing Social Protection in Europe', 22–23 November, 1999, Helsinki, Ministry of Social Affairs and Health, Finland and the European Commission.

Scholte, J. (1997) 'Global capitalism and the state', *International Affairs* 73(3): 427–52.

Sihvo, T. and Uusitalo, H. (1995) 'Welfare state opinions have several dimensions: evidence from Finland', *Scandinavian Journal of Social Welfare* 4(2): 215–23.

Sinn, H. W. (1990) 'Tax harmonization and tax competition in Europe', *European Economic Review* 34: 489–504.

Sipilä, J. (1997) *Social Care Services: The Key to the Scandinavian Model*, Aldershot: Avebury.

Sjöberg, O. (1999) 'Paying for social rights', *Journal of Social Policy* 28(2): 275–97.

Skjeie, H., Fougner Førde, B. and Lorentzen, M. (1989) *Forvaltningsanvar: Likestilling (Responsibility of the Public Administration: Gender Equality)*, Rapport 89: 3, Oslo: Institute for Social Research.

Skrede, K. (1986) 'Gifte kvinner i arbeidslivet' (Married women in the working life), in L. Allden, N. Rogoff Ramsøy and M. Vaa (eds) *Det norske samfunn (The Norwegian Society)*, Oslo: Gyldendal Norsk Forlag, 145–68.

Skrede, K. (1998) 'Shaping gender equality – the role of the state: Norwegian experiences, present policies and future challenges', paper presented at the Nordic/MIRE conference: 'Comparing social welfare systems in Nordic countries and France', Gilleleje, September.

Skrede, K. and Tornes, K. (eds) (1994a) *Den norske kvinnerevolusjonen. Kvinners arbeid 1975–85 (Women's Revolution in Norway: Women and Employment 1975–85)*, Oslo: Universitetsforlaget.

Skrede, K. and Tornes, K. (eds) (1994b) *Kan vi planlegge oss til likestilling i 2010? (Can We Plan the Way to Achieve Gender Equality in 2010?)*, Oslo: Universitetsforlaget.

Smeeding, T. M. (1992) 'Why the U.S. antipoverty system doesn't work very well', *Challenge* Jan–Feb, 30–35.

Social Protection Expenditure and Receipts 1980–1991 (1993) Eurostat, Theme Population and Social Conditions, Series Accounts and Surveys, 3 C, Luxembourg: Office for Official Publications of the European Communities.

Social Protection Expenditure and Receipts 1980–1994 (1996) Eurostat, Theme Population and Social Conditions, Series Accounts and Surveys, 3 C, Luxembourg: Office for Official Publications of the European Communities.

Social Protection Expenditure and Receipts 1980–1996 (1999) Eurostat, Theme Population and Social Conditions, Series Accounts and Surveys, 3 C, Luxembourg: Office for Official Publications of the European Communities.

Social Protection Expenditure and Receipts 1980–1997 (2000) Eurostat, Theme 3, Population and Social Conditions, Luxembourg: Office for Official Publications of the European Communities.

Socialstyrelsen (1996a) *Meddelande No. 16 (Newsletter nr 16)*, Stockholm: Socialstyrelsen.

Socialstyrelsen (1996b) *Social service, vård och omsorg i Sverige (Social Services, Care and Nursing in Sweden)*, Stockholm: Socialstyrelsen.

Sørensen, A. (1992) 'Zur geschlechtsspezifischen Struktur von Armut' (The gender-specific structure of poverty), *Kölner Zeitschrift für Soziologie und Sozialpsychologie*, Sonderheft 'Armut in modernen Wohlfahrtsstaat' 1992: 345–66.

Sørensen, A. (1994) 'Women's economic risk and the economic position of Single Mothers', *European Sociological Review* 10: 173–88.

Sørensen, A. and McLanahan, S. (1987) 'Married women's economic dependency, 1940–1980', *American Journal of Sociology* 93: 659–87.

SOU 2000, *Välfärd vid vägskäl, utvecklingen under 1990-talet* (Welfare at the Crossroads, development in the 1990s), delbetänkande från Kommittén Välfärdsbokslut SOU 2000:3, Stockholm: Fritzes.

Statistics Finland (1996) Familier 1995 (Families 1995), *Population* 1996:13.

Statistics Norway (1998a) *Aktuelle befolkningstall nr. 4/98.*

Statistics Norway (1998b) *Women and Men in Norway.*

Statistics Norway (2000) *Social Assistance Statistics 1998.*

Statistics Sweden (1997) *Kvinnor och Män på toppen. Facta om antal och lön 1995 (Women and men at the top. Facts on numbers and wages 1995).*

Stephens, J. D., Huber, E. and Ray, L. (1999) 'The welfare state in hard times', in H. Kitschelt, P. Lange, G. Marks and J. D. Stephens (eds) *Continuity and Change in Comtemporary Capitalism*, Cambridge: Cambridge University Press, 164–93.

Strange, S. (1996) *The Retreat of the State: The Diffusion of Power in the World Economy*, Cambridge: Cambridge University Press.

Streeck, W. (1995) 'From market making to state building? Reflections on the political economy of European social policy', in S. Leibfried and P. Pierson (eds) *European Social Policy: Between Fragmentation and Integration*, Washington, DC: The Brookings Institution.

Streeck, W. (1996) 'Neo-voluntarism: a new European social policy regime?', in G. Marks, F. W. Scharpf, P. Schmitter and W. Streeck (eds) *Governance in the European Union*, London: Sage, 64–94.

Structures of the Taxation Systems in the European Union, 1970–1996 (1998), Theme Economy and Finance, Series Yearbooks and Yearly Statistics, 2A, Luxembourg: Office for Official Publications of the European Communities.

Svallfors, S. (1996) *Välfärdsstatens moraliska ekonomi. Välfärdsopinionen i 90-talets Sverige (The Moral Economy of the Welfare State: Attitudes towards the Welfare State in Sweden in the 1990s)*, Umeå: Boréa bokförlag.

Swank, D. (1998) 'Funding the welfare state: globalization and the taxation of business in advanced market economies', *Political Studies* XLVI: 671–92.

Swank, D. (2000) 'Social democratic welfare states in a global economy: Scandinavia in comparative perspective', in R. Geyer, C. Ingebrigtsen and J. W. Moses (eds) *Globalization, Europeanization and the End of Scandinavian Social Democracy?*, London: Macmillan.

SZW (Ministerie van Sociale Zaken en Werkgelegenheid) (undated): *The Second Report of the Netherlands to the UN Committee for the Elimination of all Forms of Discrimination Against Women (CEDAW)*, The Hague.

Tanzi, V. (1999) 'Globalization and financing of social protection', in CD-Rom titled 'Conference on Financing Social Protection in Europe', 22–23 November, 1999, Helsinki, Ministry of Social Affairs and Health, Finland and the European Commission.

The Government Sector in the European Union: A Long-term Analysis of Receipts and Expenditures (1997) Eurostat, Theme Economy and Finance, Series Studies and Research, 2D, Luxembourg: Office for Official Publications of the European Communities.

Therborn, G. (1995) *European Modernity and Beyond*, London: Sage.

Thornton, P., Sainsbury, R. and Barnes, H. (1997) *Helping Disabled People to Work*, London: The Stationery Office.

Titmuss, R. H. (1958) *Essays on the Welfare State*, London: Allen & Unwin.

Titmuss, R. H. (1974) *Social Policy*, London: Allen & Unwin

Torp, H. (1999) 'Dagpengesystemerne i Norden' (Unemployment insurance systems in the Nordic countries) in *Dagpengesystemerne i Norden og tilpasning på arbeidsmarkedet (Nordic Unemployment insurance systems and Labour Market Adaptation)*, TemaNord Arbeidsmarked, Copenhagen: Nordisk Ministerråd (Nordic Council of Ministers), 64–97.

Townsend, P. and Davidson, N. (1982) *Inequalities in Health: The Black Report*, Harmondsworth: Penguin Books.

Trost, J. (1996) 'Family studies in Sweden', in M. B. Sussman and R. S. Hanks (eds) *Intercultural Variation in Family Research and Theory: Implications for Cross-national Studies*, Vol. 2, New York: The Hayworth Press, 723–43.

Twaddle, A. C. (1974) 'The concept of health status', *Social Science & Medicine* 8: 29–38.

UNICE (1998) *Benchmarking Europe's Competitiveness: From Analysis to Action*, Brussels: Union of Industrial and Employers' Confederations of Europe.

United Nations Development Programme (UNDP) (1998) *Human Development Report 1998*.

Uusitalo, H. (1989) *Income Distribution in Finland*, Helsinki: Central Statistical Office of Finland.

Uusitalo, H. (1999) 'Tuloerot kasvaneet jo kolmena peräkkäisenä vuonna' (Third year of growth in income differences), *Yhteiskuntapolitiikka* 5–6: 465–79.

Vågerö, D. and Erikson, R. (1997) 'Socio-economic inequalities in morbidity and mortality in western Europe', *Lancet* 350: 516.

Vågerö, D. and Gullberg, A. (1996) *Yrke och dödlighet under 1980-talet (Occupation and mortality in the 1980s)*. Stockholm: Socialstyrelsen, Rapport 1996: 3.

Vågerö, D. and Illsley, R. (eds) (1992) 'Inequality, health and policy in East and West Europe', *International Journal of Health Sciences* (special issue) 3(3/4): 114–239.

Vågerö, D. and Lundberg, O. (1989) 'Health inequalities in Britain and Sweden', *Lancet* 1989, ii: 35–6.

Valkonen, T. (1989) 'Adult mortality and level of education: a comparison of six countries', in A. J. Fox (ed.) *Health Inequalities in European Countries*, Aldershot: Gower, 142–60.

Valkonen, T. and Martelin, T. (1999) 'Social inequality in the face of death – linked registers in mortality research', in J. Alho (ed.) *Statistics, Registers, Science*, Helsinki: Statistics Finland, 213–26.

Valkonen, T., Martelin, T., Rimpelä, A., Notkola, V. and Savela, S. (1993) *Socio-economic Mortality Differences in Finland 1981–90*, Helsinki: Statistics Finland, Population 1993:1.

Vanhercke, B. (1998) 'The social stakes of economic and monetary union: an overview', in P. Pochet and B. Vanhercke (eds) *Social Challenges of Economic and Monetary Union*, Observatoire Social Européen, Brussels: European Interuniversity Press, 11–22.

Veikkola, E. S. (ed.) (1999) *Changes at the Top*, Helsinki: Statistics Finland.

Wærness, K. (1998) 'Barnet er viktigst' (The child is the main thing), *Kvinneforskning*, 2: 5–11.

Wagstaff, A., Paci, P. and van Doorslaer, E. (1991) 'On the measurement of inequalities in health', *Social Science & Medicine* 33: 545–57.

Ward, C., Dale, A. and Joshi, H. (1996) 'Income dependency within couples', in L. Morris and E. Stina Lyon (eds) *Gender Relations in Public and Private: New Research Perspectives*, London: Macmillan Press, 95–120.

Waylen, G. (1998) 'Gender, feminism and the state. An overview', see Randall and Waylen (1998), 1–18.

Weber, M. (1949) *The Methodology of the Social Sciences*, New York: The Free Press.

Webster, C. (1992) 'Beveridge after 50 years', *British Medical Journal* 305: 901–2.

Wertheimer, A. and McRae, S. (1999) *Family and Household Change in Britain*, Oxford: Centre for Family and Household Research.

Wilensky, H. (1975) *The Welfare State and Equality*, Berkeley, CA: University of California Press.

Wilensky, H. (1992) 'Active labour market policy: its contents, effectiveness, and odd relationship to evaluation research', in C. Crouch and A. Heath (eds) *Social Research and Social Reform*, Oxford: Clarendon Press.

Wilensky, H. and Lebeaux, C. (1958) *Industrial Society and Social Welfare*, New York: Russell Sage.

Wilkinson, R. (1996) *Unhealthy Societies: The Afflictions of Inequality*, London: Routledge.

Wistow, G., Knapp, M., Hardy, B., Forder, J., Kendal, J. and Manning, R. (1996) *Social Care Markets: Progress and Prospects,* Buckingham: Open University Press.

von Wright, G. H. (1972) *Varieties of Goodness*, London: Routledge & Kegan Paul.

Index